Allergy, Inflamı and Autoimmune Disorders in Emergency Medicine

Editors

R. GENTRY WILKERSON
SALVADOR SUAU

IMMUNOLOGY AND ALLERGY CLINICS OF NORTH AMERICA

https://www.immunology.theclinics.com

Consulting Editor
ROHIT KATIAL

August 2023 • Volume 43 • Number 3

ELSEVIER

1600 John F. Kennedy Boulevard • Suite 1800 • Philadelphia, Pennsylvania, 19103-2899

http://www.theclinics.com

IMMUNOLOGY AND ALLERGY CLINICS OF NORTH AMERICA Volume 43, Number 3

August 2023 ISSN 0889-8561, ISBN-13: 978-0-443-12975-9

Editor: Taylor Hayes

Developmental Editor: Nitesh Barthwal

Immunology and Allergy Clinics of North America (ISSN 0889–8561) is published quarterly by Elsevier Inc., 360 Park Avenue South, New York, NY 10010-1710. Months of issue are February, May, August, and November. Periodicals postage paid at New York, NY and additional mailing offices. Subscription prices are $365.00 per year for US individuals, $704.00 per year for US institutions, $100.00 per year for US students and residents, $445.00 per year for Canadian individuals, $100.00 per year for Canadian students, $895.00 per year for Canadian institutions, $470.00 per year for international individuals, $895.00 per year for international institutions, $220.00 per year for international students. To receive student/resident rate, orders must be accompanied by name of affiliated institution, date of term, and the *signature* of program/residency coordinator on institution letterhead. Orders will be billed at individual rate until proof of status is received. Foreign air speed delivery is included in all *Clinics* subscription prices. All prices are subject to change without notice. **POSTMASTER:** Send address changes to *Immunology and Allergy Clinics of North America,* Elsevier Health Sciences Division, Subscription Customer Service, 3251 Riverport Lane, Maryland Heights, MO 63043. **Customer Service: 1-800-654-2452 (U.S. and Canada); 314-447-8871 (outside U.S. and Canada). Fax: 314-447-8029. E-mail: journalscustomerservice-usa@elsevier.com** (for print support); journalsonlinesupport-usa@elsevier.com **(for online support).**

Reprints. For copies of 100 or more, of articles in this publication, please contact the Commercial Reprints Department, Elsevier Inc., 360 Park Avenue South, New York, New York 10010-1710. Tel. 212-633-3874, Fax: 212-633-3820, E-mail: reprints@elsevier.com.

Immunology and Allergy Clinics of North America is covered in MEDLINE/PubMed (Index Medicus), Current Contents/Life Sciences, Science Citation Index, ISI/BIOMED, Chemical Abstracts, and EMBASE/Excerpta Medica.

Contributors

CONSULTING EDITOR

ROHIT KATIAL
Division of Allergy and Clinical Immunology, Department of Medicine, National Jewish Health, Denver, Colorado, USA

EDITORS

R. GENTRY WILKERSON, MD
Associate Professor, Department of Emergency Medicine, University of Maryland School of Medicine, Baltimore, Maryland

SALVADOR SUAU, MD
Program Director, Emergency Medicine Residency, Department of Emergency Medicine, Ochsner Health System, Ochsner Emergency Department, New Orleans, Louisiana

AUTHORS

LEEN ALBLAIHED, MBBS, MHA, FAAEM
Assistant Professor, Department of Emergency Medicine, University of Maryland School of Medicine, Baltimore, Maryland, USA

RITHVIK BALAKRISHNAN, MD
Emergency Medicine Physician, Department of Emergency Medicine, Kings County Hospital, SUNY Downstate Medical Center, Kings County Hospital Center, Brooklyn, New York, USA

RONNA L. CAMPBELL, MD, PhD
Consultant, Department of Emergency Medicine, Mayo Clinic, Rochester, Minnesota, USA

DENRICK COOPER, MD, MPH
Director of International Emergency Medicine, Department of Emergency Medicine, Ochsner Health System, New Orleans, Louisiana, USA

TIMOTHY E. DRIBIN, MD
Assistant Professor, Division of Emergency Medicine, Cincinnati Children's Hospital Medical Center, Department of Pediatrics, University of Cincinnati College of Medicine, Cincinnati, Ohio, USA

SARAH B. DUBBS, MD
Assistant Professor, Department of Emergency Medicine, University of Maryland School of Medicine, Baltimore, Maryland, USA

CHEYENNE FALAT, MD
Clinical Instructor, Department of Emergency Medicine, University of Maryland School of Medicine, Baltimore, Maryland, USA

NICHOLAS P. GORHAM, MD
Emergency Medicine Physician, Ochsner Medical Center, New Orleans, Louisiana, USA

MAITE ANNA HUIS IN'T VELD, MD
Adjunct Assistant Professor, Department of Emergency Medicine, University of Maryland School of Medicine, Baltimore, Maryland, USA; Emergency Physician, Department of Emergency Medicine, Diakonessenhuis Utrecht, Utrecht, the Netherlands

THOMAS KRAJEWSKI, MD
Attending Physician, Ochsner Medical Center Emergency Department, New Orleans, Louisiana, USA

GENEVIEVE SCHULT KRAJEWSKI, MD
Attending Physician, Ochsner Medical Center Emergency Department, Core Faculty, Ochsner Emergency Medicine Residency, Senior Lecturer, Ochsner Clinical School at the University of Queensland, New Orleans, Louisiana, USA

KELLY MCHUGH, MD
Emergency Medicine Resident Physician, Department of Emergency Medicine, Lewis Katz School of Medicine, Temple University, Philadelphia, Pennsylvania, USA

JOSEPH J. MOELLMAN, MD
Professor, Department of Emergency Medicine, University of Cincinnati College of Medicine, Cincinnati, Ohio, USA

MEGAN S. MOTOSUE, MD
Allergist-Immunologist, Departments of Allergy and Immunology, and Medicine, University of Hawaii, Kaiser Honolulu Clinic, Honolulu, Hawaii, USA

ZACHARY REPANSHEK, MD
Associate Professor of Emergency Medicine; Associate Residency Program Director, Department of Emergency Medicine, Lewis Katz School of Medicine, Temple University, Philadelphia, Pennsylvania, USA

JONATHAN ROSE, MD, MBA
Residency Program Director, Department of Emergency Medicine, Memorial Healthcare System, Memorial Hospital West, Pembroke Pines, Florida, USA

LAUREN ROSENBLATT, MD
Clinical Instructor, Department of Emergency Medicine, University of Maryland School of Medicine, Baltimore, Maryland, USA

SALVADOR SUAU, MD
Program Director, Emergency Medicine Residency, Department of Emergency Medicine, Ochsner Health System, Ochsner Emergency Department, New Orleans, Louisiana, USA

HOPE A. TAITT, MD
Resident Physician, Department of Emergency Medicine, Kings County Hospital, SUNY Downstate Medical Center, Kings County Hospital Center, Brooklyn, New York, USA

DANIEL JAMES THOMAS, MD
Faculty, Department of Emergency Medicine, Ochsner Medical Center, New Orleans, Louisiana, USA

ELIZABETH G. THOMAS, MD
Emergency Medicine Physician, Department of Emergency Medicine, Ochsner Medical Center, New Orleans, Louisiana, USA

R. GENTRY WILKERSON, MD

Associate Professor, Department of Emergency Medicine, University of Maryland School of Medicine, Baltimore, Maryland, USA

MICHAEL E. WINTERS, MD, MBA

Professor, Department of Emergency Medicine, University of Maryland School of Medicine, Baltimore, Maryland, USA

Contents

Preface: Anaphylaxis, Angioedema, and Other Immunologic Emergencies   **xiii**

R. Gentry Wilkerson and Salvador Suau

Overview of Allergy and Anaphylaxis   **435**

Timothy E. Dribin, Megan S. Motosue, and Ronna L. Campbell

> Allergic reactions and anaphylaxis occur on a severity continuum from mild and self-limited to potentially life-threatening or fatal reactions. Anaphylaxis is typically a multiorgan phenomenon involving a broad range of effector cells and mediators. Emergency department visits for anaphylaxis are increasing, especially among children. There is a broad differential diagnosis for anaphylaxis, and the diagnosis of anaphylaxis can be aided by the use of the National Institutes of Allergy and Infectious Disease/Food Allergy and Anaphylaxis Network clinical diagnostic criteria. Risk factors for severe anaphylaxis include older age, delayed epinephrine administration, and cardiopulmonary comorbidities.

Anaphylaxis: Emergency Department Treatment   **453**

Kelly McHugh and Zachary Repanshek

> Anaphylaxis is a potentially life-threatening, multisystem allergic reaction that can cause airway, breathing, or circulatory compromise. Intramuscular epinephrine is the immediate treatment of all patients. Intravenous epinephrine should be used in patients in shock, either as a bolus or infusion, along with fluid resuscitation. Airway obstruction must be recognized, and early intubation may be necessary. For shock that is refractory to epinephrine, additional vasopressors may be needed. Disposition depends on patient presentation and response to treatment. Mandatory observation periods are not necessary, because biphasic reactions are difficult to predict and may occur outside of typical observation periods.

Anaphylaxis: After the Emergency Department   **467**

Nicholas P. Gorham

> After treating the acute anaphylactic reaction, the clinician's next task is to prevent a recurrence. The patient should be observed in the ED. How long this observation period should last depends on their clinical course, risk factors, and social support. All patients should be discharged with a prescription for 2 epinephrine autoinjectors and counseled on appropriate use. The patient should also receive education on the signs and symptoms of anaphylaxis and avoiding triggers. The patient should follow-up with an allergy specialist who can confirm triggers and provide immunotherapy as indicated.

Drug Hypersensitivity Reactions   473

R. Gentry Wilkerson

Drug hypersensitivity reactions are a diverse group of reactions mediated by the immune system after exposure to a drug. The Gell and Coombs classification divides immunologic DHRs into 4 major pathophysiologic categories based on immunologic mechanism. Anaphylaxis is a Type I hypersensitivity reaction that requires immediate recognition and treatment. Severe cutaneous adverse reactions (SCARs) are a group of dermatologic diseases that result from a Type IV hypersensitivity process and include drug reaction with eosinophilia and systemic symptom (DRESS) syndrome, Stevens–Johnson Syndrome (SJS), toxic epidermal necrolysis (TEN), and acute generalized exanthematous pustulosis (AGEP). Other types of reactions are slow to develop and do not always require rapid treatment. Emergency physicians should have a good understanding of these various types of drug hypersensitivity reactions and how to approach the patient regarding evaluation and treatment.

Evaluation and Management of Food Allergies in the Emergency Department   491

Genevieve Schult Krajewski and Thomas Krajewski

Food allergies are a common and serious cause of illness, accounting for an increasing number of emergency department visits annually. Although definite diagnosis lays outside of an emergency department visit, the clinical management of the most serious food allergies highlights emergency care. The staple of acute care remains epinephrine in association with antihistamines and steroids. The greatest threat remains undertreatment for this group of disorders and underutilization of epinephrine. Those who have been treated for a food allergy need a follow-up allergist evaluation, guidance of food avoidance, and avoidance of foods with cross-sensitivities as well as ready access to epinephrine.

Allergic Acute Coronary Syndrome—Kounis Syndrome   503

Leen Alblaihed and Maite Anna Huis in 't Veld

Acute coronary syndrome (ACS) in the setting of an allergic/immunologic reaction is known as Kounis syndrome. It is an underdiagnosed and underrecognized disease entity. One must keep a high index of suspicions when managing a patient presenting with cardiac as well as allergic symptoms. There are 3 main variants to the syndrome. Treating the allergic reaction may alleviate the pain; however, ACS guidelines should be followed if cardiac ischemia is present.

Angiotensin-Converting Enzyme Inhibitor–Induced Angioedema   513

R. Gentry Wilkerson and Michael E. Winters

Angioedema is a well-recognized and potentially lethal complication of angiotensin-converting enzyme inhibitor (ACEi) therapy. In ACEi-induced angioedema, bradykinin accumulates due to a decrease in its metabolism by ACE, the enzyme that is primarily responsible for this function. The action of bradykinin at bradykinin type 2 receptors leads to increased vascular permeability and the accumulation of fluid in the subcutaneous and submucosal space. Patients with ACEi-induced angioedema are at risk for airway compromise because of the tendency for the face, lips, tongue, and airway structures to be affected. The emergency physician should focus on airway evaluation and management when treating patients with ACEi-induced angioedema.

Hereditary Angioedema   533

R. Gentry Wilkerson and Joseph J. Moellman

Hereditary angioedema (HAE) is a rare autosomal dominant genetic disorder that usual results from a decreased level of functional C1-INH and clinically manifests with intermittent attacks of swelling of the subcutaneous tissue or submucosal layers of the respiratory or gastrointestinal tracts. Laboratory studies and radiographic imaging have limited roles in evaluation of patients with acute attacks of HAE except when the diagnosis is uncertain and other processes must be ruled out. Treatment begins with assessment of the airway to determine the need for immediate intervention. Emergency physicians should understand the pathophysiology of HAE to help guide management decisions.

Mimics of Allergy and Angioedema: Scombroid, Mast Cell Activation Disorders, and Hereditary Alpha Tryptasemia   553

Elizabeth G. Thomas and Daniel James Thomas

Scombroid poisoning, systemic mastocytosis, and hereditary alpha tryptasemia all present with episodes that resemble allergic reactions. Knowledge regarding systemic mastocytosis and hereditary alpha tryptasemia is quickly evolving. Epidemiology, pathophysiology, and strategies to identify and diagnose are discussed. Evidence-based management in the emergency setting and beyond is also explored and summarized. Key differences are described between these events and allergic reactions.

Immune-based Therapies—What the Emergency Physician Needs to Know   569

Sarah B. Dubbs, Cheyenne Falat, and Lauren Rosenblatt

Immunotherapy is a treatment modality that has a broad and rapidly growing range of applications to treat both chronic and acute diseases, including rheumatoid arthritis, Crohn disease, cancer, and COVID-19. Emergency physicians must be aware of the breadth of applications and be able to consider the effects of immunotherapies when patients on these treatments present to the hospital. This article provides a review of the mechanisms of action, indications for use, and potential complications of immunotherapy treatments that are relevant in the emergency care setting.

Sarcoidosis   583

Denrick Cooper and Salvador Suau

Sarcoidosis has a multitude of manifestations and affects the human body widely. Pulmonary complaints are most common; however, cardiac, optic, and neurologic manifestations carry high mortality and morbidity. Acute presentations in the emergency room can cause life-altering effects if not appropriately diagnosed and treated. Generally, less severe cases of sarcoidosis have a favorable prognosis and can be treated with steroid therapy. Resistant and more severe cases of the disease carry high mortality and morbidity. It is incredibly important to arrange specialty follow-up for these patients when needed. This review focuses on the acute presentations of sarcoidosis.

Spondyloarthritides   593

Hope A. Taitt and Rithvik Balakrishnan

The spondyloarthritides are a diverse group of distinct yet interrelated disease processes with overlapping clinical features. They are ankylosing spondylitis, reactive arthritis, inflammatory bowel disease–associated arthritis, and psoriatic arthritis. Genetically, these disease processes have been linked by the presence of HLA-B27. They manifest with axial and peripheral symptoms, such as inflammatory back pain, enthesitis, oligoarthritis, and dactylitis. The onset of symptoms can begin before the age of 45; however, because of the wide range of signs and symptoms, diagnosis can be delayed, leading to unchecked inflammation, structural damage, and later, restriction in physical mobility.

Autoimmune Connective Tissue Diseases: Systemic Lupus Erythematosus and Rheumatoid Arthritis   613

Jonathan Rose

Systemic lupus erythematosus and rheumatoid arthritis are just 2 of several autoimmune connective tissue diseases that are primarily chronic in nature but can present to the emergency department by virtue of an acute exacerbation of disease. Beyond an acute exacerbation of disease, their predilection for invading multiple organ systems lends itself to the potential for patients presenting to the emergency department with either a single or isolated symptom or a myriad of signs and/or symptoms indicative of a degree of disease complexity and severity that warrant timely recognition and resuscitation.

IMMUNOLOGY AND ALLERGY CLINICS OF NORTH AMERICA

FORTHCOMING ISSUES

November 2023
Mast Cell Disorders
Cem Akin, *Editor*

February 2024
Climate Change and Allergy
Rosalind Wright and Jeffrey G. Demain, *Editors*

May 2024
Eosinophilic Gastrointestinal Diseases
Glenn T. Furuta and Dan Atkins, *Editors*

RECENT ISSUES

May 2023
Interstitial Lung Disease
Joshua Solomon and Kevin K. Brown, *Editors*

February 2023
Pregnancy and Allergy
Edward S. Schulman, *Editor*

November 2022
Environmental Issues and Allergy
Jill A. Poole, *Editor*

SERIES OF RELATED INTEREST

Medical Clinics
https://www.medical.theclinics.com/

THE CLINICS ARE AVAILABLE ONLINE!
Access your subscription at:
www.theclinics.com

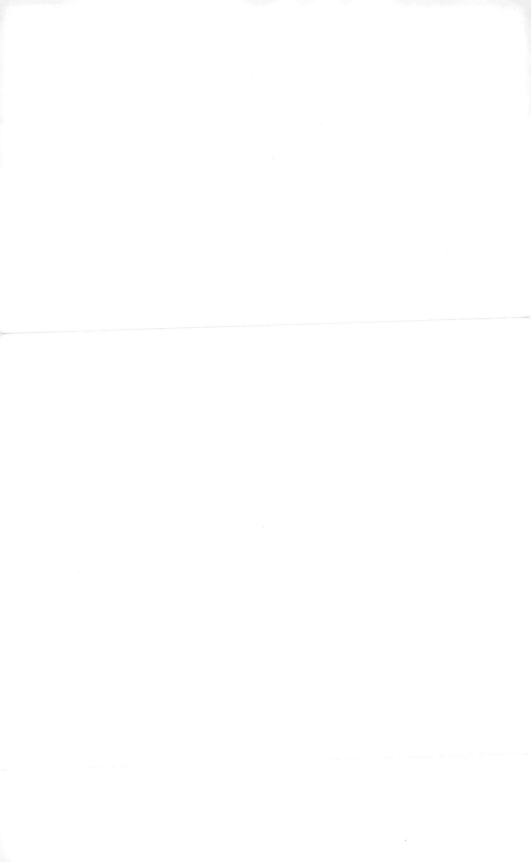

Preface

Anaphylaxis, Angioedema, and Other Immunologic Emergencies

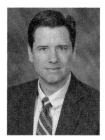 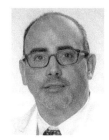

R. Gentry Wilkerson, MD   Salvador Suau, MD
Editors

We are honored that this issue of *Immunology and Allergy Clinics of North America* consists of the articles that we curated for the February 2022 issue of *Emergency Medicine Clinics of North America.* The topics contained within this issue are of great importance to emergency medicine practitioners as well as to allergists and immunologists. Our specialties share a dedication to providing up-to-date, evidence-based medical care to patients, which is highlighted by the conditions covered in this issue: anaphylaxis, angioedema, immune-based therapies, and other immunologic disorders.

Anaphylaxis has been described by the World Allergy Organization as a "serious systemic hypersensitivity reaction that is usually rapid in onset and may cause death," which captures the essence of emergency medicine. Patients with anaphylaxis require prompt recognition and treatment to prevent morbidity and mortality. The first group of articles in this issue focuses on allergies and anaphylaxis. A common thread throughout these articles is the importance of epinephrine as the first-line treatment for anaphylaxis. In this group of articles, two focus on major causes of allergic reactions and anaphylaxis—drugs and food. The last article in this group focuses on Kounis syndrome, an underrecognized form of allergic acute coronary syndrome.

The second set of articles in this issue focuses on angioedema, the physical finding of swelling of the subcutaneous layer of skin or submucosal swelling of the respiratory or gastrointestinal tract. Angioedema may result from several distinct processes. Knowledge of the underlying pathophysiology responsible for an individual patient's presentation is key to guiding appropriate therapy for treatment. Two articles in this section focus on forms of angioedema that are primarily due to accumulation of bradykinin. Hereditary angioedema is a rare disease that affects approximately 5000 individuals in the United States. In recent years, there have been major advances in the

Immunol Allergy Clin N Am 43 (2023) xiii–xiv
https://doi.org/10.1016/j.iac.2023.04.007
0889-8561/23/© 2023 Published by Elsevier Inc.

prevention and treatment of hereditary angioedema attacks. Another form is bradykinin-mediated angioedema, which is associated with the use of ACE inhibitor medications. Despite the similarity in the mechanism of hereditary angioedema, a proven treatment for ACE inhibitor-induced angioedema remains elusive. Last, there is an article that details some other conditions that can be confused with allergic reactions and angioedema, such as scombroid, mast cell activation disorders, and hereditary alpha tryptasemia.

The use of immune-based therapies has exploded in recent years even though it has been around for much longer. William Bradley Coley, known as the Father of Immunotherapy, first attempted to use the immune system to treat bone cancer in 1891 after observing several patients who went into remission after developing the streptococcal skin infection erysipelas. These new immune-based therapies have revolutionized the treatment of multiple conditions but come with their own set of complications. It is important for practitioners caring for patients on these therapies to be familiar with their indications for use and potential complications associated with them.

The issue concludes with three articles focused on some of the important diseases of the immune system. Sarcoidosis is a "chameleon" disease, which can affect numerous organ systems and manifest in protean ways. The different forms of spondyloarthritides require special attention so that potential new cases or flares of existing cases can be identified. The treatment of spondyloarthritides is also associated with a distinct set of possible complications that the practitioner should be vigilant for recognizing. Systemic lupus erythematosus and rheumatoid arthritis are two autoimmune connective tissue diseases that lead to multiple complications. It is important to recognize that patients with lupus and rheumatoid arthritis are at increased risk for other common complications, such as coronary artery disease and venous thromboembolism.

We are thankful for the excellent authors who contributed their time and expertise in writing the articles within this issue. We hope that this issue becomes a valuable resource for the readers of *Immunology and Allergy Clinics of North America.* Most importantly, we are thankful for our patients, who have entrusted us with their care. We are obligated to be lifelong learners so that the care that we provide is making a positive impact on the lives of our patients.

R. Gentry Wilkerson, MD
Department of Emergency Medicine
University of Maryland School of Medicine
110 South Paca Street 6th Floor, Suite 200
Baltimore, MD 21201, USA

Salvador Suau, MD
Department of Emergency Medicine
Ochsner Health System
Ochsner Emergency Department
1514 Jefferson Highway
New Orleans, LA 71021, USA

E-mail addresses:
gwilkerson@som.umaryland.edu (R.G. Wilkerson)
salvador.suau@ochsner.org (S. Suau)

Overview of Allergy and Anaphylaxis

Timothy E. Dribin, MD[a], Megan S. Motosue, MD[b,c], Ronna L. Campbell, MD, PhD[d,*]

KEYWORDS

- Anaphylaxis • Epinephrine • Epidemiology • Diagnosis • Risk factors

KEY POINTS

- Allergic reactions and anaphylaxis occur on a severity continuum from mild and self-limited to potentially life-threatening or fatal reactions.
- The clinical diagnosis of anaphylaxis can be aided by the use of diagnostic criteria.
- Prompt treatment with epinephrine is necessary to prevent progression to a potentially life-threatening reaction.
- Risk factors for increased anaphylaxis severity include older age, cardiopulmonary co-morbidities, and delayed epinephrine administration.

INTRODUCTION

The term anaphylaxis was originally coined by Charles Richet and Paul Portier in 1902 based on experiments intended to immunize dogs against toxins from the Mediterranean snakelocks sea anemone (*Anemonia sulcata*).[1] However, in contrast to expectations, subsequent vaccinations caused the dogs to react with wheezing, vomiting, and death. Richet and Portier labeled this lack of protection as anaphylaxis (ana = absence + phylaxis = protection in Greek).

ANAPHYLAXIS DIAGNOSIS

Although anaphylaxis is a potentially life-threatening allergic reaction, reactions can range in severity from mild and self-limited to fatal. Although allergic reactions are

This article originally appeared in Emergency Medicine Clinics, Volume 40 Issue 1, February 2022.

[a] Division of Emergency Medicine, Department of Pediatrics, Cincinnati Children's Hospital Medical Center, University of Cincinnati College of Medicine, 3333 Burnet Avenue, MLC 2008, Cincinnati, OH 45229-3039, USA; [b] Department of Allergy and Immunology, University of Hawaii, Kaiser Honolulu Clinic, 1010 Pensacola Street, Honolulu, HI 96814, USA; [c] Department of Medicine, University of Hawaii, Kaiser Honolulu Clinic, 1010 Pensacola Street, Honolulu, HI 96814, USA; [d] Department of Emergency Medicine, Mayo Clinic, 200 First Street Southwest, Generose Building G-410, Rochester, MN, USA
* Corresponding author.
E-mail address: Campbell.ronna@mayo.edu

typically limited to a single organ system (eg, skin), anaphylaxis typically, although not always, involves multiple organ systems. The diagnosis of anaphylaxis is challenging because of the wide range of potential clinical manifestations and the fact that the line differentiating an allergic reaction and anaphylaxis is not always easily discernible. The difficulty in diagnosing anaphylaxis has resulted in under-recognition and undertreatment in the emergency department.[2]

The clinical diagnosis of anaphylaxis can be aided by the use of diagnostic criteria. Currently, the most widely accepted clinical diagnostic criteria are the National Institutes of Allergy and Infectious Disease/Food Allergy and Anaphylaxis Network (NIAID/FAAN) criteria (**Box 1**).[3] The NIAID/FAAN criteria were proposed by an international multidisciplinary symposium in 2005 and consist of 3 criteria. Only 1 criterion needs to be met for the clinical diagnosis of anaphylaxis to be highly likely. The first criterion requires the acute onset of signs or symptoms associated with mucocutaneous manifestations along with signs or symptoms of respiratory system involvement and/or cardiovascular involvement. For example, a patient who experiences the sudden onset of hives associated with difficulty breathing would fulfill the first criterion even in the absence of a clear inciting allergen. The second criterion requires sudden onset of symptoms after exposure to a likely allergen or other trigger along with signs

---

Box 1
National Institutes of Allergy and Infectious Disease/Food Allergy and Anaphylaxis Network clinical criteria for diagnosing anaphylaxis

Anaphylaxis is highly likely when any of the following 3 criteria are fulfilled:

1. Acute onset of an illness (minutes to several hours) with involvement of the skin, mucosal tissue, or both (eg, generalized hives, pruritus or flushing, swollen lips-tongue-uvula)

And at least one of the following
   a. Respiratory compromise (eg, dyspnea, wheeze-bronchospasm, stridor, reduced peak expiratory flow [PEF], hypoxemia)
   b. Reduced blood pressure (BP) or associated symptoms of end-organ dysfunction (eg, hypotonia [collapse], syncope, incontinence)

2. Two or more of the following that occur rapidly after exposure to a likely allergen for that patient (minutes to several hours)
   a. Involvement of the skin-mucosal tissue (eg, generalized hives, itch-flush, swollen lips-tongue-uvula)
   b. Respiratory compromise (eg, dyspnea, wheeze-bronchospasm, stridor, reduced PEF, hypoxemia)
   c. Reduced BP or associated symptoms (eg, hypotonia [collapse], syncope, incontinence)
   d. Persistent gastrointestinal symptoms (eg, crampy abdominal pain, vomiting)

3. Reduced BP after exposure to known allergen for that patient (minutes to several hours)
   a. Infants and children: low systolic BP (age specific) or greater than 30% decrease in systolic BP[a]
   b. Adults: systolic BP of less than 90 mm Hg or greater than 30% decrease from that person's baseline

[a]Low systolic blood pressure for children is defined as less than 70 mm Hg from 1 month to 1 year, less than (70 mm Hg + [2 × age]) from 1 to 10 years, and less than 90 mm Hg from 11 to 17 years.

From Sampson HA, Muñoz-Furlong A, Campbell RL, et al. Second symposium on the definition and management of anaphylaxis: summary report–second National Institute of Allergy and Infectious Disease/Food Allergy and Anaphylaxis Network symposium. Ann Emerg Med 2006;47(4):373 to 80; with permission.

or symptoms involving 2 organ systems, including mucocutaneous, respiratory, cardiovascular, or gastrointestinal. The third criterion requires sudden onset of hypotension after exposure to a known allergen.

The NIAID/FAAN criteria have been widely adopted[4] and both retrospectively[5] and prospectively studied. They were found to be 95% sensitive and 71% specific in a prospective validation study among emergency department patients.[6] This means that for every 100 patients with anaphylaxis, 95 will meet one of the criteria. But that among 100 patients who meet NIAID/FAAN criteria, only 71 will have anaphylaxis. Thus, it is remains imperative that clinicians use clinical judgment when diagnosing anaphylaxis.

In 2019, the World Allergy Organization proposed a revision to the NIAID/FAAN criteria (**Box 2**).[7] The rationale for the proposed refinement was to simplify the existing criteria and recognize that some cases of anaphylaxis may involve primarily respiratory (eg, wheezing), laryngeal (eg, stridor, vocal changes or odynophagia), or cardiovascular symptoms (eg, hypotension) in the absence of other organ system involvement. Although this is likely to be a small subset of patients, this is a critical subset to recognize. Furthermore, the revision recognizes the potential for delayed presentations that can occur with alpha-Gal mediated reactions or with

---

Box 2
Amended criteria for the diagnosis of anaphylaxis, proposed by the WAO Anaphylaxis Committee, 2019

Anaphylaxis is highly likely when any of the following 2 criteria are fulfilled:

1. Acute onset of an illness (minutes to several hours) with involvement of the skin, mucosal tissue, or both (eg, generalized hives, pruritus or flushing, swollen lips-tongue-uvula)

And at least one of the following:
a. Respiratory compromise (eg, dyspnea, wheeze-bronchospasm, stridor, reduced PEF, hypoxemia)
b. Reduced BP or associated symptoms of end-organ dysfunction (eg, hypotonia [collapse], syncope, incontinence)
c. Severe gastrointestinal symptoms (eg, severe crampy abdominal pain, repetitive vomiting), especially after exposure to nonfood allergens

2. Acute onset of hypotension[a] or bronchospasm[b] or laryngeal involvement[c] after exposure to a known or highly probable allergen[d] for that patient (minutes to several hours[e]), even in the absence of typical skin involvement

[a]Hypotension defined as a decrease in systolic BP greater than 30% from that person's baseline, or. i. Infants and children under 10 y: systolic BP less than (70 mm Hg + [2 x age in years]). ii. Adults: systolic BP less than less than 90 mm Hg.

[b]Excluding lower respiratory symptoms triggered by common inhalant allergens or food allergens perceived to cause inhalational reactions in the absence of ingestion.

[c]Laryngeal symptoms include: stridor, vocal changes, odynophagia.

[d]An allergen is a substance (usually a protein) capable of triggering an immune response that can result in an allergic reaction. Most allergens act through an IgE-mediated pathway, but some non-allergen triggers can act independent of IgE (for example, via direct activation of mast cells).

[e]Most allergic reactions occur rapidly, but delayed reactions, with onset up to 10 hours after ingestion, may occur for some food allergens (eg, alpha-Gal) or secondary to immunotherapy.

Adapted from Cardona V, Ansotegui IJ, Ebisawa M, et al. World Allergy Organization anaphylaxis guidance 2020. World Allergy Organ J 2020;13(10):100472; with permission.

immunotherapy. Future studies are needed to determine the clinical utility of the revised criteria.

Fortunately, most allergic and anaphylactic reactions are self-limited and not life-threatening. However, the inability to predict when a reaction will become life-threatening necessitates early recognition and prompt treatment with epinephrine to prevent progression. Furthermore, some allergic reactions should be treated with epinephrine before anaphylaxis diagnostic clinical criteria are met. For example, a patient who has a history of a peanut allergy with prior severe anaphylactic reactions and develops hives after a peanut exposure should be treated promptly to halt reaction progression. Conversely, a patient whose symptoms have resolved by the time of his or her emergency department evaluation may no longer require epinephrine even if the initial symptoms met anaphylaxis diagnostic criteria. In a study of epinephrine administration for emergency department anaphylaxis patients, allergist-immunologists agreed with the emergency department management for 98% of patients despite the fact that only 70% of patients received epinephrine either before or during their emergency department evaluation.[8] These findings demonstrate that some patients who have experienced resolution of their anaphylactic reaction prior to emergency department arrival do not require epinephrine administration. However, even if patients do not require epinephrine administration in the emergency department, they should still receive the diagnosis of anaphylaxis, a prescription for self-injectable epinephrine, education regarding risk of biphasic and future reactions, and referral for follow-up with an allergist-immunologist.[2,9]

DEFINITIONS OF PERSISTENT, REFRACTORY, AND BIPHASIC ANAPHYLAXIS

Following treatment with intramuscular epinephrine, many patients with anaphylaxis experience symptom resolution. However, some patients have persistent symptoms necessitating treatment with additional epinephrine doses or life-saving resuscitative interventions (eg, positive pressure ventilation for patients with respiratory failure or vasopressors for those in shock).[10] On the other hand, some patients may develop recurrent symptoms following an initial asymptomatic period and without repeat exposure to the original trigger, referred to as biphasic or late phase reactions.[10,11] Taking into account the possibility that symptoms may return, ED clinicians must determine the need for prolonged observation or whether to hospitalize patients for monitoring.

Until recently, there were inconsistent definitions used to describe these disparate clinical courses, thus making it challenging to conduct comparative studies to identify the prevalence and risk factors for these outcomes, or to standardize ED management guidelines including optimal lengths of observation or hospitalization criteria. To account for the lack of standardized anaphylaxis outcome definitions, a multidisciplinary group of researchers developed consensus definitions for persistent, refractory, and biphasic anaphylaxis (**Box 3**) to harmonize outcomes in clinical care and research.[10] Application of the definitions in clinical care will help standardize communication among providers, patients, and families, and their use in research will help elucidate the true prevalence and risk factors for these outcomes with the ultimate goal of optimizing and standardizing emergency department management guidelines.

SEVERITY GRADING SYSTEM FOR ACUTE ALLERGIC REACTIONS

As noted previously, anaphylaxis occurs on a severity continuum from mild (requiring minimal interventions) to potentially life-threatening or fatal reactions. Unfortunately, clinical care and research are hampered by the lack of a uniformly accepted grading system to measure reaction severity during the course of reactions, including for initial,

---

Box 3
Clinical criteria for diagnosing persistent, refractory, and biphasic anaphylaxis

Persistent anaphylaxis is highly likely when there is[a] presence of symptoms/examination findings that fulfill the 2006 NIAID/FAAN anaphylaxis criteria that persist for at least 4 hours[1]

Refractory anaphylaxis is highly likely when both of the following 2 criteria are fulfilled:[b]

1. Presence of anaphylaxis following appropriate epinephrine dosing and symptom-directed medical management (eg, intravenous fluid bolus for hypotension)

2. The initial reaction must be treated with 3 or more appropriate doses of epinephrine (or initiation of an intravenous epinephrine infusion)[c]

Biphasic anaphylaxis is highly likely when all of the following 4 criteria are fulfilled[d]:

1. New/recurrent symptoms/examination findings must fulfill the 2006 NIAID/FAAN anaphylaxis criteria[1]

2. Initial symptoms/examination findings must completely resolve prior to the onset of new/recurrent symptoms/examination findings

3. There cannot be allergen repeat exposure prior to the onset of new/recurrent symptoms/examination findings

4. New/recurrent symptoms/examination findings must occur within 1 to 48 hours from complete resolution of initial symptoms/examination findings.

[a]The diagnosis of persistent anaphylaxis is independent of the management of the initial reaction.

[b]Refractory anaphylaxis is not dependent on the duration of symptoms/examination findings.

[c]Appropriate epinephrine dosing: 0.01 mg/kg intramuscular epinephrine, maximum single dose 0.5 mg. Also includes manufacturer recommended dosing for epinephrine autoinjectors.

[d]The diagnosis of biphasic anaphylaxis is independent of the management of the initial reaction.

From Dribin TE, Sampson HA, Camargo Jr CA, et al. Persistent, refractory, and biphasic anaphylaxis: A multidisciplinary Delphi study. J Allergy Clin Immunol 2020;146(5):1089-96; with permission.

---

persistent, and recurrent/new symptoms. This makes it difficult to evaluate the true prevalence of severe reactions, and to tailor management and therapeutic strategies accordingly. To account for this gap, researchers recently developed a consensus severity grading system for acute allergic reactions to standardize research outcomes and communication among providers, patients, and families (**Fig. 1**).[12] The grading system is optimal, because it can be used to measure reaction severity for anaphylactic and nonanaphylactic reactions, for all patient ages (children and adults), and it accounts for subjective symptoms (eg, throat tightness) in addition to symptoms specific to infants and young children. Before the grading system can be applied in clinical care, it must be validated prospectively; therefore, it is not intended to be used to inform management decisions including whether to administer epinephrine.

ANAPHYLAXIS PATHOPHYSIOLOGY

Anaphylaxis is typically a multiorgan phenomenon involving a broad range of effector cells including mast cells, basophils, neutrophils, macrophages, and platelets. From a mechanistic standpoint, anaphylaxis can be categorized as immunologic, nonimmunologic, or idiopathic, with the latter category caused by an unidentified allergen or

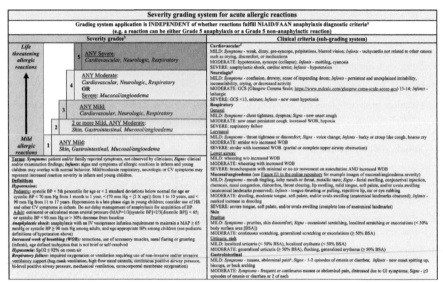

Fig. 1. Severity grading system for acute allergic reactions. [a]For patients with multiple symptoms, reaction severity is based on the most severe symptom; symptoms that constitute more severe grades always supersede symptoms from less severe grades. The grading system can be used to assign reaction severity at any time during the course of reactions; reactions may progress rapidly (within minutes) from one severity grade to another. The grading system does not dictate management decisions; reactions of any severity grade may require treatment with epinephrine. [b]Patients with severe cardiovascular and/or neurologic involvement may have urinary or stool incontinence. However, the significance of incontinence as an isolated symptom is unclear, and it is therefore not included as a symptom in the subgrading system. [c]Abdominal pain may also result from uterine cramping. (*From* Dribin TE, Schnadower D, Spergel JM, et al. Severity grading system for acute allergic reactions: a multidisciplinary Delphi study J Allergy Clin Immunol 2021;148(1):173-181: with permission.)

underlying mastocytosis (clonal mast cell disorder) (**Fig. 2**).[13] Immunologic anaphylaxis can be further subcategorized to immunoglobulin E (IgE)-mediated (eg, food, drugs, and insect stings) and IgE-independent forms, which include immunoglobulin G (IgG)-dependent anaphylaxis (eg, high molecular weight iron dextran, infusion of human monoclonal antibodies such as infliximab) and complement-mediated (eg, oversulfated chondroitin sulfate-contaminated heparin and polyethylene glycols). Mixed reactions involving both IgE and non-IgE mediated pathways can also occur with chemotherapy. Nonimmunologic anaphylaxis may be caused by direct mediator release from mast cells and basophils (eg, opioids), physical factors (eg, exercise, heat, and sunlight/UV radiation), contact system activation (eg, dialysis membranes), and arachidonic acid metabolism disruptions (eg, nonsteroidal anti-inflammatory drugs [NSAIDs]).

The degranulation of mast cells and basophils leads to the release of mediators that orchestrate the various systemic manifestations that define anaphylaxis. Such mediators include histamine, platelet-activating factor (PAF), cysteinyl leukotrienes (CysLTs), and anaphylatoxins. Histamine targets multiple organ systems and triggers various signs and symptoms involving the upper respiratory (sneezing and angioedema), lower respiratory (cough and wheezing), digestive (vomiting and diarrhea), cardiovascular (tachycardia and hypotension), and skin systems (flushing and urticaria)

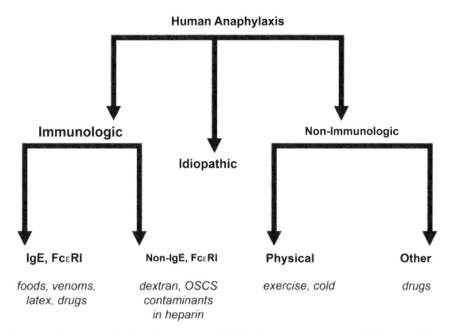

Fig. 2. Mechanisms underlying human anaphylaxis. (*From* Simons FE. Anaphylaxis. J Allergy Clin Immunol 2010;125(2 Suppl 2):S161-8; with permission.)

(Fig. 3).[14] PAF is a lipid-derived mediator of anaphylaxis produced by platelets, neutrophils, mast cells, and macrophages. PAF has effects on the skin and cardiovascular systems, and its effects are thought to be independent of mast cell degranulation.[15] Increased levels of PAF have been shown to correlate with increasing anaphylaxis grade severity.[16] CysLTs represent a third mediator category and include LTB4, LTC4, and LTD4.[17] CysLTs are produced from arachidonic acid by mast cells, basophils, and macrophages. CysLTs and their metabolites are increased during anaphylaxis and have been shown to induce wheal and flare reactions along with bronchoconstriction.[18] Anaphylatoxins (C3a, C4a, and C5a) represent the fourth category of mediators. These are small polypeptides that are potent inflammatory mediators that activate mast cells and basophils. Elevated levels of anaphylatoxins have also been correlated with anaphylaxis severity.[14] Based on mouse models, anaphylatoxins may mediate similar effects as other mediators and work in a redundant fashion.[14] Anaphylaxis may also induce changes in other mediators including prostaglandins, chemokines/cytokines, and tryptase. With regards to the latter, tryptase is a serine protease released by mast cells and basophils that possesses pro-inflammatory effects triggering tissue edema, chemokine secretion, and subsequent neutrophil recruitment. Tryptase is a biomarker that can be measured 15 minutes to 180 minutes after symptom onset, and, although timely results may not be available during the emergency department evaluation, it may aid in the final diagnosis of anaphylaxis. Elevated tryptase of more than 12.4 ng/mL in the emergency department has a positive predictive value of up to 93% and negative predictive value as low as 17%.[19] An elevated tryptase may support the clinical diagnosis of anaphylaxis, although it may not be elevated in all cases, particularly in cases of food-induced anaphylaxis.[20] Of note, recent research has linked a similar group of mediators (histamine, tryptase, interleukin (IL)-16, IL-10, and tumor necrosis factor [TNF]-receptor 1), with both

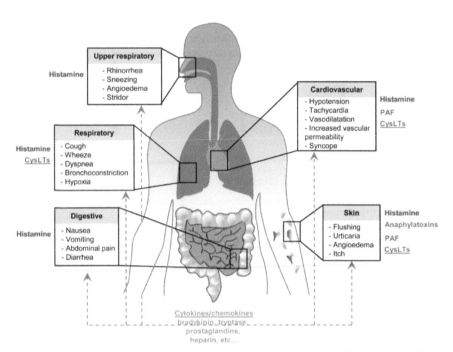

Fig. 3. Pathophysiological changes in anaphylaxis and mediators that have been implicated in these processes. (*From* Reber LL, Hernandez JD, Galli SJ. The pathophysiology of anaphylaxis. J Allergy Clin Immunol 2017;140(2):335-48; with permission.)

reaction severity and protracted reactions suggesting that protracted reactions may be closely linked to initial reaction severity.[21]

ANAPHYLAXIS EPIDEMIOLOGY

The lifetime prevalence of anaphylaxis in the general population (from all triggers) has been estimated to be between 0.05% and 2%.[22] Numerous studies have demonstrated increasing rates of anaphylaxis in Western countries, including the United States, Canada, Australia, Finland, Sweden, the United Kingdom, as well as in Asia, including Korea and Hong Kong.[23] Among children under 10 years of age, boys have higher incidence rates of anaphylaxis than girls.[23] However, after age 10, girls have comparable or higher rates of anaphylaxis. Among adults, anaphylaxis rates are higher among women than men.[23,24]

Time Trends

In the United States, anaphylaxis-related ED visits are increasing.[25] Based on a large national administrative claims database study, the overall rate of anaphylaxis per 100,000 enrollees increased by 101% from 2005 to 2014. Similar results were published in a recent national cross-sectional study that revealed a 3.2-fold increase in anaphylaxis-related emergency department visits from 2008 to 2016.[26]

Triggers

Food represents the leading cause of pediatric anaphylaxis and is the leading cause of anaphylaxis presenting to emergency departments in the United States, with about 30,000 cases per year. The most common specific food trigger varies by age group, with cow's milk more common in infants, peanuts in children, and shellfish and tree nuts in young adults and adults.[27] In an observational study examining national time trends of pediatric food-induced anaphylaxis-related emergency department visits from 2005 to 2014, anaphylaxis caused by a food trigger increased by 214%, with infants and toddlers (0–2 years of age) comprising most of those visits.[28] A retrospective cohort study examining 37 pediatric hospitals from 2007 to 2012 reported a similar trend of increasing rates of food-induced anaphylaxis emergency department visits.[29] However, there was no increase in the proportion of patients admitted to the hospital or intensive care unit (ICU) for food-related anaphylaxis.

A novel food allergy syndrome was recently defined over the past decade. Referred to as alpha-Gal syndrome, it is associated with 2 distinct presentations: (1) delayed allergic reaction, typically 2 to 6 hours after ingestion of mammalian meat; and (2) anaphylaxis immediately upon receiving the chemotherapy agent cetuximab commonly used to treat colorectal and head and neck cancers.[30] Patients are typically adults, many of whom tolerated meats previously and who present with symptoms ranging from localized urticaria and angioedema to severe anaphylaxis requiring emergency department management and hospital admission. The reactions are caused by the development of a novel IgE antibody response to galactose-alpha-1,3-galactose (alpha-Gal). Alpha-Gal is an oligosaccharide epitope present in the saliva of some ticks, mammalian meat, and on the antigen-binding fragment (Fab) portion of the cetuximab heavy chain. It is hypothesized that the introduction of alpha-Gal that occurs with a tick bite results in the production of IgE, which later causes anaphylaxis to mammalian meat or cetuximab (**Fig. 4**).[30] The distinctive delay between ingestion of mammalian meat and symptom onset is because of the time required for digestion and then presentation of the antigen to mast cells in peripheral tissues. In the United States, the Lone Star tick (*Amblyomma americanum*) is the primary cause of alpha-Gal syndrome, whereas different species of ticks are responsible for this disease in other countries. Management of alpha-Gal syndrome involves avoidance of red meat and mammalian organs, with up to 20% of patients also needing to avoid gelatin and dairy products. Patients are also advised to avoid tick bites, as further tick bites may maintain or increase the titer of IgE specific to alpha-Gal.

Stinging insect venom are a major cause of adult and pediatric anaphylaxis including children and adolescents. Although insect allergy is more common in young adults, fatal anaphylaxis caused by insect stings are more likely to occur in older adults, a likely consequence of underlying comorbidities and impaired compensatory physiologic responses.[31] The most common venom triggers include hymenopterans (yellow jacket, hornet, wasp, and honeybee) and the imported fire ant (*Solenopsis invicta* and *Solenopsis richteri*). Among the stinging insects, yellow jackets cause the most frequent insect sting reactions in the United States. More than 10% of all anaphylaxis-related emergency department visits are caused by insect allergy. Systemic reactions to insect stings may affect up to 0.8% of children and 3% of adults, with at least 40 fatal stings per year nationally.[32] For patients, the first sting related reaction may be fatal. Venom content varies among the different stinging insect families and demonstrates seasonal and geographic variation, which may explain the variability of allergic reactions with individual stings.

Medications represent the third most common anaphylaxis trigger. Generally, adverse drug reactions occur in up to 10% of the general population, and of those, 10% are drug hypersensitivity reactions.[33] The incidence of anaphylaxis caused by medication triggers is increasing.[25,34] In the United States, the most commonly identified drug culprits include antibiotics (penicillin, cephalosporins, and sulfonamides), along with aspirin and other NSAIDs. In the United States as well as globally in

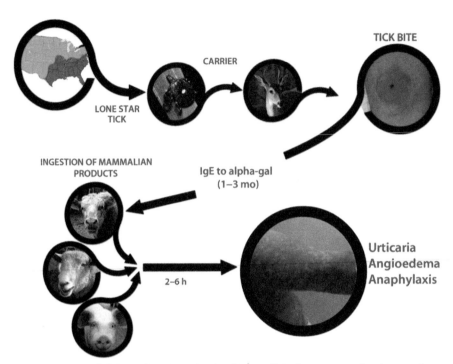

Fig. 4. Summary of alpha-Gal sensitization leading to clinical symptoms of red meat allergy. The southeastern section of the United States is where most of the reactions to red meat have been reported. This region overlaps with the distribution of the lone star tick. The current hypothesis is that persons are bitten by lone star ticks carried by deer into rural and urban areas. After a period of time, IgE to alpha-Gal develops. Once IgE to alpha-Gal reaches sufficient levels, ingestion of red meat can trigger reactions. Several of the images used in this figure are licensed under a Creative Commons CC BY-NC 2.0 (Attribution-NonCommercial 2.0 Generic) license (Cow: https://flic.kr/p/adgjhp by user Plashing Vole; Deer: https://flic.kr/p/jeZwq7 by user Cherry Bream; Sheep: https://flic.kr/p/4WirD by user Lauren; Tick: https://flic.kr/p/cdnNaY by user Katja Schulz; Pig: https://flic.kr/p/N7gpc by user Anne). (*From* Steinke JW, Platts-Mills TA, Commins SP. The alpha-Gal story: lessons learned from connecting the dots. J Allergy Clin Immunol 2015;135(3):589-96; with permission.)

Australia, the United Kingdom, and New Zealand, medications are a common cause of fatal anaphylaxis.[35]

In the emergency department, the exact trigger can often be difficult to identify, and thus referral to an allergist-immunologist specialist is recommended. In a prior retrospective study, more than one-third of patients with suspected anaphylaxis in the emergency department had a change in the diagnosis or suspected trigger after allergy consultation.[36] Moreover, for those with suspected venom-induced anaphylaxis, allergy specialists can offer venom immunotherapy, which may not only help to reduce a patient's risk of subsequent anaphylaxis from 30% to 60% to less than 5%, but also improve quality of life by reducing anxiety related to risk of future reactions.[37–39]

RISK FACTORS FOR SEVERE, BIPHASIC, AND FATAL ANAPHYLAXIS
Severe Anaphylaxis

It is challenging to evaluate risk factors for severe anaphylaxis given the preponderance of research related to this topic uses inconsistent outcome definitions (eg, need for ICU admission, hospitalization, or repeat epinephrine administration) and study designs. Despite this, recent research has identified several potential risk factors for severe anaphylaxis (**Box 4**): older patient age (>65 years), history of mastocytosis, medication trigger, and comorbidities including pulmonary (eg, asthma) and cardiac disease (coronary disease, heart failure).[40,41] Although history of asthma may be a risk factor for severe reactions, it is unclear whether patients with a history of asthma should be managed more conservatively (eg, extended observation periods, hospital admission) than patients without asthma to monitor for biphasic reactions.[40,42]

Biphasic Anaphylaxis

Although there is wide variability in the reported prevalence (1% to 20%) and risk factors for biphasic reactions, it is important for emergency department clinicians to be aware of potential risk factors when making management decisions including determining the length of emergency department observation or need for hospitalization (see **Box 4**).[11] Recently published anaphylaxis guidelines recommend (albeit a weak recommendation based on low evidence) extended observation periods to monitor for biphasic reactions for patients with resolved severe anaphylaxis (eg, hypotension) and those who receive greater than 1 dose of epinephrine.[42] Although antihistamines and systemic steroids are commonly used to treat anaphylaxis and have a theoretic role in preventing biphasic reactions, the same guidelines recommend against their routine use to prevent biphasic reactions given insufficient supporting data.[42]

Fatal Anaphylaxis

Despite an apparent increase in the prevalence of anaphylaxis globally (reflected in rising emergency department visits and hospitalizations),[25,26] there does not appear to

---

Box 4
Potential risk factors for severe, biphasic, and fatal anaphylaxis

Severe anaphylaxis[40,41,45–47]

- Patient factors: age ≥65 years, male sex

- Comorbidities: cardiac or lung disease (eg, chronic obstructive pulmonary disease [COPD], asthma), prior emergency department visit or hospitalization for anaphylaxis, mastocytosis

- Triggers: medication, insect venom, iatrogenic

- P factors: use of beta blockers or angiotensin-converting enzyme (ACE) inhibitors in proximity to allergen exposure, vigorous physical activity

Biphasic anaphylaxis[48–52]

- Comorbidities: prior anaphylaxis

- Triggers: unknown trigger

- Examination findings: wide pulse pressure, hypotension, wheezing, diarrhea

- Reaction features: delayed epinephrine administration, greater than 1 dose of epinephrine

Fatal anaphylaxis[7,35,53–55]

- Patient factors: elderly patients, male sex

- Comorbidities: asthma, cardiovascular disease, mastocytosis

- Reaction features: delayed epinephrine administration

Box 5
Differential diagnosis of anaphylaxis

Tissue swelling

- Idiopathic urticaria
- Isolated angioedema[a]
- Idiopathic
- ACE inhibitor-induced
- Acquired or hereditary C1 esterase inhibitor deficiency

Conditions mimicking upper airway edema

- Dystonic reactions mimicking symptoms of a swollen tongue after taking metoclopramide, prochlorperazine, or antihistamines
- Acute esophageal reflux (sudden onset of painful throat swelling)

Endocrine/flushing syndromes

- Peptide-secreting tumors (eg, carcinoid syndrome, VIPomas[b])
- Alcohol-related
- Medullary carcinoma of thyroid
- Vancomycin Infusion Syndrome[c]
- Menopause (flushing, hot flashes)
- Hypoglycemia

Neurologic syndromes

- Seizure
- Stroke

Other causes of syncope

- Vasovagal episodes
- Sepsis
- Shock (septic, cardiogenic, hypovolemic, hemorrhagic, neurologic)

Acute respiratory distress

- Asthma
- Panic disorders
- Globus hystericus
- Laryngospasm
- Vocal cord dysfunction

Medications

- Vancomycin (vancomycin infusion syndrome)
- Niacin (flushing)
- General anesthetics (hypotension)

Psychosomatic/functional disorders

- Panic disorders
- Factitious anaphylaxis
- Undifferentiated somatoform anaphylaxis

- Vocal cord dysfunction

Miscellaneous

- Scombroid fish poisoning

- Serum sickness

- Pheochromocytoma

- Systemic mastocytosis

- Urticaria pigmentosa

- Basophil leukemia

- Acute promyelocytic leukemia with tretinoin treatment

[a]Isolated angioedema lacks any other organ or systemic features and thus by definition is not anaphylaxis

[b]Neuroendocrine tumors that secrete vasoactive intestinal polypeptide

[c]Vancomycin infusion syndrome is flushing and erythema associated with infusion of vancomycin (or occasionally other antibiotics); it is thought to be caused by histamine release, and may be related to dose or infusion rate

Adapted from Brown SG, Mullins RJ, Gold MS. Anaphylaxis: diagnosis and management. Med J Aust 2006;185(5):283-9; LoVerde D, Iweala OI, Eginli A, et al. Anaphylaxis. Chest 2018;153(2):528-43; with permission.

be a parallel increase in anaphylaxis fatalities, which fortunately remain rare events. Recent studies report population fatality rates between 0.47 and 0.69 per million persons, and emergency department and inpatient fatality rates between 0.25% and 0.33%.[35,42] Establishing the true prevalence and risk factors for fatal anaphylaxis is challenging given the preponderance of data are from retrospective registries and case series from which it is difficult to develop reliable predictive models. Still, clinicians must be knowledgeable of potential risk factors for this rare outcome, and optimize management strategies to mitigate patient risk. This is challenging given risk factors for fatal anaphylaxis vary by allergen.[35,43] Potential risk factors for drug-induced fatalities include underlying cardiovascular disease and older age (age >65), whereas delayed epinephrine administration may be a risk factor for food-induced fatalities and cardiovascular disease and mastocytosis for inset sting fatalities.[35] Given the unpredictable nature of fatal anaphylaxis, it is essential that patients adhere to strict allergen avoidance. Likewise, clinicians should seek to optimize the management of predisposing comorbidities (eg, asthma, immunotherapy for sting allergy), and ensure patients have access to epinephrine autoinjectors and are educated on their use.[42]

DIFFERENTIAL DIAGNOSIS

Clinicians must maintain a broad differential when treating patients with suspected anaphylaxis (**Box 5**), especially for patients who do not respond to standard anaphylaxis management. Additionally, because anaphylaxis is under-recognized and undertreated (specifically around treatment with epinephrine),[2] it is critical for emergency department providers to consider anaphylaxis in the differential diagnosis for patients whose symptoms overlap with those of anaphylaxis (eg, upper airway obstruction, wheezing, angioedema, flushing, syncope, hypotension) given delayed treatment with epinephrine may be a risk factor for adverse outcomes including biphasic and fatal anaphylaxis. Likewise, recognition of anaphylaxis may be especially challenging for noncommunicative patients including infants and young children who may present with nonspecific symptoms that overlap with normal infant behavior (eg, fussiness, drooling, spitting up).[44]

CLINICS CARE POINTS

- Epinephrine is indicated for patients with potentially life-threatening allergic manifestations even if multiple organ systems are not involved.
- Consider alpha-Gal syndrome in patients without a clear inciting allergic trigger.
- Inform patients of their risk of a biphasic reaction and ensure that they are adequately prepared to manage it.
- Refer patients with anaphylaxis to an allergist for confirmation of the diagnosis and trigger and for possible immunotherapy.

DISCLOSURE

Dr. Campbell is an author for UpToDate and a consultant for Bryn Pharma. Dr. Dribin has received research funding from the National Center for Advancing Translational Sciences of the National Institutes of Health under Award Number 2UL1TR001425-05A1 and Award Number 2KL2TR001426-05A1.

REFERENCES

1. Bergmann K-C, Ring J. History of allergy. Chemical immunology and allergy, vol. 100. Basel: Karger; 2014.
2. Fineman SM, Bowman SH, Campbell RL, et al. Addressing barriers to emergency anaphylaxis care: from emergency medical services to emergency department to outpatient follow-up. Ann Allergy Asthma Immunol 2015;115(4):301–5.
3. Sampson HA, Muñoz-Furlong A, Campbell RL, et al. Second symposium on the definition and management of anaphylaxis: summary report–second National Institute of Allergy and Infectious Disease/Food Allergy and Anaphylaxis Network symposium. Ann Emerg Med 2006;47(4):373–80.
4. Simons FE, Ebisawa M, Sanchez-Borges M, et al. 2015 update of the evidence base: World Allergy Organization anaphylaxis guidelines. World Allergy Organ J 2015;8(1):32.
5. Campbell RL, Hagan JB, Manivannan V, et al. Evaluation of national institute of allergy and infectious diseases/food allergy and anaphylaxis network criteria for the diagnosis of anaphylaxis in emergency department patients. J Allergy Clin Immunol 2012;129(3):748–52.
6. Loprinzi Brauer CE, Motosue MS, Li JT, et al. Prospective validation of the NIAID/FAAN criteria for emergency department diagnosis of anaphylaxis. J Allergy Clin Immunol Pract 2016;4(6):1220–6.
7. Cardona V, Ansotegui IJ, Ebisawa M, et al. World Allergy Organization anaphylaxis guidance 2020. World Allergy Organ J 2020;13(10):100472.
8. Baalmann DV, Hagan JB, Li JT, et al. Appropriateness of epinephrine use in ED patients with anaphylaxis. Am J Emerg Med 2016;34(2):174–9.
9. Campbell RL, Li JT, Nicklas RA, et al. Emergency department diagnosis and treatment of anaphylaxis: a practice parameter. Ann Allergy Asthma Immunol 2014;113(6):599–608.

10. Dribin TE, Sampson HA, Camargo CA Jr, et al. Persistent, refractory, and biphasic anaphylaxis: a multidisciplinary Delphi study. J Allergy Clin Immunol 2020;146(5):1089–96.
11. Lee S, Sadosty AT, Campbell RL. Update on biphasic anaphylaxis. Curr Opin Allergy Clin Immunol 2016;16(4):346–51.
12. Dribin TE, Schnadower D, Spergel JM, et al. Severity grading system for acute allergic reactions: a multidisciplinary Delphi study. J Allergy Clin Immunol 2021; 148(1):173–81.
13. Simons FE. Anaphylaxis. J Allergy Clin Immunol 2010;125(2 Suppl 2):S161–81.
14. Reber LL, Hernandez JD, Galli SJ. The pathophysiology of anaphylaxis. J Allergy Clin Immunol 2017;140(2):335–48.
15. Vadas P, Perelman B, Liss G. Platelet-activating factor, histamine, and tryptase levels in human anaphylaxis. J Allergy Clin Immunol 2013;131(1):144–9.
16. Vadas P, Gold M, Perelman B, et al. Platelet-activating factor, PAF acetylhydrolase, and severe anaphylaxis. N Engl J Med 2008;358(1):28–35.
17. Austen KF. The cysteinyl leukotrienes: where do they come from? What are they? Where are they going? Nat Immunol 2008;9(2):113–5.
18. Weiss JW, Drazen JM, Coles N, et al. Bronchoconstrictor effects of leukotriene C in humans. Science 1982;216(4542):196–8.
19. Buka RJ, Knibb RC, Crossman RJ, et al. Anaphylaxis and clinical utility of real-world measurement of acute serum tryptase in UK Emergency Departments. J Allergy Clin Immunol Pract 2017;5(5):1280–7.e2.
20. Lin RY, Schwartz LB, Curry A, et al. Histamine and tryptase levels in patients with acute allergic reactions: an emergency department-based study. J Allergy Clin Immunol 2000;106(1 Pt 1):65–71.
21. Brown SG, Stone SF, Fatovich DM, et al. Anaphylaxis: clinical patterns, mediator release, and severity. J Allergy Clin Immunol 2013;132(5):1141–9.e5.
22. Lieberman P, Camargo CA Jr, Bohlke K, et al. Epidemiology of anaphylaxis: findings of the American College of Allergy, Asthma and Immunology Epidemiology of Anaphylaxis Working Group. Ann Allergy Asthma Immunol 2006;97(5): 596–602.
23. Wang Y, Allen KJ, Suaini NHA, et al. The global incidence and prevalence of anaphylaxis in children in the general population: a systematic review. Allergy 2019;74(6):1063–80.
24. Jensen-Jarolim E, Untersmayr E. Gender-medicine aspects in allergology. Allergy 2008;63(5):610–5.
25. Motosue MS, Bellolio MF, Van Houten HK, et al. Increasing emergency department visits for anaphylaxis, 2005-2014. J Allergy Clin Immunol Pract 2017;5(1): 171–5.e3.
26. Michelson KA, Dribin TE, Vyles D, et al. Trends in emergency care for anaphylaxis. J Allergy Clin Immunol Pract 2020;8(2):767–8.e2.
27. Poowuttikul P, Seth D. Anaphylaxis in children and adolescents. Pediatr Clin North Am 2019;66(5):995–1005.
28. Motosue MS, Bellolio MF, Van Houten HK, et al. National trends in emergency department visits and hospitalizations for food-induced anaphylaxis in US children. Pediatr Allergy Immunol 2018;29(5):538–44.
29. Parlaman JP, Oron AP, Uspal NG, et al. Emergency and hospital care for food-related anaphylaxis in children. Hosp Pediatr 2016;6(5):269–74.
30. Steinke JW, Platts-Mills TA, Commins SP. The alpha-gal story: lessons learned from connecting the dots. J Allergy Clin Immunol 2015;135(3):589–96 [quiz 597].

31. Tankersley MS, Ledford DK. Stinging insect allergy: state of the art 2015. J Allergy Clin Immunol Pract 2015;3(3):315–22 [quiz 323].

32. Graft DF. Insect sting allergy. Med Clin North Am 2006;90(1):211–32.

33. Lazarou J, Pomeranz BH, Corey PN. Incidence of adverse drug reactions in hospitalized patients: a meta-analysis of prospective studies. JAMA 1998;279(15): 1200–5.

34. Lee S, Hess EP, Lohse C, et al. Trends, characteristics, and incidence of anaphylaxis in 2001-2010: a population-based study. J Allergy Clin Immunol 2017; 139(1):182–8.e2.

35. Turner PJ, Jerschow E, Umasunthar T, et al. Fatal anaphylaxis: mortality rate and risk factors. J Allergy Clin Immunol Pract 2017;5(5):1169–78.

36. Campbell RL, Park MA, Kueber MA Jr, et al. Outcomes of allergy/immunology follow-up after an emergency department evaluation for anaphylaxis. J Allergy Clin Immunol Pract 2015;3(1):88–93.

37. Dhami S, Zaman H, Varga EM, et al. Allergen immunotherapy for insect venom allergy: a systematic review and meta-analysis. Allergy 2017;72(3):342–65.

38. Lange J, Cichocka-Jarosz E, Marczak H, et al. Natural history of Hymenoptera venom allergy in children not treated with immunotherapy. Ann Allergy Asthma Immunol 2016;116(3):225–9.

39. Confino-Cohen R, Melamed S, Goldberg A. Debilitating beliefs and emotional distress in patients given immunotherapy for insect sting allergy: a prospective study. Allergy Asthma Proc 2009;30(5):546–51.

40. Motosue MS, Bellolio MF, Van Houten HK, et al. Risk factors for severe anaphylaxis in the United States. Ann Allergy Asthma Immunol 2017;119(4):356–61.e2.

41. Worm M, Francuzik W, Renaudin JM, et al. Factors increasing the risk for a severe reaction in anaphylaxis: an analysis of data from The European Anaphylaxis Registry. Allergy 2018;73(6):1322–30.

42. Shaker MS, Wallace DV, Golden DBK, et al. Anaphylaxis-a 2020 practice parameter update, systematic review, and Grading of Recommendations, Assessment, Development and Evaluation (GRADE) analysis. J Allergy Clin Immunol 2020; 145(4):1082–123.

43. Pumphrey R. Anaphylaxis: can we tell who is at risk of a fatal reaction? Curr Opin Allergy Clin Immunol 2004;4(4):285–90.

44. Greenhawt M, Gupta RS, Meadows JA, et al. Guiding principles for the recognition, diagnosis, and management of infants with anaphylaxis: an expert panel consensus. J Allergy Clin Immunol Pract 2019;7(4):1148–56.e5.

45. Brown SG. Clinical features and severity grading of anaphylaxis. J Allergy Clin Immunol 2004;114(2):371–6.

46. Calvani M, Cardinale F, Martelli A, et al. Risk factors for severe pediatric food anaphylaxis in Italy. Pediatr Allergy Immunol 2011;22(8):813–9.

47. Clark S, Wei W, Rudders SA, et al. Risk factors for severe anaphylaxis in patients receiving anaphylaxis treatment in US emergency departments and hospitals. J Allergy Clin Immunol 2014;134(5):1125–30.

48. Alqurashi W, Stiell I, Chan K, et al. Epidemiology and clinical predictors of biphasic reactions in children with anaphylaxis. Ann Allergy Asthma Immunol 2015;115(3):217–23.e2.

49. Lee JM, Greenes DS. Biphasic anaphylactic reactions in pediatrics. Pediatrics 2000;106(4):762–6.

50. Lee S, Bellolio MF, Hess EP, et al. Predictors of biphasic reactions in the emergency department for patients with anaphylaxis. J Allergy Clin Immunol Pract 2014;2(3):281–7.

51. Lee S, Bellolio MF, Hess EP, et al. Time of Onset and Predictors of Biphasic Anaphylactic Reactions: A Systematic Review and Meta-analysis. J Allergy Clin Immunol Pract 2015;3(3):408–16, e401-402.
52. Lee S, Peterson A, Lohse CM, et al. Further evaluation of factors that may predict biphasic reactions in emergency department anaphylaxis patients. J Allergy Clin Immunol Pract 2017;5(5):1295–301.
53. Pouessel G, Claverie C, Labreuche J, et al. Fatal anaphylaxis in France: analysis of national anaphylaxis data, 1979-2011. J Allergy Clin Immunol 2017;140(2): 610–2.e2.
54. Pouessel G, Turner PJ, Worm M, et al. Food-induced fatal anaphylaxis: from epidemiological data to general prevention strategies. Clin Exp Allergy 2018; 48(12):1584–93.
55. Turner PJ, Gowland MH, Sharma V, et al. Increase in anaphylaxis-related hospitalizations but no increase in fatalities: an analysis of United Kingdom national anaphylaxis data, 1992-2012. J Allergy Clin Immunol 2015;135(4):956–63.e1.

Anaphylaxis
Emergency Department Treatment

Kelly McHugh, MD, Zachary Repanshek, MD*

KEYWORDS

- Anaphylaxis • Epinephrine • Anaphylactic shock • Airway management
- Awake intubation

KEY POINTS

- Anaphylaxis is a life-threatening allergic reaction that requires the management of airway, breathing, and circulation.
- Intramuscular epinephrine is the mainstay of anaphylaxis treatment. There are no absolute contraindications to administration of epinephrine.
- Intravenous epinephrine is the treatment of anaphylactic shock and should be given as an infusion along with intravenous crystalloids.
- When upper airway obstruction necessitates intubation, awake intubation may be safer than rapid sequence intubation.
- There is no best practice for the amount of observation required after treatment, and this should be tailored to the individual patient, because biphasic reactions often occur outside of traditional observation periods.

INTRODUCTION

Anaphylaxis is a serious systemic allergic reaction which, if not treated quickly, can lead to cardiovascular collapse.[1] Emergency department (ED) care involves appropriate triage, administration of epinephrine, and general management of the airway, breathing, and circulation. Intramuscular (IM) epinephrine is the mainstay of anaphylaxis treatment. For patients in shock, intravenous (IV) epinephrine is necessary. Adjunctive medications include bronchodilators, corticosteroids, and antihistamines. Glucagon and additional vasopressors should be used when anaphylaxis is refractory to epinephrine. Airway management is key if there are signs of airway obstruction.

This article originally appeared in Emergency Medicine Clinics, Volume 40 Issue 1, February 2022.
Department of Emergency Medicine, Lewis Katz School of Medicine, Temple University, 3401 North Broad Street, Philadelphia, PA 19140, USA
* Corresponding author.
E-mail address: zachary.repanshek2@tuhs.temple.edu

INITIAL EVALUATION AND MANAGEMENT

The patient with severe allergic symptoms should be triaged to a monitored bed and evaluated by a physician immediately, because the initial symptoms of anaphylaxis can progress rapidly to cardiopulmonary instability (**Fig. 1**). In 1 study, the mean time from onset of anaphylaxis to cardiac arrest by trigger was 30 minutes for food, 15 minutes for venom, and 5 minutes for medication.[2] IM epinephrine should be administered as soon as anaphylaxis is identified, which may be done concurrently with the primary assessment. Risk factors for fatal anaphylaxis should be assessed if possible. These include a history of cardiopulmonary disease, history of asthma, peanut or tree nut allergy, advanced age, delayed presentation, and mast cell disease.[3]

Respiratory distress may be secondary to bronchospasm or upper airway obstruction. Stridor, drooling, and tongue or facial edema are ominous signs, suggestive of impending airway obstruction, and there should be a low threshold to secure the airway. The physician should expect and prepare for a difficult intubation.

Hypotension should alert the provider of the potential for circulatory collapse. The patient should be placed in the supine position to increase cerebral and cardiac

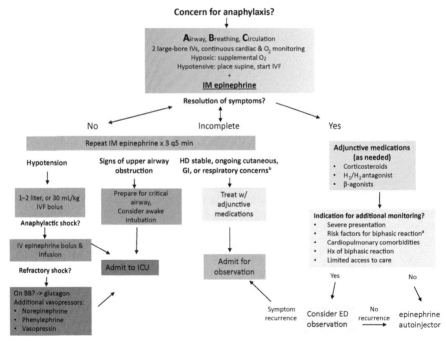

Fig. 1. Overview of anaphylaxis management in the ED. [a]Risk factors for biphasic reaction include, initial presentation with severe features or hypotension, multiple doses of epinephrine required, delayed administration of epinephrine 60 minutes to 190 minutes after symptom onset, onset of symptoms greater than 30 minutes after the initial exposure, or an unknown trigger—note that these are not consistent across studies [b]For minor gastrointestinal symptoms, such as ongoing nausea or diarrhea, or minor cutaneous symptoms, such as residual urticaria or pruritis, patients can be discharged home with good follow-up. BB, β-blocker; GI, gastrointestinal; HD, hemodynamically; H$_1$, histamine 1; H$_2$, histamine 2; Hx, history; ICU, intensive care unit; IVF, IV fluids; w/, with.

perfusion. Standing has been associated with cardiovascular arrest, likely secondary to the profound vasodilation that occurs in anaphylaxis.[4] In patients who are hypotensive, IV crystalloids should be initiated immediately; 1 L to 2 L or 20 mL/kg of isotonic fluids for adult and pediatric patients, respectively, should be bolused, unless there is a history of heart failure or end-stage renal disease. Life-sustaining equipment, such as a code cart and defibrillator, should be readily available, and providers should be ready to proceed to advanced cardiac life support in the event of cardiac arrest.

The cause of anaphylaxis may not always be known. It is important, however, to consider ongoing exposures to the trigger. If anaphylaxis develops while the patient is already in the ED, stop all potential offending medications immediately. For those who have been envenomated, attempt to remove any stingers that still are imbedded in the skin. In cases of food allergy, there is no role for gastric lavage.[5]

FIRST-LINE THERAPY: EPINEPRHINE

Epinephrine is the mainstay of anaphylaxis management and is widely accepted by major guidelines as first-line therapy.[1,3,6–10] Because anaphylaxis is rapid in onset and potentially fatal, and epinephrine has such a long history of effectiveness, a randomized controlled trial (RCT) comparing another intervention is ethically questionable. Thus, there is a lack of prospective data that demonstrate the benefits of epinephrine.[11] Experience has shown it to be effective, however, and most cases of fatal anaphylaxis are associated with delayed or failure to provide epinephrine.[2,11] Epinephrine acts on α_1-adrenergic, β_1-adrenergic, and β_2-adrenergic receptors to counteract anaphylactic physiology. Stimulation of the α_1-adrenergic receptor leads to decreased mucosal edema and increased systemic vascular resistance, thereby decreasing airway obstruction and improving hypotension. Stimulation of the β_1-receptor leads to increased inotropy and chronotropy, also improving hypotension. Stimulation of the β_2-receptor causes bronchodilation and decreased production of inflammatory mediators that otherwise would increase vascular permeability and smooth muscle contraction as well as attract additional inflammatory cells.[12]

Despite the many benefits of epinephrine, studies show that it is underutilized in the emergency setting. One retrospective study found that only 16% of patients presenting with anaphylaxis received epinephrine.[13] Epinephrine is often withheld in the older population, especially in those with coronary disease, due to concern for precipitating ischemia or arrythmia. There are no absolute contraindications to epinephrine, however, which, when given IM, exhibits a wide safety profile.[3,8,11] Most adverse events have occurred after use of IV epinephrine, especially when administered incorrectly.[2] It is now recognized that there may be direct cardiotoxic effects from anaphylaxis as well as the potential for ischemia from hypotension.[14] Thus, epinephrine should not be withheld from anyone presenting with severe allergic symptoms.

In patients presenting with anaphylaxis who are not in cardiac arrest, the optimal administration route of IM epinephrine is in the anterolateral thigh, at a dose of 0.01 mg/kg, with a maximum of 0.5 mg in adults and 0.3 mg in children (**Table 1**).[12] Doses can be repeated at 5-minute intervals as needed for symptom control. Patients already may have received epinephrine via autoinjector prior to arrival in a dose of 0.1 mg, 0.15 mg, or 0.3 mg. Patients who received epinephrine en route without resolution of symptoms should be treated immediately with an additional dose of IM epinephrine. There are limited pharmacokinetic data on epinephrine in anaphylaxis, and those studies that have been conducted have been on healthy patients. One study in children with a history of anaphylaxis found that peak levels of epinephrine were

Table 1 Epinephrine dosing for anaphylaxis		
Epinephrine dose	Adults	Pediatrics
Initial dosing		
	0.3–0.5 mg IM 1:1000 (max 0.5 mg) q5 min	0.01 mg/kg IM 1:1000 (max 0.3 mg) q5 min
Severe hypotension/shock		
IV bolus	10–20 μg IV push q 2–5 min	
Add 1 mL of 1:10,000 epi to 9 mL syringe of NS = 10-μg/mL solution		
Infusion[a]	0.1–1 μg/kg/min	0.01–1 μg/kg/min IV
Add 1 mg epi (1 mL of 1:1000 or 10 mL of 1:10,000) to 1L NS = 1 μg/mL solution		

Abbreviations: epi, epinephrine; max, maximum; NS, normal saline; peds, pediatrics.
[a] Epinephrine infusion should be titrated to achieve MAP greater than 65; increase by half the starting dose every 2 min to 3 min.

higher and achieved faster when it was given IM compared with subcutaneously.[15] Another study in adults found similar results when epinephrine was administered in the thigh as opposed to the deltoid.[16] For patients requiring more than 2 doses of IM epinephrine because of either ongoing respiratory symptoms or hypotension, IV epinephrine as a bolus or infusion should be considered.

ANAPHYLACTIC SHOCK
Definition and Mechanisms

Shock occurs when circulation is inadequate to meet the oxygen requirement of tissues, leading to cellular and end organ dysfunction.[17] There are multiple mechanisms by which distributive shock develops in anaphylaxis. IgE-mediated release of vasoactive mediators from mast cells and basophils leads to decreased systemic vascular resistance with resultant hypotension.[18] There also is significant capillary leak, leading to intravascular volume depletion. Decreased coronary perfusion may cause myocardial depression, further exacerbating hypotension. There also is growing evidence that inflammatory mediators may lead to coronary vasoconstriction and direct myocardial injury.[14]

Intravenous Epinephrine

For patients presenting in shock, IM epinephrine may be given while IV access is being obtained. IM epinephrine alone, however, is unlikely to be adequate, and IV epinephrine should be used. In 1 canine study of anaphylactic shock, IM epinephrine had no effect on mean arterial pressure (MAP), but IV epinephrine was effective at increasing MAP.[19] Compared with IM, IV epinephrine is faster in onset, has a more predictable effect, and is more easily titratable, all of which are favorable in the critically ill patient.

An infusion of epinephrine should be started at 1 μg/min to 10 μg/min and titrated up as needed to achieve a MAP of 65.[3] If an epinephrine infusion is not immediately available, this can be made by adding 1 mg of epinephrine, either 1 mL of the 1:1000 solution, or 10 mL of 1:10,000 solution, to a 1-L bag of normal saline. This creates a 1-μg/mL solution of epinephrine. Starting the infusion at a rate of 60 mL per hour gives a dose of 1 μg/min. The infusion should be titrated to achieve a MAP of 65 by increasing by one-half of the starting dose every 2 minutes to 3 minutes. This typically is achieved in a range from 10 μg/min to 20 μg/min, but a higher dose may be utilized if there is not adequate response. A bolus of epinephrine can also be given while the infusion is being prepared. Bolus-dose epinephrine can be created by adding 0.1 mg of epinephrine (1 mL of code dose [1:10,000] epinephrine) to a 9-mL syringe of normal saline to create a 10 μg/mL solution.[20,21] Small aliquots of 10 μg to 20 μg can be given every few minutes to achieve MAPs above 65. This dose also could be given in the setting of extreme hemodynamic instability in an attempt to avoid cardiac arrest.

Caution should be taken when administering IV epinephrine as a bolus or infusion. Although IM epinephrine is relatively safe, adverse cardiac events, including ischemia and arrythmias, have been observed with IV epinephrine, usually when it is given at the incorrect dose.[2] Additionally, observational studies have shown that adverse events are not uncommon when bolus-dose vasopressors are utilized in the ED.[22] There is potential for error both because of confusion over dosing and from mistakes when mixing the medications. Importantly, code dose epinephrine (1 mg) never should be given to a patient with a pulse, because this can lead to fatal arrythmias.

Fluids

Fluid resuscitation is an important part of anaphylaxis management, because significant intravascular volume can be lost due to increased capillary permeability. One study in patients in the operating room with anaphylaxis estimated that 35% of plasma volume can be lost from capillary leak within minutes.[23] Patients also may lose volume through vomiting and diarrhea from anaphylaxis. Patients presenting in shock may require large volumes of fluid to restore intravascular volume, in addition to IV epinephrine. Boluses of isotonic crystalloid, 30 mL/kg for adults or 20 mL/kg for pediatric patients, can be given to those presenting with hypotension or hypovolemia and without a clear contraindication to volume. Boluses can be repeated as necessary to maintain perfusion.[1,3,6,9,24] By contrast, those who are normotensive, with primarily respiratory symptoms, may not need aggressive fluid resuscitation. It is important to monitor all patients receiving large volumes of fluids for signs of volume overload. Lung and inferior vena cava ultrasound can be useful adjuncts to the physical examination when assessing volume status.

SECOND-LINE THERAPY
Inhaled Bronchodilators

Short-acting inhaled β-agonists can be used to treat bronchospasm associated with anaphylaxis.[1,3,6,9] Although there are no high-quality data suggesting that inhaled β-agonists are effective in this setting, they may benefit patients with significant wheezing that persists after epinephrine is given. Albuterol can be given via nebulizer or metered dose inhaler, similarly to its use in asthma. Inhaled anticholinergics, such as ipratropium, although not consistently recommended, also can be given if wheezing is significant (**Table 2**). Importantly, inhaled β-agonists and anticholinergics have no role in the treatment of upper airway edema, which typically presents as stridor and is a more concerning sign of impending airway compromise. For any patient with anaphylaxis presenting with respiratory symptoms, airway obstruction should be first ruled out as the potential cause before treating pulmonary disease.

Corticosteroids

Corticosteroids frequently are given in the ED for the treatment of anaphylaxis. The benefits are theoretical, however, and there are no high-quality data showing that they are effective for the acute management of anaphylaxis.[25] Despite this, some

Table 2
Second-line therapies for anaphylaxis with adult and pediatric dosing

Second Line Agents	Adult Dosing	Pediatric Dosing
Corticosteroids[a]		
Dexamethasone	8–16 mg IV/IM/PO	0.3 mg/kg PO/IV/IM (max 8 mg)
Prednisone	1mg/kg (max 50 mg) PO	1-2 mg/kg (max 50 mg) PO
Methylprednisolone	1–2 mg/kg (max 125 mg) IV	1-2 mg/kg (max 60 mg) IV
Hydrocortisone	200–500 mg IM or IV	5–10 mg/kg (max 500 mg) IM, IV
H_1 antagonists[b]		
Diphenhydramine	25–50 mg IV/IM/PO over 5 min	1 mg/kg IM/IV/PO over 5 min
Cetirizine	10 mg PO/IV over 1–2 min	<6 yo 2.5 mg IV/PO 6–11 yo 5–10 mg IV/PO
H_2 antagonists[b]		
Ranitidine	50 mg IV/PO	1 mg/kg (max 50 mg) IV/PO
Famotidine	20 mg IV/PO	0.25 mg/kg (max 20 mg) IV/PO
Bronchodilators		
Albuterol	2.5–5 mg nebulized q20 min × 3 4–8 puffs MDI q20 min ×3 15 mg continuous nebulized	1.25–5.0 mg nebulized q20 min ×3 2–8 puffs MDI q20 min × 3 5–15 mg continuous nebulized
Ipratropium	500 µg nebulized	250–500 µg nebulized

Abbreviations: max, maximum; MDI, metered dose inhaler;.

[a] Given lack of evidence that prolonged steroid course is effective in preventing recurrence, a 1-time dose of dexamethasone is recommended for patients with uncomplicated presentation.

[b] No proved benefit of IV over PO antihistamines; consider PO unless severe nausea/vomiting, airway/respiratory compromise.

studies show that corticosteroids still are used as first-line therapy over epinephrine.[25] Corticosteroids act by modulation of transcription, leading to decreased production of inflammatory cytokines, with an onset of action of approximately 4 hours to 6 hours.[26] They are ineffective, therefore, for the immediate treatment of anaphylaxis. In theory, by decreasing inflammatory mediators, corticosteroids may lessen the chance of symptom return after initial resolution, referred to as a biphasic reaction. There are no compelling data, however, showing this to be true. Major guidelines recommend corticosteroids be given as second-line therapy or not at all.[1,6,9,10,24,26] A single dose of corticosteroids is unlikely to have significant adverse effects; therefore, if steroids are to be used at all, a 1-time dose of dexamethasone in the ED may be given only after epinephrine is administered. For patients whose symptoms have resolved, there is no need for additional steroids at discharge. For those with residual symptoms or who are admitted to the hospital, a 3-day to 5-day course of oral steroids may be considered. **Table 2** lists the recommended agents and doses.

Antihistamines

Similar to corticosteroids, antihistamines have no role in the primary management of life-threatening signs and symptoms of anaphylaxis, including upper airway edema and shock. The rationale for their use stems from the effectiveness of antihistamines in other allergic disorders, but there are no data that suggest benefit in anaphylaxis.[27,28] Histamine 1 and Histamine 2 antagonist are most helpful for relieving cutaneous symptoms, including urticaria, pruritis, flushing, and rhinorrhea.[29] H_1 blockers and H_2 blockers also have been shown to be more effective when used together, compared with when either is used alone.[30] Most major guidelines recommend that both H_1 blockers and H_2 blockers be given as adjunctive therapy after the administration of epinephrine. H_1 blockers and H_2 blockers are recommended if there are significant cutaneous or gastrointestinal symptoms, but this should not delay the administration of epinephrine. **Table 2** lists recommended agents and dosing.

REFRACTORY ANAPHYLAXIS

A majority of anaphylactic reactions respond to epinephrine. On occasion, however, patients may have shock or airway compromise that is refractory to initial treatment. Glucagon may be effective in these instances, especially if the patient is on a β-blocker. Additional vasopressors also may be required for refractory shock. For severe airway obstruction, intubation is necessary.

Glucagon

β-Blocker use has been associated with increased incidence of severe, protracted anaphylaxis.[31–33] Intrinsic β-adrenergic effects blunt production of inflammatory mediators, whereas α-adrenergic effects increase production.[31] Thus β-blockade would be expected to shift the balance in favor of anaphylactic mediators. The effects of epinephrine also are likely to be blunted in those taking β-blockers, and unopposed alpha stimulation may result in a reflex increase in vagal tone, causing bradycardia and increased inflammatory mediator release.[31] Several case reports have shown glucagon to be effective in patients on β-blockers with refractory anaphylaxis.[32,34,35] Similar to use in β-blocker overdose, glucagon bypasses the β-receptor and activates adenyl cyclase, thereby increasing inotropy and chronotropy. Glucagon also may be effective in those who are not taking β-blockers and should be given to patients who are not responding to epinephrine, regardless of medication history.[3] The recommended dose of glucagon in adults is 1 mg to 5 mg over 5 minutes, followed by an infusion of 5 μg/min to 15 μg/min, titrated to clinical response.[3] For pediatrics, 20 μg/kg to 30 μg/kg can be given over 5 minutes followed by infusion of 5 μg/min to 15 μg/min. Vomiting is a frequent adverse reaction to glucagon, so patients should have a secure airway and antiemetics should be considered prior to administration.

Vasopressors

If hypotension persists despite escalating doses of epinephrine, additional vasopressors should be added. Tachycardia and arrythmias may limit the doses of epinephrine that can be used to maintain acceptable blood pressure. Although there are no data to indicate when to add a second vasopressor, if 15 μg/min to 20 μg/min of epinephrine is not adequate, likely another agent is needed. This may include norepinephrine, phenylephrine, or vasopressin. Norepinephrine is the vasopressor of choice in septic shock, which, like anaphylaxis, is a distributive form of shock. Norepinephrine has both α_1-adrenergic and β_1-adrenergic effects. It is a more potent vasoconstrictor compared with epinephrine but is less likely to cause tachyarrhythmias, making it a reasonable agent to add. Phenylephrine, an α_1-agonist, also may be used. The successful use of α-agonists to treat refractory anaphylactic shock in the operating room has been described and may counteract the tachycardia induced by epinephrine.[36]

There is limited evidence that vasopressin may be effective in catecholamine-resistant anaphylactic shock. In several case reports, vasopressin improved hypotension refractory to multiple vasopressors, including epinephrine.[37–40] Vasopressin works through multiple mechanisms independent of catecholamine receptors.

Vasopressin binds to the vasopressin-1 receptor on vascular smooth muscle, which leads to vasoconstriction.[40] It also inactivates ATP sensitive potassium channels on the endothelium, leading to increased influx of calcium and increased smooth muscle tone.[40] Finally, vasopressin inhibits cyclic GMP and nitric oxide production, thereby inhibiting further vasodilation.[40] Although evidence is limited, vasopressin is a reasonable addition when hypotension is refractory to other vasopressors because of its unique mechanisms of action.

AIRWAY MANAGEMENT

One of the most dangerous manifestations of anaphylaxis is airway edema. The presentation may range from minor lip swelling to stridor, drooling, and asphyxia. Patients with any signs of obstruction should be treated with IM epinephrine, and airway management quickly should become the priority.

Patients with stridor or respiratory distress due to airway obstruction should be intubated emergently. In those with facial or tongue swelling who are not in distress, clues to airway involvement include edema of the posterior oropharyngeal structures, voice changes, and inability to handle secretions. Those with any of these symptoms should be monitored closely and, if symptoms progress, require definitive airway management. The rapidity of onset also is an important consideration when determining need for intubation. Symptoms of airway compromise that start minutes after an exposure suggest a rapidly progressing process, and early intubation is advised. Someone with mild tongue swelling that has not progressed multiple hours after exposure, however, likely does not require intubation.

Whether to perform rapid-sequence intubation (RSI) or an awake intubation depends on the clinical scenario and provider comfort level. Paralysis may result in complete loss of an airway that otherwise was obstructed only partially. RSI medications also can cause hypotension and may precipitate cardiovascular collapse in the patient in shock. If a patient is deteriorating rapidly and the airway must be secured immediately, however, RSI still may be preferred because most providers are more experienced with this technique, it does not require patient cooperation, and it is likely to be performed faster than awake intubation. A video laryngoscope, bougie, and multiple smaller-sized endotracheal tubes should be at bedside. The neck should be prepped prior to intubation, and the provider should be prepared to proceed immediately to cricothyrotomy if intubation is unsuccessful. Fluids should be running and bolus-dose pressors or an epinephrine infusion should be available to counteract hypotension. For a patient with a more stable airway, who requires intubation for progressive airway edema, awake intubation is recommended. Awake intubation allows the for preservation of airway tone and respiratory drive and generally is the preferred method of intubation when the airway is predicted to be difficult.[41] Adequate topical anesthesia is paramount for the success of this procedure. Lidocaine is the agent of choice and has a greater safety profile compared with cocaine or benzocaine.[42] **Table 3** lists the various methods and dosing for topical anesthesia. If nasal intubation is to be performed, a topical vasoconstrictor, such as phenylephrine, can be applied along with an anesthetic to prevent bleeding. If stability allows, light sedation may be administered so that the patient is comfortable, but spontaneously breathing, to help facilitate the procedure. **Table 4** details the recommended agents and dosing. Intubation then can be performed using the fiberoptic bronchoscope, direct laryngoscope, or video laryngoscope. A smaller-sized endotracheal tube may be necessary, depending on the degree of airway edema. Once the patient is intubated, adequate placement of the tube should be confirmed, and standard sedation and analgesia should be provided.

Table 3
Topical anesthesia for awake intubation

Application	Dose[a]	Technique
Atomized	10 mL of 4% lidocaine solution	Commercial devices: EZ Atomizer (Alcove Medical Inc.), mucosal atomized device. Spray into the back of the oropharynx prior to procedure, and spray down to vocal cords during the procedure
Nebulized	4 mL of 4% lidocaine solution at 4 L/min	Nebulizer with mask
Direct application		
Oropharyngeal	2% viscous lidocaine, 5% lidocaine ointment	Lidocaine lollipop—apply a blob of viscous or lidocaine ointment to a tongue depressor, insert the tongue depressor as posterior into the oropharynx as possible; instruct patient to hold it but not to swallow; lidocaine drips down into the trachea
Nasal	4% lidocaine solution, 2% viscous lidocaine	For nasal intubation; soak multiple cotton swabs or nasal airway in solution and insert into the nose. Alternatively, may inject viscous into nasal passage using 10-mL syringe and have patient sniff back into throat.

[a] Dosing is listed for adult patients, and should be modified for the pediatric patient; recommended max weight-based dose of topical lidocaine is 8.2 mg/kg.

Table 4
Adjunctive agents for sedation and analgesia in awake intubation

Medication	Initial Dose[a]	Dose in Average Adult	Use	Comments
Ketamine	0.1–0.3 mg/kg IV	20 mg, may repeat 10-mg boluses	Sedation, analgesia	Preferred agent, does not cause hypotension, preserves respiratory drive, may increase secretions
Propofol	0.5–1 mg/kg IV	50–100 mg	Sedation	Caution if hypotensive, can cause over-sedation or respiratory depression
Midazolam	20–40 µg/kg IV/IM	2–4 mg	Sedation	Benzodiazepine of choice due to rapid on and off, can cause over-sedation and respiratory depression
Fentanyl	0.5–2 µg/kg IV	50–100 µg	Analgesia	Rapid on and off, can cause respiratory depression, reversible with naloxone

[a] Initial doses are lower than for typical procedural sedation; start low and repeat doses with goal to keep patient relaxed, but spontaneously breathing and arousable.

OBSERVATION AND DISPOSITION

The disposition of patients with anaphylaxis depends on the severity of the reaction, the resolution of symptoms, patient history, and access to care. Patients with ongoing symptoms requiring epinephrine infusion or intubation should be admitted to an intensive care unit. Patients with symptoms that have not completely resolved, other than mild cutaneous or gastrointestinal symptoms, may require admission for observation. Most patients whose symptoms have resolved completely can be discharged home. Many guidelines recommend an observation period of 4 hours to 6 hours in the ED after the resolution of anaphylaxis in order to watch for recurrence of symptoms. This recommendation is not evidence based, however.

Biphasic Reactions

A biphasic anaphylactic reaction refers to the recurrence of symptoms after the initial episode of anaphylaxis has resolved without any further exposure to the trigger.[43] The pathogenesis behind biphasic reactions is not understood completely. Several theorized mechanisms include delayed release of inflammatory mediators, activation of secondary inflammatory pathways, prolonged absorption of antigen in oral ingestions, or simply recurrence of a temporarily interrupted reaction after treatment has worn off.[43,44] Unfortunately, it is difficult to predict who will develop a biphasic reaction. Clinical predictors have been proposed, but they are not consistent across studies. Several risk factors for a biphasic response that have been described include an initial presentation with severe features or hypotension, multiple doses of epinephrine required, delayed administration of epinephrine (60–190 minutes after symptom onset), onset of symptoms greater than 30 minutes after the initial exposure, or an unknown trigger.[10,43,44] There is no consistent evidence that shows that the use of glucocorticoids decreases the likelihood of a biphasic reaction.[45]

The incidence of biphasic reactions had been previously described to be as high as 20%.[43,46] In more recent, larger studies, the incidence ranges between 0.4% and 4.5%.[47,48] The incidence of clinically significant reactions also is low and there have been no reported deaths due to biphasic reactions.[43,48] The time of onset of biphasic reactions reported is variable, between 1 hour and 72 hours, with a majority occurring outside of the typical 4-hour to 6-hour ED observation period.[43,48] This calls into question the utility of any standard length of ED observation. The period of observation should be tailored to the individual patient, and mandatory durations should be abandoned. For example, a patient presenting with severe symptoms requiring multiple doses of epinephrine whose symptoms are resolved may be observed for several hours after symptom resolution. A patient with less severe symptoms resolving after 1 dose of epinephrine, however, may be discharged soon after symptom resolution. Other reasons to consider observation include significant cardiopulmonary comorbidities, history of biphasic reactions, and limited access to medical care. All patients should be warned of the potential for recurrence of symptoms and instructed to return to the ED promptly if they do occur.

Discharge Medications

All patients should be discharged home with a prescription for an epinephrine autoinjector and instructed to have it on their person at all times. Unfortunately, multiple observational studies have shown rates of epinephrine prescription at discharge to be less than ideal.[13,49–51] This is a potentially life-saving intervention, and its importance cannot be stressed enough.

It is not uncommon for patients to be discharged with several days of antihistamines and corticosteroids. This has not been shown, however, to reduce potential symptom recurrence and it is not uniformly recommended across guidelines.[3] Corticosteroids, even in short courses, are not benign and may have adverse effects, including hyperglycemia and neuropsychiatric symptoms. Additionally, antihistamines can cause drowsiness and delirium, especially in the elderly population. The routine prescription of corticosteroids and standing-dose antihistamines at discharge is not recommended if symptoms are resolved. Patients can be advised to take antihistamines as needed for cutaneous symptoms. The benefit of a short course of oral steroids in those with residual symptoms should be weighed against the potential harms.

FUTURE DIRECTIONS

ED protocols may help improve compliance with best practices and improve care of patients with anaphylaxis. In 1 retrospective observational study, patients were more likely to receive epinephrine after the implementation of an anaphylaxis ED order set.[52] Quality control benchmarks of 100% utilization of epinephrine to treat anaphylaxis should be set and measured. Additionally, RCTs regarding the utility of adjunctive agents are needed. Because antihistamines and corticosteroids are not lifesaving and have little proved benefit, it is not unreasonable to have control groups who do not receive these medications. This would help elucidate if there is any role for adjunctive treatments.

SUMMARY

Anaphylaxis is a potentially deadly condition that, when treated correctly, can be reversed rapidly. Although randomized controlled data regarding treatment are lacking, consensus regarding management exists. As in any resuscitation, airway, breathing, and circulation are essential. Epinephrine should be administered immediately. Epinephrine possesses the ideal pharmacologic actions to counteract the pathologic processes at play. Adjunctive agents include inhaled bronchodilators, corticosteroids, and antihistamines but epinephrine administration should not be delayed. Airway management is necessary when there are severe obstructive or respiratory symptoms, and awake intubation may be the safest and preferred method. Anaphylactic shock should be treated with IV epinephrine and isotonic fluids, and refractory shock may require additional vasopressors. Biphasic reactions are relatively rare and difficult to predict, and any observation period should be tailored to the individual patient. Extended observation for uncomplicated cases with complete resolution is unnecessary. Patients should be educated about the signs and treatment of anaphylaxis, and all patients should be discharged with an epinephrine autoinjector and strict return precautions.

CLINICS CARE POINTS

- Anaphylaxis can progress to cardiac arrest rapidly and thus must be triaged and treated promptly.
- IM epinephrine is the core of anaphylaxis treatment, but it is underutilized due to concerns for precipitating arrythmia or ischemia.
- Failure to provide epinephrine may result in worse outcomes.
- Corticosteroids, antihistamines, and inhaled bronchodilators never should be given in place of or prior to the administration of epinephrine.

- IV epinephrine bolus or infusion should be used for patients in shock; however, providers should familiarize themselves with dosing, because errors in administration can lead to significant adverse outcomes including arrythmias and myocardial infarction.
- Intubation may be necessary in the case of severe airway obstruction but comes with the risks of worsening hypotension and a difficult airway.
- Awake intubation may be the safest and preferred method for patients with progressive airway obstruction.

DISCLOSURE

The authors have no financial disclosures to report.

REFERENCES

1. Sampson HA, Munoz-Furlong A, Campbell RL, et al. Second symposium on the definition and management of anaphylaxis: summary report–second National Institute of Allergy and Infectious Disease/Food Allergy and Anaphylaxis Network symposium. Ann Emerg Med 2006;47(4):373–80.
2. Pumphrey RS. Lessons for management of anaphylaxis from a study of fatal reactions. Clin Exp Allergy 2000;30(8):1144–50.
3. Campbell RL, Li JT, Nicklas RA, et al, Members of the Joint Task Force, Practice Parameter Workgroup. Emergency department diagnosis and treatment of anaphylaxis: a practice parameter. Ann Allergy Asthma Immunol 2014;113(6): 599–608.
4. Pumphrey RS. Fatal posture in anaphylactic shock. J Allergy Clin Immunol 2003; 112(2):451–2.
5. Howe B, Gaeta T. Anaphylaxis, allergies, and angioedema. In: Tintinalli J, ed. Tintinallis emergency medicine a comprehansive study guide 8th edition; 2016.
6. Muraro A, Roberts G, Worm M, et al. Anaphylaxis: guidelines from the European Academy of Allergy and Clinical Immunology. Allergy 2014;69(8):1026–45.
7. Alrasbi M, Sheikh A. Comparison of international guidelines for the emergency medical management of anaphylaxis. Allergy 2007;62(8):838–41.
8. Simons FE, Ebisawa M, Sanchez-Borges M, et al. 2015 update of the evidence base: World Allergy Organization anaphylaxis guidelines. World Allergy Organ J 2015;8(1):32.
9. Soar J, Pumphrey R, Cant A, et al. Emergency treatment of anaphylactic reactions–guidelines for healthcare providers. Resuscitation 2008;77(2):157–69.
10. Shaker MS, Wallace DV, Golden DBK, et al. Anaphylaxis-a 2020 practice parameter update, systematic review, and Grading of Recommendations, Assessment, Development and Evaluation (GRADE) analysis. J Allergy Clin Immunol 2020; 145(4):1082–123.
11. Sheikh A, Shehata YA, Brown SG, et al. Adrenaline (epinephrine) for the treatment of anaphylaxis with and without shock. Cochrane Database Syst Rev 2008;(4):CD006312.
12. Kemp SF, Lockey RF, Simons FE, World Allergy Organization ad hoc Committee on Epinephrine in Anaphylaxis. Epinephrine: the drug of choice for anaphylaxis. A statement of the World Allergy Organization. Allergy 2008;63(8):1061–70.
13. Clark S, Bock SA, Gaeta TJ, et al. Multicenter study of emergency department visits for food allergies. J Allergy Clin Immunol 2004;113(2):347–52.

14. Kounis NG, Cervellin G, Koniari I, et al. Anaphylactic cardiovascular collapse and Kounis syndrome: systemic vasodilation or coronary vasoconstriction? Ann Transl Med 2018;6(17):332.
15. Simons FE, Roberts JR, Gu X, et al. Epinephrine absorption in children with a history of anaphylaxis. J Allergy Clin Immunol 1998;101(1 Pt 1):33–7.
16. Simons FE, Gu X, Simons KJ. Epinephrine absorption in adults: intramuscular versus subcutaneous injection. J Allergy Clin Immunol 2001;108(5):871–3.
17. Cecconi M, De Backer D, Antonelli M, et al. Consensus on circulatory shock and hemodynamic monitoring. Task force of the European Society of Intensive Care Medicine. Intensive Care Med 2014;40(12):1795–815.
18. LoVerde D, Iweala OI, Eginli A, et al. Anaphylaxis. Chest 2018;153(2):528–43.
19. Bautista E, Simons FE, Simons KJ, et al. Epinephrine fails to hasten hemodynamic recovery in fully developed canine anaphylactic shock. Int Arch Allergy Immunol 2002;128(2):151–64.
20. Holden D, Ramich J, Timm E, et al. Safety considerations and guideline-based safe use recommendations for "bolus-dose" vasopressors in the emergency department. Ann Emerg Med 2018;71(1):83–92.
21. Tilton LJ, Eginger KH. Utility of push-dose vasopressors for temporary treatment of hypotension in the emergency department. J Emerg Nurs 2016;42(3):279–81.
22. Rotando A, Picard L, Delibert S, et al. Push dose pressors: experience in critically ill patients outside of the operating room. Am J Emerg Med 2019;37(3):494–8.
23. Fisher MM. Clinical observations on the pathophysiology and treatment of anaphylactic cardiovascular collapse. Anaesth Intensive Care 1986;14(1):17–21.
24. Simons FE, Ardusso LR, Bilo MB, et al. World allergy organization guidelines for the assessment and management of anaphylaxis. World Allergy Organ J 2011;4(2):13–37.
25. Choo KJ, Simons E, Sheikh A. Glucocorticoids for the treatment of anaphylaxis: cochrane systematic review. Allergy 2010;65(10):1205–11.
26. Liyanage CK, Galappatthy P, Seneviratne SL. Corticosteroids in management of anaphylaxis; a systematic review of evidence. Eur Ann Allergy Clin Immunol 2017;49(5):196–207.
27. Sheikh A, Ten Broek V, Brown SG, et al. H1-antihistamines for the treatment of anaphylaxis: cochrane systematic review. Allergy 2007;62(8):830–7.
28. Nurmatov UB, Rhatigan E, Simons FE, et al. H2-antihistamines for the treatment of anaphylaxis with and without shock: a systematic review. Ann Allergy Asthma Immunol 2014;112(2):126–31.
29. Runge JW, Martinez JC, Caravati EM, et al. Histamine antagonists in the treatment of acute allergic reactions. Ann Emerg Med 1992;21(3):237–42.
30. Lin RY, Curry A, Pesola GR, et al. Improved outcomes in patients with acute allergic syndromes who are treated with combined H1 and H2 antagonists. Ann Emerg Med 2000;36(5):462–8.
31. Toogood JH. Beta-blocker therapy and the risk of anaphylaxis. CMAJ 1987;137(7):587–8, 590–81.
32. Thomas M, Crawford I. Best evidence topic report. Glucagon infusion in refractory anaphylactic shock in patients on beta-blockers. Emerg Med J 2005;22(4):272–3.
33. Lang DM, Alpern MB, Visintainer PF, et al. Elevated risk of anaphylactoid reaction from radiographic contrast media is associated with both beta-blocker exposure and cardiovascular disorders. Arch Intern Med 1993;153(17):2033–40.
34. Zaloga GP, DeLacey W, Holmboe E, et al. Glucagon reversal of hypotension in a case of anaphylactoid shock. Ann Intern Med 1986;105(1):65–6.

35. Javeed N, Javeed H, Javeed S, et al. Refractory anaphylactoid shock potentiated by beta-blockers. Cathet Cardiovasc Diagn 1996;39(4):383–4.
36. Heytman M, Rainbird A. Use of alpha-agonists for management of anaphylaxis occurring under anaesthesia: case studies and review. Anaesthesia 2004; 59(12):1210–5.
37. Schummer C, Wirsing M, Schummer W. The pivotal role of vasopressin in refractory anaphylactic shock. Anesth Analg 2008;107(2):620–4.
38. Schummer W, Schummer C, Wippermann J, et al. Anaphylactic shock: is vasopressin the drug of choice? Anesthesiology 2004;101(4):1025–7.
39. Meng L, Williams EL. Case report: treatment of rocuronium-induced anaphylactic shock with vasopressin. Can J Anaesth 2008;55(7):437–40.
40. Di Chiara L, Stazi GV, Ricci Z, et al. Role of vasopressin in the treatment of anaphylactic shock in a child undergoing surgery for congenital heart disease: a case report. J Med Case Rep 2008;2:36.
41. Ahmad I, El-Boghdadly K, Bhagrath R, et al. Difficult Airway Society guidelines for awake tracheal intubation (ATI) in adults. Anaesthesia 2020;75(4):509–28.
42. Simmons ST, Schleich AR. Airway regional anesthesia for awake fiberoptic intubation. Reg Anesth Pain Med 2002;27(2):180–92.
43. Pourmand A, Robinson C, Syed W, et al. Biphasic anaphylaxis: a review of the literature and implications for emergency management. Am J Emerg Med 2018;36(8):1480–5.
44. Tole JW, Lieberman P. Biphasic anaphylaxis: review of incidence, clinical predictors, and observation recommendations. Immunol Allergy Clin North Am 2007; 27(2):309–26, viii.
45. Alqurashi W, Ellis AK. Do corticosteroids prevent biphasic anaphylaxis? J Allergy Clin Immunol Pract 2017;5(5):1194–205.
46. Stark BJ, Sullivan TJ. Biphasic and protracted anaphylaxis. J Allergy Clin Immunol 1986;78(1 Pt 1):76–83.
47. Rohacek M, Edenhofer H, Bircher A, et al. Biphasic anaphylactic reactions: occurrence and mortality. Allergy 2014;69(6):791–7.
48. Lee S, Sadosty AT, Campbell RL. Update on biphasic anaphylaxis. Curr Opin Allergy Clin Immunol 2016;16(4):346–51.
49. Owusu-Ansah S, Badaki O, Perin J, et al. Under prescription of epinephrine to medicaid patients in the pediatric emergency department. Glob Pediatr Health 2019;6. 2333794X19854960.
50. Nakajima M, Ono S, Michihata N, et al. Epinephrine autoinjector prescription patterns for severe anaphylactic patients in Japan: a retrospective analysis of health insurance claims data. Allergol Int 2020;69(3):424–8.
51. Waserman S, Avilla E, Ben-Shoshan M, et al. Epinephrine autoinjectors: new data, new problems. J Allergy Clin Immunol Pract 2017;5(5):1180–91.
52. Manivannan V, Hess EP, Bellamkonda VR, et al. A multifaceted intervention for patients with anaphylaxis increases epinephrine use in adult emergency department. J Allergy Clin Immunol Pract 2014;2(3):294–9.e1.

Anaphylaxis:
After the Emergency Department

Nicholas P. Gorham, MD

KEYWORDS

- Biphasic anaphylaxis • Protracted anaphylaxis • Anaphylaxis management plans
- Allergy testing

KEY POINTS

- Clinically significant biphasic reactions are rare and typically occur after the traditional 4-hour observation period.
- All patients who are discharged from the Emergency Department (ED) should be prescribed or provided with 2 epinephrine autoinjectors and shown how to use them appropriately.
- Glucocorticoids have not shown clinical efficacy in preventing biphasic anaphylaxis.
- Patient education following an anaphylactic reaction should start before discharge from the ED. A written action plan should be used to help guide patients, families, teachers, and community medical personnel.
- Patients should be referred to an allergy specialist who is able to confirm triggers and perform immunotherapy as indicated.

ANAPHYLAXIS: AFTER THE ED

After the emergency clinician has successfully resuscitated a patient suffering from an allergic reaction, several steps should be taken to assure they do not have a return of symptoms. Some period of observation is recommended and is discussed in detail later in the discussion. The clinician can also make a significant impact by prescribing outpatient medications, providing education, and arranging appropriate follow-up.

BIPHASIC ANAPHYLAXIS

Following the acute management of anaphylaxis in the ED, many patients are observed for a return of symptoms. Biphasic anaphylaxis is where symptoms recur within 1 to 72 hours after initial symptoms have resolved despite no further exposure to the trigger.[1] The incidence of biphasic anaphylaxis is reported to range from 0.4%

This article originally appeared in Emergency Medicine Clinics, Volume 40 Issue 1, February 2022.

Ochsner Medical Center, 1514 Jefferson Hwy, New Orleans, LA 70121, USA

E-mail address: Nicholas.Gorham@ochsner.org

Immunol Allergy Clin N Am 43 (2023) 467–471
https://doi.org/10.1016/j.iac.2022.10.008

immunology.theclinics.com

to 23% with most recent studies reporting a rate of around 5%.[1–6] The rate of clinically significant biphasic reactions is reported to be less than 2%.[2] The pathophysiology of these reactions is not well understood.[7] Risk factors for having a biphasic reaction include delayed administration of epinephrine and anaphylaxis requiring more than 1 dose of epinephrine. Other risk factors may include a prior history of anaphylaxis, unknown precipitant, diarrhea, and wheezing (**Box 1**).[4] No laboratory test exists that helps predict or aids in the management of these patients.[3]

The duration of monitoring following an anaphylactic reaction varies with the patient's severity of symptoms, social support, level of health literacy, and local conditions like hospital bed and staff capacity. Historic consensus guidelines recommend at least 4 hours of monitoring for patients with moderate symptoms and 8 to 10 hours for more severe symptoms.[1,8] Several studies looking into the appropriate time needed to observe a postanaphylactic patient have found that greater than 8 hours is needed to assure full resolution of symptoms.[4,7,9] However, most of these reactions after discharge are not clinically significant.[2] The emergency department physician should reevaluate these patients frequently and use their best judgment in determining how much observation time is needed on a case-by-case basis.

PROTRACTED AND REFRACTORY ANAPHYLAXIS

Anaphylaxis lasting greater than 4 hours is considered protracted.[10] Two small studies have found that protracted anaphylaxis occurs in around 4% of cases.[11,12] Refractory anaphylaxis occurs when the symptoms of anaphylaxis persist despite fluid resuscitation and 3 or more doses of epinephrine.[10] This is a rare condition and warrants even more aggressive resuscitative measures, such as IV epinephrine. A 1:10,000 concentration is used for IV dosing. A titratable, continuous infusion, or a bolus dose formulation can be used. Large volumes of IV fluids may be required to fill the increased intravascular volume caused by systemic vasodilation. If hypotension persists despite these measures, a secondary vasopressor should be added. There is no specific agent that has shown clear superiority in these cases.[1] Patient who can no longer protect their airway or who have progressive angioedema should be intubated for airway protection. Glucagon should be considered for patients who take beta-blockers. Patients on an epinephrine infusion should be admitted to the ICU and invasive monitoring should be considered.

PRESCRIPTIONS AT ED DISCHARGE

Patients who have had one anaphylactic event are at much greater risk to have another in their lifetime. The use of epinephrine is the mainstay of anaphylaxis

---

Box 1
Risk factors for biphasic anaphylaxis[4,7]

Delayed epinephrine administration

Multiple doses of epinephrine

History of prior anaphylaxis

Unknown precipitant

Diarrhea

Wheezing

treatment. All patients who are discharged from the ED after an episode of anaphylaxis should be provided with prescribed 2 epinephrine autoinjectors and given training on proper use.[1,8] Patients who have a return of symptoms following ED discharge should use their injector in the lateral thigh and then return to the ED. Glucocorticoids have been routinely prescribed to try and prevent biphasic anaphylaxis. However, current data does not show that glucocorticoids prevent a return of symptoms.[7,13–15] Their role in anaphylaxis is controversial and unclear. H_1-antihistamines are another second-line medication that is sometimes prescribed or recommended at discharge. These medications help relieve the symptoms of itching and urticaria, but do not prevent upper airway obstruction, hypotension, or shock. They can be added for symptom relief but should not delay the administration of epinephrine.[1]

ANAPHYLAXIS MANAGEMENT PLAN

Anaphylaxis education and risk reduction should begin before ED discharge. Patients and their families should be counseled on the signs and symptoms of anaphylaxis so that they will know when and how to administer an epinephrine autoinjector correctly. Education should include recognizing triggers so they can avoid exposure. National and international guidelines recommend a written action plan.[1,15–17] The American Academy of Pediatrics has tried to standardize this form and published a consensus plan in 2017.[16] Such a plan has shown to improve outcomes in asthma, but has yet to

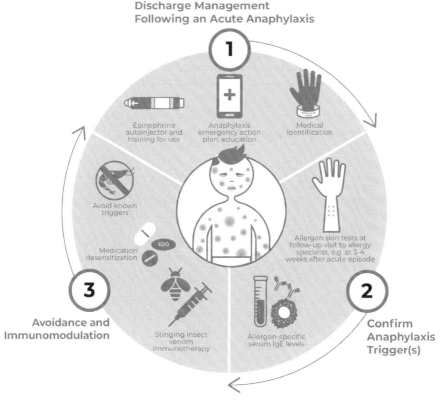

Fig. 1. Discharge management following acute anaphylaxis. (© 2020 World Allergy Organization; Reused with permission from Cardona et al, 2020[15])

have been shown to be effective for anaphylaxis in large prospective trials.[18–20] A written action plan may be especially helpful for school-aged children so that teachers and school nurses have guidance from a physician on the child's allergic triggers, reactions, and care needs.

OUTPATIENT FOLLOW-UP

Patients seen in the ED and diagnosed with anaphylaxis should be referred to an allergy specialist for outpatient follow-up.[1] This specialist will be able to confirm anaphylaxis triggers and initiate desensitization protocols as clinically indicated. They may also help manage concomitant asthma which can be exacerbated by allergen exposure. Yearly follow-up is recommended to renew epinephrine autoinjector prescriptions and review techniques on allergen avoidance.[1,15] The full continuum of postanaphylaxis care has been summarized by the World Allergy Organization since 2010 and illustrated in **Fig. 1**.

CLINICS CARE POINTS

- Many biphasic anaphylactic reactions occur after the traditional 4-hour observation period, but very few are clinically significant.[2,7]
- Data do not support the use of glucocorticoids to prevent biphasic reactions.[7,13–15]
- All patients should be discharged with a prescription for an epinephrine autoinjector and provided training on proper use.[1,8]
- A written action plan may assist in the outpatient management of anaphylaxis, but further study is needed to determine the efficacy of this practice.[1,15–17]
- ED physicians should refer and recommend outpatient follow-up for patients who have recovered from anaphylaxis with an allergy specialist.[1,15]

DISCLOSURE

The author has nothing to disclose.

REFERENCES

1. Simons FE, Ardusso LR, Bilò MB, et al. World allergy organization guidelines for the assessment and management of anaphylaxis. World Allergy Organ J 2011; 4(2):13–37. Epub 2011 Feb 23. PubMed PMID: 23268454; PubMed Central PMCID: PMC3500036.
2. Grunau BE, Li J, Yi TW, et al. Incidence of clinically important biphasic reactions in emergency department patients with allergic reactions or anaphylaxis. Ann Emerg Med 2014;63(6):736–44.e2. Epub 2013 Nov 13. PubMed PMID: 24239340.
3. Kraft M, Scherer Hofmeier K, Ruëff F, et al. Risk factors and characteristics of biphasic anaphylaxis. J Allergy Clin Immunol Pract 2020;8(10):3388–95.e6. Epub 2020 Aug 4. PubMed PMID: 32763470.
4. Lee S, Bellolio MF, Hess EP, et al. Predictors of biphasic reactions in the emergency department for patients with anaphylaxis. J Allergy Clin Immunol Pract 2014;2(3):281–7. Epub 2014 Apr 2. PubMed PMID: 24811018.
5. Lee S, Peterson A, Lohse CM, et al. Further evaluation of factors that may predict biphasic reactions in emergency department anaphylaxis patients. J Allergy Clin Immunol Pract 2017;5(5):1295–301. PubMed PMID: 28888253.

6. Liu X, Lee S, Lohse CM, et al. Biphasic reactions in emergency department anaphylaxis patients: a prospective cohort study. J Allergy Clin Immunol Pract 2020;8(4):1230–8. Epub 2019 Nov 6. PubMed PMID: 31704438.
7. Pourmand A, Robinson C, Syed W, et al. Biphasic anaphylaxis: a review of the literature and implications for emergency management. Am J Emerg Med 2018;36(8):1480–5. Epub 2018 May 9. Review. PubMed PMID: 29759531.
8. Campbell RL, Li JT, Nicklas RA, et al. Emergency department diagnosis and treatment of anaphylaxis: a practice parameter. Ann Allergy Asthma Immunol 2014;113(6):599–608. PubMed PMID: 25466802.
9. Kim TH, Yoon SH, Hong H, et al. Duration of observation for detecting a biphasic reaction in anaphylaxis: a meta-analysis. Int Arch Allergy Immunol 2019;179(1): 31–6. Epub 2019 Feb 14. PubMed PMID: 30763927.
10. Dribin TE, Sampson HA, Camargo CA Jr, et al. Persistent, refractory, and biphasic anaphylaxis: A multidisciplinary Delphi study. J Allergy Clin Immunol 2020;146(5):1089–96. https://doi.org/10.1016/j.jaci.2020.08.015. Epub 2020 Aug 24. PubMed PMID: 32853640.
11. Oya S, Nakamori T, Kinoshita H. Incidence and characteristics of biphasic and protracted anaphylaxis: evaluation of 114 inpatients. Acute Med Surg 2014; 1(4):228–33. PubMed PMID: 29930853; PubMed Central PMCID: PMC5997245.
12. Kim TH, Yoon SH, Lee SY, et al. Biphasic and protracted anaphylaxis to iodinated contrast media. Eur Radiol 2018;28(3):1242–52. Epub 2017 Sep 27. PubMed PMID: 28956131.
13. Shaker MS, Wallace DV, Golden DBK, et al. Anaphylaxis-a 2020 practice parameter update, systematic review, and Grading of Recommendations, Assessment, Development and Evaluation (GRADE) analysis. J Allergy Clin Immunol 2020; 145(4):1082–123. Epub 2020 Jan 28. PubMed PMID: 32001253.
14. Simons FE, Ebisawa M, Sanchez-Borges M, et al. 2015 update of the evidence base: World Allergy Organization anaphylaxis guidelines. World Allergy Organ J 2015;8(1):32. PubMed PMID: 26525001; PubMed Central PMCID: PMC4625730.
15. Cardona V, Ansotegui IJ, Ebisawa M, et al. World allergy organization anaphylaxis guidance 2020. World Allergy Organ J 2020;13(10):100472. PubMed PMID: 33204386; PubMed Central PMCID: PMC7607509.
16. Wang J, Sicherer SH. Guidance on completing a written allergy and anaphylaxis emergency plan. Pediatrics 2017;139(3). https://doi.org/10.1542/peds.2016-4005. Epub 2017 Feb 13. PubMed PMID: 28193793.
17. Muraro A, Werfel T, Hoffmann-Sommergruber K, et al. EAACI food allergy and anaphylaxis guidelines: diagnosis and management of food allergy. Allergy 2014;69(8):1008–25. Epub 2014 Jun 9. PubMed PMID: 24909706.
18. Gibson PG, Powell H, Coughlan J, et al. Self-management education and regular practitioner review for adults with asthma. Cochrane Database Syst Rev 2003;1: CD001117.
19. Choo K, Sheikh A. Action plans for the long-term management of anaphylaxis: systematic review of effectiveness. Clin Exp Allergy 2007;37(7):1090–4. PubMed PMID: 17581204.
20. Nurmatov U, Worth A, Sheikh A. Anaphylaxis management plans for the acute and long-term management of anaphylaxis: a systematic review. J Allergy Clin Immunol 2008;122(2):353–61. Epub 2008 Jun 24. Review. PubMed PMID: 18572231.

Drug Hypersensitivity Reactions

R. Gentry Wilkerson, MD

KEYWORDS

- Drug hypersensitivity • Drug allergy • Adverse drug reaction
- Hypersensitivity reactions • Anaphylaxis • Severe cutaneous adverse reactions

KEY POINTS

- Drug hypersensitivity reactions result from various immune system-mediated responses to exposure to a drug.
- The Gell and Coombs classification divides immunologic drug hypersensitivity reactions into 4 major categories based on immunologic mechanism.
- Dermatologic manifestations are the most common clinical finding of a drug allergy.
- Type IV hypersensitivity reactions include severe cutaneous adverse reactions (SCARs) such as drug reaction with eosinophilia and systemic symptom (DRESS) syndrome, Stevens–Johnson Syndrome (SJS), toxic epidermal necrolysis (TEN), and acute generalized exanthematous pustulosis (AGEP).
- Epinephrine is the first-line treatment of anaphylaxis. Antihistamines may be given to alleviate cutaneous manifestations but, they do not treat the underlying process of anaphylaxis.

INTRODUCTION

Drug hypersensitivity reactions (DHRs) are a diverse group of reactions mediated by the immune system after exposure to a drug. The mechanisms underlying the development of a hypersensitivity reaction are complex and not always fully characterized. Anaphylaxis is a DHR that requires immediate recognition and treatment. Other types of reactions are slow to develop and do not always require rapid treatment. Emergency physicians should have a good understanding of these various types of DHRs and how to approach the patient regarding evaluation and treatment.

This article originally appeared in Emergency Medicine Clinics, Volume 40 Issue 1, February 2022.

Department of Emergency Medicine, University of Maryland School of Medicine, 110 South Paca Street, 6th Floor, Suite 200, Baltimore, MD 21201, USA

E-mail address: gwilkerson@som.umaryland.edu

Twitter: @gentrywmd (R.G.W.)

Immunol Allergy Clin N Am 43 (2023) 473–489
https://doi.org/10.1016/j.iac.2022.10.005
0889-8561/23/© 2022 Elsevier Inc. All rights reserved.

EPIDEMIOLOGY

The true burden of disease due to allergic reactions is difficult to determine because epidemiologic data are limited in quality due to variations in terminology used, different methodological approaches for determining the prevalence of disease, and different outcomes used to determine the presence of an allergy. Overall, adverse drug reactions (ADRs) have been estimated to affect up to approximately 15% of hospitalized patients.[1] In a 2013 study using random digit dialing to survey members of the general public, the prevalence of anaphylaxis using the most stringent criteria was at least 1.6%, whereas the prevalence was 7.7% using the least stringent criteria. Respondents in the survey attributed episodes of anaphylaxis to drugs in 35% of cases.[2] From 2001 to 2012, there was an increase in the percentage of emergency department (ED) visits due to allergic drug reactions—from 0.49% to 0.94%.[3] In New York City between 2004 and 2008, anaphylaxis accounted for 0.18% of pediatric ED visits.[4] Overall, medications are the leading cause of anaphylaxis that results in death.[5] In children, however, exposure to food causes the greatest number of anaphylaxis fatalities.[6] In contrast to anaphylaxis in general, whereby there has been a rise in hospital admissions without a rise in fatalities, for drug-induced anaphylaxis, one study of an Australian database found a threefold increase in deaths due to anaphylaxis but only a 1.5x increase in the number of hospital admissions between 1997 and 2005. In this study, over half of all the fatalities due to anaphylaxis were likely caused by drug allergies.[7] The risk of anaphylaxis to drugs increases with age.[8] The United States Food and Drug Administration (FDA) Adverse Event Reporting System (FAERS) is a web-based system used to compile adverse event reports to assist with postmarketing surveillance of drugs to identify potential safety concerns. Analysis of FAERS data demonstrated that the rate of anaphylaxis due to monoclonal antibodies (mAbs) is rising faster than any other class of drug. In 1999, mAbs accounted for 2% of all reported cases of anaphylaxis, but this had risen to 17.37% in 2019.[9]

RISK FACTORS

Most ADRs are an extension of the usual pharmacologic effect of the drug. Factors that increase the risk of ADRs include the type of drug, the dose of the drug, specific pharmacokinetic properties of the drug, and other factors that play a role in the metabolism and action of the drug. A study by Gurwitz and colleagues in 2003 found that ADRs were common in the elderly population and that as many as one-fourth were preventable.[10] The elderly experience age-related changes in drug metabolism but also are subject to polypharmacy and inappropriate prescribing.[11] At the other end of the age spectrum, Clavenna and Bonati found that the incidence of ADRs in pediatric patients was 10.9% for in-hospital patients and 1.0% for outpatients.

The risk of having an allergic reaction to a drug is greatest when there is a history of allergic relation to the same or closely related compounds. Drug-specific factors influence the likelihood of developing an allergy. Large molecular weight compounds such as proteins and polysaccharides have increased rates of allergic reactions. The route of administration of a drug may influence the likelihood of developing an allergic reaction although the data supporting these statements is weak. Some polymorphisms of human leukocyte antigen (HLA) region carry a higher risk of certain forms of allergic reaction.[12]

The risk of anaphylaxis increases with age, presence of comorbid conditions, and the use of angiotensin-converting enzyme (ACE) inhibitors.[13,14] A retrospective analysis of a European registry of anaphylaxis cases found that age was the greatest risk factor for having severe cardiovascular complications from anaphylaxis (adjusted odds ratio 6.08).[15] Asthma and other respiratory conditions have been associated with greater severity of anaphylactic reactions.[14,16,17]

CLASSIFICATION & MECHANISMS

Multiple systems have been developed to characterize and classify different reactions to drugs. These reactions may occur as the result of a multitude of different pathways with an immunologic basis being just one. In 1955, Brown wrote that the use of the term drug allergy was used "as a sort of wastepaper basket into which are cast many unexplained phenomena."[18] The FDA defines an adverse event as "any untoward medical occurrence associated with the use of a drug in humans, whether or not considered drug related."[19] In the report published in 1972, International Drug Monitoring: The Role of National Centers, the World Health Organization (WHO) defined an ADR as "one that is noxious, is unintended, and occurs at doses normally used in man."[20]

The Rawlins–Thompson classification of ADRs was proposed in 1977.[21] The system broke ADRs into Type A, which are dose-dependent and predictable and Type B, which are not dose-dependent or predictable. Type A reactions make up 85% to 90% of all ADRs and have been referred to as "augmented" as these reactions are an extension of the normal pharmacologic properties of the drug. Prolongation of the QRS complex in tricyclic antidepressant overdose is an example of a Type A reaction. Type B reactions comprise 10% to 15% of ADRs and have been referred to as "bizarre" because they are not a normal, expected property of the drug. Anaphylaxis resulting from exposure to penicillin is an example of a Type B reaction. Subsequently, additional categories have been added by some to further characterize different types of ADRs. These include: Type C (dose-related and time-related), Type D (time-related), Type E (withdrawal), and Type F (unexpected failure of efficacy).[22]

A DHR is a response to a drug that results in symptoms or signs due to exposure to a drug at a dose normally tolerated by nonhypersensitive people and is induced by immunologic or inflammatory pathways. The term DHR is preferred in cases of suspected drug allergy because clinically it is difficult to distinguish between a true drug allergy and nonallergic DHR. In its International Consensus on Drug Allergy, the World Allergy Organization classified DHRs based on the timing of onset of symptoms after exposure. Immediate DHRs such as urticaria, anaphylaxis, and bronchospasm, typically occur within 1 to 6 hours of exposure although usually within 1 hour. Nonimmediate or delayed DHRs occur after 1 hour of exposure and frequently many days later.[23]

Gell and Coombs Classification of Hypersensitivity Reactions

The Gell and Coombs classification divides immunologic DHRs into 4 major pathophysiologic categories based on the immunologic mechanism (**Table 1**). In this classification which was first proposed in 1963, each reaction has a distinct and mutually exclusive mechanism. In the following years, advances in the understanding of various immunologic effectors and pathways have exploded and it is now known that there may be overlap across different Gell and Coombs reaction types.[24]

Type I, or immediate-type hypersensitivity reactions occur when exposure to a previously encountered antigen causes crosslinking of IgE bound to high-affinity receptors (FcϵRI) on the surface of sensitized mast cells and basophils leading to release of preformed vasoactive mediators such as histamine, tryptase, and chymase.[25,26] These mediators cause vasodilation and increased capillary permeability. The initial reaction is followed 4 to 8 hours later by a late phase release of cytokines such as IL-1, IL-4, IL-5, granulocyte monocyte colony-stimulating factor (GM-CSF), and tumor

Table 1
Gell and coombs classification of hypersensitivity reactions

Type		Reactant	Mechanism	Clinical Symptoms
I (Immediate)		IgE	Antigen-induced crosslinking of IgE bound to FcεRI receptors on mast cells and basophils leads to release of vasoactive mediators	Anaphylaxis, angioedema, urticaria, bronchospasm, hypotension
II (cytotoxic)		IgG	IgG recognition of cell surface epitopes leads to the assembly of the complement C5–C9 membrane attack complex (MAC) and subsequent lysis of the cell or, antibody-dependent cell-mediated cytotoxicity (ADCC) whereby natural killer (NK) cells recognize IgG attached to target cells bearing these antigens leading to perforin release and NK cell-mediated lysis	Autoimmune hemolytic anemia and Rh incompatibility
III (Immune Complex Disease)		IgG or IgM	IgM or IgG and complement or FcR	Serum sickness, vasculitis
IV (cell-mediated)	IVa	IFN-γ, TNF-α, T$_H$1 cells	Antigen is presented by cells or there is direct T-cell stimulation	Eczema
	IVb	IL-5, IL-4/IL-13, T$_H$2 cells	Antigen is presented by cells or there is direct T-cell stimulation	Maculopapular exanthema with eosinophilia, DRESS
	IVc	Perforin and Granzyme B, Cytotoxic T Cells	Cell associated antigen or direct T-cell stimulation	SJS/TEN, pustular exanthema
	IVd	CXCL8, GM-CSF, T Cells	Soluble antigen presented by cells or direct T-cell stimulation	AGEP

Adapted from: Pichler WJ, Adam J, Daubner B, Gentinetta T, Keller M, Yerly D. Drug Hypersensitivity Reactions: Pathomechanism and Clinical Symptoms. Med Clin N Am. 2010;94(4):645 to 664.[34]

necrosis factor (TNF)-α. Type I hypersensitivity reactions lead to the development of urticaria, angioedema, bronchospasm, and hypotension.[27]

Type II hypersensitivity reactions are delayed cytotoxic reactions in which host cells are destroyed through complement-mediated reactions, antibody-dependent cell-mediated cytotoxicity, or antibody-mediated cellular dysfunction. Host cells coated with antigen bind to IgG, or less commonly, IgM antibodies. This can lead to the activation of the classic complement pathway leading to the assembly of the membrane attack complex (C5–C9) and subsequent lysis of the host cell. Natural killer cells and macrophages can also be activated by binding antibodies to FcγRIIb receptors expressed on their surface. Examples of Type II hypersensitivity reactions include autoimmune hemolytic anemia, Rh-incompatibility, and Goodpasture syndrome (antiglomerular basement membrane disease).[28]

In Type III hypersensitivity reactions, IgG or IgM form immune complexes with antigens and activate the complement system. This leads to inflammation and tissue injury by activated neutrophils. The clinical manifestations of this process result from the site whereby the immune complexes deposit rather than the specific antigen or antibody and usually take at least a week to appear.[29] Serum sickness and Arthus reactions are examples of Type III hypersensitivity reactions.[30,31]

Type IV hypersensitivity reactions are distinct from Types I through III in that Type IV reactions are not mediated by antibodies but instead involve the activation and expansion of T cells. This process is not immediate and sometimes takes days to weeks to develop. Since the original classification by Gell and Coombs, Type IV reactions have been further characterized into 4 subclasses based on the cytokines produced and the cells involved.[32] There is a strong link to T cell-mediated hypersensitivity reactions and specific HLA risk alleles.[33] Stevens–Johnson syndrome/toxic epidermal necrolysis (SJS/TEN), acute generalized exanthema pustulosis (AGEP), and drug reaction with eosinophilia and systemic symptoms (DRESS) are examples of Type IV hypersensitivity reactions.

DHRs have also been classified based on the mode of action of the drug with immune/inflammatory cells. In this system, there are 3 types of reactions-allergic/immune, pseudoallergic, and pharmacologic stimulation of immune receptors (p-i concept). Large molecular weight drugs can be recognized directly by immune cells and antibodies. However, most drugs act as haptens in that they are too small (<1000 Da) to elicit an immune response and must bind covalently to a protein to form an antigen.[26] In the pseudoallergic class, drugs cause the release of mediators from mast cells, basophils, and other effector cells without the involvement of immunoglobulins or T cells. In the p-i concept, some drugs may bind noncovalently to nonactive sites of HLA molecules or T cell receptors to cause activation. The drugs are thus not acting as antigens.[35]

CLINICAL MANIFESTATIONS

Patients experiencing an allergic reaction to a drug may have a wide variety of clinical presentations based on the immunologic mechanism underlying the drug allergy. Within the same mechanism, there may be substantial differences in presentation and organ systems involved from patient to patient. Dermatologic manifestations are the most commonly seen presentation in allergic reactions to drugs.[36,37]

The manifestations of Type I (immediate) hypersensitivity reactions are a direct result of the actions of the vasoactive mediators that are released from mast cells and basophils. Common dermatologic manifestations include urticaria and angioedema associated with flushing and pruritus. The classic description of this swelling associated with vasodilation-induced erythema is the wheal-and-flare response.[38] The respiratory system may be involved resulting in wheezing due to bronchoconstriction and stridor due to edema of the upper airway including the vocal cords. Death due to asphyxiation may occur in severe cases.[39] Gastrointestinal involvement may present with crampy abdominal pain, nausea, and vomiting, as well as diarrhea although these may also be attributable to a non–immune-mediated ADR. Vasoplegia and third-spacing of fluids may result in hypotension and loss of consciousness. Anaphylaxis is the most severe presentation of an IgE-mediated allergic reaction. The clinical presentation of Type I hypersensitivity reactions usually occurs within minutes to hours of the exposure.

The clinical presentation of Type II (cytotoxic) hypersensitivity reactions is usually the result of anemia, thrombocytopenia, or neutropenia, as these are the most common cell types involved. Symptoms most commonly occur within days of exposure. When red blood cells are targeted, drug-induced immune hemolytic anemia (DIIHA) occurs. The drugs most frequently associated with the development of DIIHA are antimicrobials (mostly penicillin and cephalosporins), anti-inflammatories, and antineoplastic agents.[40] Patients will present with typical signs and symptoms of anemia including fatigue, pallor, jaundice, darkened urine due to bilirubinuria, tachycardia, tachypnea, and hypotension. Destruction of platelets via this mechanism leads to drug-induced immune thrombocytopenia (DIITP). This is a secondary form of immune thrombocytopenia (ITP). In this condition, low platelet counts lead to easy bruising and bleeding. In one review of 309 cases, the median time between exposure to the offending drug and development of DIITP was 21 days and the median minimum platelet count was 11,000/μL.[41] Drug-induced immune neutropenia (DIIN) occurs when exposure to a drug results in the development of antibodies that cross-react with glycoproteins on neutrophil cell walls leading to their destruction and placing the patient at risk for infection.[42]

In Type III (immune complex) hypersensitivity reactions, there is an abnormal formation of antigen–antibody complexes that are deposited in tissues and result in the activation of the complement system. Diseases that are the result of Type III hypersensitivity reactions include poststreptococcal glomerulonephritis, serum sickness, hypersensitivity pneumonitis (also called extrinsic allergic alveolitis), and systemic lupus erythematosus (SLE). The clinical presentation depends on the disease. SLE is a prototypical Type III hypersensitivity reaction whereby antibodies develop to components of the cellular nucleus—antinuclear antibodies (ANA). The type of ANA that develops often has a strong association with the patient's clinical presentation. For example, anti-Smith antibodies are frequently associated with kidney disease.[43] Drug-induced lupus (DIL) occurs when exposure to a drug leads to the development of autoantibodies and loss of self-tolerance. The use of procainamide and hydralazine is associated with a high risk of the development of DIL. DIL may not develop until after years of use of the associated drug. Patients with DIL most commonly present with fatigue, low-grade fever, and other systemic symptoms. Generally, DIL tends to present with more mild symptoms than SLE. Development of major organ system involvement is less frequent in DIL than in SLE.[44]

Type IV hypersensitivity reactions occur as a result of T cell response to an antigen leading to an inflammatory response. These reactions are further subdivided (IVa through IVd) based on the type of T cells involved. The clinical presentation is based on the distinct condition that develops. The skin is a depository for a large number of T cells so dermatologic involvement is common in Type IV hypersensitivity reactions. Contact dermatitis is a very common Type IV hypersensitivity reaction. During the sensitization (afferent) stage, a hapten contacts the skin and leads to the formation of hapten-specific T cells. During the elicitation (efferent) phase, re-exposure to the same hapten causes the release of mediators that are responsible for the clinical presentation including the development of an erythematous, pruritic rash with swelling. Severe cutaneous adverse reactions (SCARs) are a group of dermatologic diseases that result from a Type IV hypersensitivity process.

Drug Reaction with Eosinophilia and Systemic Symptoms Syndrome

DRESS syndrome, also known as drug-induced hypersensitivity syndrome (DIHS), is a SCAR that has a long latency period before the development of clinical symptoms which include fever, adenopathy, hematologic abnormalities, and multiorgan system involvement. The onset of disease usually occurs within 3 weeks of exposure to the drug but may be delayed by as much as 3 months.[45] Reactions to the medication phenytoin were described soon after its introduction in the 1930s. Over time various terms were used to describe similar reactions including anticonvulsant hypersensitivity syndrome and drug-induced pseudolymphoma. In 1996, Bocquet and colleagues introduced the term drug rash with eosinophilia and systemic symptoms.[46] Due to variations in dermatologic involvement the word "rash" in the name was subsequently replaced with "reaction." Different diagnostic criteria have been proposed to define disease patterns that are likely a continuum of DRESS (**Table 2**). A Japanese consensus group proposed a set of diagnostic criteria in 2006 and later developed a scoring system.[47,48] In 2007, the RegiSCAR group, a multinational effort that collects data on cases of SCAR, proposed a similar set of diagnostic criteria and a scoring system to help classify cases as definite, probable, or not DRESS.[49] DRESS is associated with the reactivation of human herpes virus (HHV), especially HHV-6, HHV-7, Epstein–Barr virus (EBV), varicella-zoster virus (VZV), and cytomegalovirus (CMV).[50] Aromatic anticonvulsant medications such as phenytoin, carbamazepine, and phenobarbital have classically been associated with DRESS. Several other drug classes have now been implicated as causative agents including antidepressants, sulfonamides and sulfones, nonsteroidal anti-inflammatories (NSAIDs), antibiotics, ACE inhibitors, and beta-blockers.[51] The overall mortality of DRESS is approximately 5% to 10%.[52] In cases with cardiac involvement, one retrospective analysis demonstrated the mortality increases to 37.5%.[53]

Stevens–Johnson Syndrome and Toxic Epidermal Necrolysis

SJS and TEN are SCARs with skin necrosis and detachment that represent different points on a continuum of severity based on the percentage involvement of body surface area (BSA). SJS involves less than 10% BSA, whereas TEN involves more than 30%. SJS/TEN overlap describes cases whereby there is between 10% and 30% BSA involved.[54] Previously considered to be on the continuum of the same disease, erythema multiforme is now thought to be a distinct entity. Drugs are the most common triggers for the development of SJS/TEN with aromatic antiepileptics, NSAIDs, and antibacterial sulfonamides frequently implicated. Infections are also implicated in the development of SJS/TEN. Cases associated with *Mycoplasma pneumoniae* often have a less severe presentation.[55]

Patients with SJS/TEN initially present with an influenza-like prodromal phase which may include fever and burning sensation. This prodrome precedes the development of skin findings by 1 to 3 days.[56] The rash of SJS/TEN typically begins as erythematous macules with purpuric centers and ill-defined borders. Lesions are first present on the face and thorax before spreading to other areas. The distribution is symmetric and usually spares the scalp, palms, and soles. Over time, sometimes within hours, vesicles and bullae form, and then the skin begins to slough off. The blisters will demonstrate Nikolsky sign whereby the application of lateral pressure results in

Table 2
Diagnostic criteria for DRESS syndrome, also known as drug-induced hypersensitivity syndrome (DIHS)

Bocquet et al[46]	Japanese Consensus Group[47]	RegiSCAR[48]
Presence of a cutaneous drug eruption	Maculopapular rash developing > 3 wk after starting drug	Acute rash
Systemic involvement: Lymphadenopathy ≥2 cm in diameter, hepatitis (transaminase ≥2 times upper limit of normal), interstitial nephritis, or interstitial pneumonitis or carditis	Clinical manifestation of reaction continuing >2 wk after discontinuing drug	Hospitalization
Hematologic abnormalities eosinophilia ≥1.5 × 10⁹/L or presence of atypical lymphocytes	Fever (>38°C)	Fever (>38°C)
	Hepatic involvement with ALT > 100 or other organ involvement	Lymphadenopathy at ≥ 2 sites
All 3 criteria must be present for diagnosis	At least 1 abnormality of leukocytes • Leukocytosis (>11 × 10⁹/L) • Atypical lymphocytosis (>5%) • Eosinophilia (>1.5 × 10⁹/L)	Involvement of at least 1 internal organ system
	Lymphadenopathy	Blood count abnormalities • Lymphocytosis or lymphopenia • Eosinophilia • Thrombocytopenia
	HHV-6 reactivation	
		* A scoring system is available for classifying HSS/DRESS cases as definite, probable, possible, or no case
	*Typical DIHS occurs with all 7 criteria. Atypical form is when only the first 5 are present.	

Abbreviations: SJS, Stevens–Johnson syndrome; TEN, toxic epidermal necrolysis.

sloughing. The Asboe-Hansen sign may also be present whereby lateral pressure on the edge of a blister will cause the blister to spread into previously uninvolved skin.[57] Greater than 90% of cases of SJS/TEN will have mucosal involvement with erythema and erosions of the buccal, genital, and ocular tissue. The eyes may demonstrate conjunctival erythema, periorbital edema, discharge, crusting, and development of a pseudomembrane.[58]

The severity-of-illness score for toxic epidermal necrolysis (SCORTEN) was developed to assess the severity and predict prognosis. Using logistic regression techniques, 7 independent variables were identified and assigned a value of either 1 or 0 based on the presence or absence of the variable. These variables included age $\geq$40, associated cancer, heart rate $\geq$120 beats per minute, serum blood urea nitrogen greater than 28 mg/dL, BSA $\geq$10%, serum bicarbonate less than 20 mEq/L, and serum glucose greater than 250 mg/dL. With increasing scores, the mortality rate increases. A score of 5 or more is associated with a greater than 90% mortality.[59] Recently, another scoring system was derived from an international dataset, the ABCD-10 Score, named for age, bicarbonate, cancer, dialysis, and 10% BSA.[60] Recent comparisons of the 2 scores have demonstrated better performance of SCORTEN than ABCD-10.[61,62]

Acute Generalized Exanthematous Pustulosis

Acute generalized exanthematous pustulosis (AGEP) is a SCAR that is almost exclusively caused by exposure to a drug with a very short latency period, frequently less than 2 days.[63] It presents with numerous nonfollicular pustules on an erythematous base. The multinational EuroSCAR group found that the medications most often implicated in the development of AGEP were pristinamycin, ampicillin and amoxicillin, quinolones, chloroquine and hydroxychloroquine, anti-infective sulfonamides, terbinafine, and diltiazem.[64] The rash tends to first appear in the axillary, submammary, and inguinal intertriginous regions. Mucosal involvement is limited and only seen in about one-fourth of patients.[62] Evidence of systemic inflammation includes the development of fever, leukocytosis with elevated neutrophils, and elevated C-reactive protein. The lesions of AGEP typically spontaneously regress after 2 weeks with the development of collarette desquamation in previously affected areas. The mortality rate of AGEP is about 5% and death usually occurs in patients with significant comorbidities.[65]

EVALUATION

In the ED, the initial evaluation of a patient with a possible DHR focuses on the clinical stability of the patient by assessing the airway, breathing, and circulation. Once the patient is stable, clinical evaluation of a patient with a possible DHR focuses on the drug and on the patient. Information to gather include the name of the medication, the timing from drug exposure to the development of symptoms, a history of similar reactions especially in the absence of the suspected drug, and the signs and symptoms of the reaction. Clearly delineating the timing of all symptoms and the timing of drug exposure can help to avoid protopathic bias. In this form of bias, a symptom occurs for which the patient takes a drug which is followed by the full development of the disease. The disease is erroneously thought to be caused by the drug even though the exposure actually occurred after the onset of disease.[66]

Type I hypersensitivity reactions are acute in onset after exposure to the offending agent. Evaluation of patients in the ED is often conducted without the aid of laboratory or radiographic testing. Clinical evaluation is what is used to differentiate a simple allergic reaction from life-threatening anaphylaxis. The National Institutes of Allergy and Infectious Disease/Food Allergy and Anaphylaxis Network (NIAID/FAAN) criteria are used to determine the presence of anaphylaxis based on the presence of any one of the 3 clinical scenarios. The first criterion requires the presence of mucocutaneous findings coupled with either respiratory or cardiovascular involvement. In the second criterion, there is the involvement of any 2 of the following 4 organ systems after exposure to a *likely* allergen—mucocutaneous, respiratory, cardiovascular, and gastrointestinal. For the final criterion, hypotension develops after exposure to a *known* allergen for the patient.[67]

Evaluating a patient with a Type II hypersensitivity reaction requires laboratory evaluation with a complete blood count. Considering DIIHA, DIITP, and DIIN as a diagnosis requires a high degree of suspicion and is made by the demonstration of reduced red blood cells, platelets, or neutrophils in the setting of drug administration. Similarly, when patients present with a Type III hypersensitivity reaction, the signs and symptoms are nonspecific and require a high degree of suspicion. The diagnosis is usually made during an admission whereby other possible etiologies can be ruled out.

The SCARs that develop as a result of a Type IV hypersensitivity reaction carry a high risk of mortality and thus rapid evaluation is paramount to ensure that the patient receives proper treatment. Usually, patients that present with DRESS, SJS/TEN, or AGEP have such profound skin findings that suspicion is easily raised for these diagnoses. The patient may present early whereby the full clinical picture has not yet evolved making the diagnosis that much harder to make. Early involvement of a dermatologist to facilitate histopathologic analysis is recommended. Laboratory studies are used to assess the severity of illness and to help guide supportive care.

TREATMENT

The first step in the treatment of any DHR is discontinuing the offending agent. Further treatment is dictated by the acuity and severity of the reaction. All patients should be assessed for clinical stability by first evaluating the ABCs—patency of the airway, ensuring breathing is adequate, and assessing for the effectiveness of cardiac output.

For cases of anaphylaxis, epinephrine is the first-line medication.[68] For patients not in cardiac arrest, epinephrine should be administered intramuscularly in the anterolateral thigh—at the location of the vastus lateralis muscle, a large, highly vascularized muscle. Administration in the thigh leads to better absorption than either subcutaneous injection or intramuscular injection into the deltoid muscle.[69] The concentration of epinephrine used for intramuscular injection is 1:1000 (1 mg/mL). The dose is 0.01 mg/kg to a maximum of 0.5 mg for adults and 0.3 mg for children. This can be repeated every 5 to 15 minutes as needed for persistent symptoms of anaphylaxis.[70] Epinephrine can be given as a continuous infusion using a 1:10,000 (0.1 mg/mL) concentration for patients that fail to respond to intramuscular doses. In cases of severe anaphylaxis, patients can lose up to one-third of their intravascular volume through plasma extravasation into surrounding tissue leading to cardiovascular collapse.[71] Patients should have adequate intravenous access established with 2 large-bore IV catheters. In the anticipation of intravascular volume loss, crystalloids should be administered. Supplemental oxygen should be administered to all patients in respiratory distress, those requiring multiple doses of epinephrine, and patients with chronic cardiac or respiratory diseases.[72] Antihistamines may be given for the treatment of pruritus and cutaneous signs in anaphylaxis. It is important to realize the limits of antihistamine treatment, specifically that it lacks the bronchodilatory, inotropic, vasoconstrictive, and mast cell stabilization properties of epinephrine. Glucocorticoid steroids are also frequently given in cases of anaphylaxis. These have a slow onset of action and there is no compelling evidence that their use reduces the occurrence of biphasic reactions.[73] Some guidelines now recommend against the routine use of steroids for the treatment of anaphylaxis.[74]

Patients with drug-induced Type II hypersensitivity reactions will need treatment tailored to the abnormalities that are specific to the reaction. In severe cases of DIIHA, transfusion of packed red blood cells may be required. In cases of DIITP, there is limited evidence for the use of immunosuppressive therapy; however, because DIITP may not be distinguished from ITP, intravenous immune globulin (IVIG) may be administered. Transfusion with platelets should be given in cases of severe thrombocytopenia.[75] Patients with DIIN who develop infections should be treated aggressively with broad-spectrum antibiotics and possibly antifungal agents. Administration of recombinant granulocyte colony-stimulating factor (G-CSF) may shorten the time to recovery of normal neutrophil counts. Transfusion of granulocyte concentrates are generally reserved for cases of severe, life-threatening infection.[76]

The treatment of drug-induced Type III hypersensitivity reactions is generally more long-term management options. Acute presentations due to infections or organ damage (eg, acute kidney injury) may occur. The treatment will need to be directed to the presenting problem.

Patients with a Type IV hypersensitivity reaction will be managed based on the severity of the presentation. For minor reactions such as contact dermatitis, the only treatment required may be the removal of the offending agent. More severe presentations such as a SCAR like SJS or TEN will need aggressive resuscitation and often transfer to a specialty center that cares for burn patients as many of the principles of therapy are similar to that patient population.[77] Other than the initial resuscitation, most treatment decisions will be made by the specialist. There is no clear consensus on the use of debridement or treatment with either steroids or IVIG.[78]

DISPOSITION

The disposition of patients who present to the ED for a DHR depends on the severity of the reaction and the response to treatment. For mild cases such as contact dermatitis, patients can be discharged once they have been evaluated and a treatment plan has been developed and explained to the patient. For cases of anaphylaxis, patients can be discharged home if they have a rapid response to treatment and complete resolution of symptoms. There should be some period of observation in the ED after an episode of anaphylaxis; however, the duration of this observation is based on limited evidence. The Resuscitation Council UK updated guidelines for anaphylaxis released in 2021 suggests a 2 hour observation for patients who responded to epinephrine treatment within 5 to 10 minutes, had complete resolution of symptoms, and who have adequate outpatient resources including an epinephrine autoinjector. A longer observation period of 6 hours is recommended if more than one dose of epinephrine is administered or if there is a history of a previous biphasic reaction. More severe cases require longer periods of observation.[73] The Joint Task Force on Practice Parameters comprised of members from the American Academy of Allergy, Asthma & Immunology and the American College of Allergy, Asthma and Immunology state that it may be reasonable to discharge low-risk patients after a 1 hour period of asymptomatic observation.[69] All patients with anaphylaxis should receive education about the avoidance of triggers, indications for return to the ED, and the use of epinephrine auto-injectors. Patients should be discharged with a prescription for an appropriate epinephrine auto-injector and a referral to an allergist.[69]

For other types of DHRs, the disposition will be determined by the presenting signs and symptoms, the clinical status of the patient, and the treatment needs of the patient. As mentioned previously, patients with SJS or TEN should be considered for transfer to a burn center for specialized treatment. A delay of greater than 7 days in the transfer of care of patients with TEN to a burn center has been associated with increased mortality.[79]

DELABELING OF DRUG ALLERGIES

Many patients are given a label of having a drug allergy despite not actually having an episode of a DHR. This can lead to substandard care due to the withholding of optimal treatments. Many of these reactions are patient reported and do not meet the clinical criteria for an allergic reaction.[80] Since 2013, there has been an increased focus on the problems of misattributed drug allergies with a push to "de-label" these patients.[81] This issue is commonly encountered with patients who are identified as being allergic to penicillin. In the US, approximately 8% of the population or 25 million individuals carry the label of being allergic to penicillin. In one study of 500 patients who were identified as being allergic to penicillin, only 4 patients (0.8%, 95% confidence interval (CI): 0.32% to 2.03%) had a positive reaction on gold standard testing.[82] A penicillin and cephalosporin testing pathway was implemented at a large academic hospital in Boston whereby patients identified as having an allergy to these antibiotics could undergo test dosing in the ED. Of the 310 test doses given, hypersensitivity reactions occurred in only 10 patients (3.2%; 95% CI: 1.6%–5.9%). In 5 of those cases, the pathway was not followed correctly. This led to a change in allergy labeling for 146 (47%) of the patients.[83] Programs to perform confirmatory testing for patients labeled as having a penicillin allergy may have substantial cost-benefit through improved utilization of resources and selection of treatment options.[84] There should also be an effort to ensure greater accuracy of allergy labeling in the first place.

SUMMARY

The immune system, the body's defense against foreign substances which may be harmful, can respond to the administration of drugs leading to the development of a wide variety of DHRs. These are a form of unpredictable events that have been classified as Type B ADRs. Clinical presentations are heterogeneous, and the exact diagnosis is often beyond the scope of the ED. Care of patients who present to the ED focuses on stabilization, providing supportive care, and, in cases of anaphylaxis, administering epinephrine, the first-line treatment.

CLINICS CARE POINTS

- Patients with new clinical symptoms after the administration of a drug must be carefully evaluated for timing, associated symptoms, and type of drug to help determine if the patient is having a DHR.
- When the possibility of a DHR is being considered, all possible causes of the reaction should be discontinued.
- Initially focus on the tenets of good resuscitation, such as airway, breathing, and circulation as anaphylaxis is a potentially fatal reaction.
- Cutaneous signs and symptoms are the most common manifestation of an allergic reaction to a drug, but one should carefully assess for the involvement of the respiratory and gastrointestinal systems as well as signs of poor circulation resulting in hypotension or loss of consciousness.
- Patients presenting with severe rashes should be queried about the use of drugs, even if the drug was not started recently. These rashes could be a manifestation of SCARs, which has a high mortality rate.

DISCLOSURE

The authors have nothing to disclose.

REFERENCES

1. Lazarou J, Pomeranz BH, Corey PN. Incidence of adverse drug reactions in hospitalized patients: a meta-analysis of prospective studies. JAMA 1998;279: 1200–5.
2. Wood RA, Camargo CA Jr, Lieberman P, et al. Anaphylaxis in America: the prevalence and characteristics of anaphylaxis in the United States. J Allergy Clin Immunol 2014;133(2):461–7.
3. Saff R, Camargo C, Rudders SA, et al. Utility of ICD-9-CM codes for identification of allergic drug reactions. J Allergy Clin Immunol Pract 2014;133:AB271.
4. Huang F, Chawla K, Järvinen KM, et al. Anaphylaxis in a New York City pediatric emergency department: Triggers, treatments, and outcomes. J Allergy Clin Immunol 2012;129:162–8.e3.
5. Jerschow E, Lin RY, Scaperotti MM, et al. Fatal anaphylaxis in the United States, 1999-2010: Temporal patterns and demographic associations. J Allergy Clin Immun 2014;134:1318–28.e7.
6. Tanno LK, Demoly P. Epidemiology of anaphylaxis. Curr Opin Allergy Clin Immunol 2021;21:168–74.
7. Liew WK, Williamson E, Tang MLK. Anaphylaxis fatalities and admissions in Australia. J Allergy Clin Immunol 2009;123:434–42.
8. Turner PJ, Gowland MH, Sharma V, et al. Increase in anaphylaxis-related hospitalizations but no increase in fatalities: An analysis of United Kingdom national anaphylaxis data, 1992-2012. J Allergy Clin Immunol 2015;135(4):956–63.e1. https://doi.org/10.1016/j.jaci.2014.10.021.
9. Yu RJ, Krantz MS, Phillips EJ, et al. Emerging causes of drug-induced anaphylaxis: a review of anaphylaxis-associated reports in the FDA adverse event reporting system (FAERS). J Allergy Clin Immunol Pract 2021;9:819–29.e2.
10. Gurwitz JH, Field TS, Harrold LR, et al. Incidence and preventability of adverse drug events among older persons in the ambulatory setting. JAMA 2003;289: 1107–16.
11. Lavan AH, Gallagher P. Predicting risk of adverse drug reactions in older adults. Ther Adv Drug Saf 2016;7:11–22.
12. Alfirevic A, Pirmohamed M. Drug induced hypersensitivity and the HLA Complex. Pharmacogenomics 2010;4:69–90.
13. Clark S, Wei W, Rudders SA, et al. Risk factors for severe anaphylaxis in patients receiving anaphylaxis treatment in US emergency departments and hospitals. J Allergy Clin Immunol 2014;134:1125–30.
14. Motosue MS, Bellolio MF, Houten HKV, et al. Risk factors for severe anaphylaxis in the United States. Ann Allergy Asthma Immunol 2017;119:356–61.e2.
15. Worm M, Francuzik W, Renaudin J-M, et al. Factors increasing the risk for a severe reaction in anaphylaxis: An analysis of data from The European Anaphylaxis Registry. Allergy 2018;73(6):1322–30.
16. Calvani M, Cardinale F, Martelli A, et al. Risk factors for severe pediatric food anaphylaxis in Italy. Pediatr Allergy Immu 2011;22(8):813–9.
17. Iribarren C, Tolstykh IV, Miller MK, et al. Asthma and the prospective risk of anaphylactic shock and other allergy diagnoses in a large integrated health care delivery system. Ann Allergy Asthma Immunol 2010;104:371–7.e2.
18. Brown EA. Problems of Drug Allergy. J Am Med Assoc 1955;157:814–9.

19. Available at: https://www.accessdata.fda.gov/scripts/cdrh/cfdocs/cfcfr/CFRSearch.cfm?CFRPart=312&showFR=1. Accessed July 23, 2021.

20. WHO. International drug monitoring: the role of national centres. World Health Organ Tech Rep Ser 1972;498:1–25.

21. Rawlins MD, Thompson JW. Pathogenesis of adverse drug reactions. In: Davies DM, editor. Textbook of adverse drug reactions. Oxford: Oxford University Press; 1977. p. 10.

22. Edwards IR, Aronson JK. Adverse drug reactions: definitions, diagnosis, and management. Lancet 2000;356:1255–9.

23. Demoly P, Adkinson NF, Brockow K, et al. International Consensus on drug allergy. Allergy 2014;69:420–37.

24. Gell PGH, Coombs RRA. The classification of allergic reactions underlying disease. In: Coombs RRA, Gells PGH, editors. Clinical aspects of immunology. Oxford: Blackwell; 1963.

25. Siraganian RP. Mast cell signal transduction from the high-affinity IgE receptor. Curr Opin Immunol 2003;15:639–46.

26. Dispenza MC. Classification of hypersensitivity reactions. Allergy Asthma Proc 2019;40:470–3.

27. Limsuwan T, Demoly P. Acute symptoms of drug hypersensitivity (urticaria, angioedema, anaphylaxis, anaphylaxis shock). Med Clin North Am 2010;94(4):691–710.

28. Dimenstein IB. The road from cytotoxins to immunohistochemistry. J Histotechnol 2021;44(4):164–72. https://doi.org/10.1080/01478885.2020.1804234.

29. Uzzaman A, Cho SH. Chapter 28: classification of hypersensitivity reactions. Allergy Asthma Proc 2012;33:96–9.

30. Karmacharya P, Poudel DR, Pathak R, et al. Rituximab-induced serum sickness: A systematic review. Semin Arthritis Rheum 2015;45:334–40.

31. Peng B, Wei M, Zhu F-C, et al. The vaccines-associated Arthus reaction. Hum Vaccin Immunother 2019;15:2769–77.

32. Pavlos R, Mallal S, Ostrov D, et al. T Cell–Mediated Hypersensitivity Reactions to Drugs. Annu Rev Med 2015;66:1–16.

33. Redwood AJ, Pavlos RK, White KD, et al. HLAs: Key regulators of T-cell-mediated drug hypersensitivity. HLA 2018;91:3–16.

34. Pichler WJ, Adam J, Daubner B, et al. Drug Hypersensitivity Reactions: Pathomechanism and Clinical Symptoms. Med Clin North Am 2010;94(4):645–64.

35. Pichler WJ, Hausmann O. Classification of Drug Hypersensitivity into Allergic, p-i, and Pseudo-Allergic Forms. Int Arch Allergy Immunol 2017;171:166–79.

36. Riedl MA, Casillas AM. Adverse drug reactions: types and treatment options. Am Fam Physician 2003;68:1781–90.

37. Khan DA, Solensky R. Drug allergy. J Allergy Clin Immun 2010;125:126–37.e1.

38. Monroe EW, Daly AF, Shalhoub RF. Appraisal of the validity of histamine-induced wheal and flare to predict the clinical efficacy of antihistamines. J Allergy Clin Immunol 1997;99:S798–806.

39. Greenberger PA, Ditto AM. Chapter 24: Anaphylaxis. Allergy Asthma Proc 2012;33:80–3.

40. Garratty G. Drug-induced immune hemolytic anemia. Hematology Am Soc Hematol Educ Program 2009;73–9.

41. Pedersen-Bjergaard U, Andersen M, Hansen PB. Drug-induced thrombocytopenia: clinical data on 309 cases and the effect of corticosteroid therapy. Eur J Clin Pharmacol 1997;52:183–9.

42. Curtis BR. Drug-induced immune neutropenia/agranulocytosis. Immunohematology 2014;30:95–101.
43. Maidhof W, Hilas O. Lupus: an overview of the disease and management options. P T 2012;37(4):240–9.
44. Vaglio A, Grayson PC, Fenaroli P, et al. Drug-induced lupus: Traditional and new concepts. Autoimmun Rev 2018;17:912–8.
45. Miyagawa F, Asada H. Current Perspective Regarding the Immunopathogenesis of Drug-Induced Hypersensitivity Syndrome/Drug Reaction with Eosinophilia and Systemic Symptoms (DIHS/DRESS). Int J Mol Sci 2021;22:2147.
46. Bocquet H, Bagot M, Roujeau JC. Drug-induced pseudolymphoma and drug hypersensitivity syndrome (drug rash with eosinophilia and systemic symptoms: DRESS). Semin Cutan Med Surg 1996;15:250–7.
47. Shiohara T, Inaoka M, Kano Y. Drug-induced Hypersensitivity Syndrome(DIHS): A Reaction Induced by a Complex Interplay among Herpesviruses and Antiviral and Antidrug Immune Responses. Allergol Int 2006;55:1–8.
48. Mizukawa Y, Hirahara K, Kano Y, et al. Drug-induced hypersensitivity syndrome/drug reaction with eosinophilia and systemic symptoms severity score: A useful tool for assessing disease severity and predicting fatal cytomegalovirus disease. J Am Acad Dermatol 2019;80:670–8.e2.
49. Kardaun SH, Sidoroff A, Valeyrie-Allanore L, et al. Variability in the clinical pattern of cutaneous side-effects of drugs with systemic symptoms: does a DRESS syndrome really exist? Br J Dermatol 2007;156:609–11.
50. Shiohara T, Mizukawa Y. Drug-induced hypersensitivity syndrome (DiHS)/drug reaction with eosinophilia and systemic symptoms (DRESS): An update in 2019. Allergol Int 2019;68:301–8.
51. Criado PR, Avancini J, Santi CG, et al. Drug reaction with eosinophilia and systemic symptoms (DRESS): a complex interaction of drugs, viruses and the immune system. Isr Med Assoc J 2012;14(9):577–82.
52. Cacoub P, Musette P, Descamps V, et al. The DRESS syndrome: a literature review. Am J Med 2011;124(7):588–97.
53. Intarasupht J, Kanchanomai A, Leelasattakul W, et al. Prevalence, risk factors, and mortality outcome in the drug reaction with eosinophilia and systemic symptoms patients with cardiac involvement. Int J Dermatol 2018;57(10):1187–91.
54. Bastuji-Garin S, Rzany B, Stern RS, et al. Clinical classification of cases of toxic epidermal necrolysis, Stevens-Johnson syndrome, and erythema multiforme. Arch Dermatol 1993;129(1):92–6.
55. Wetter DA, Camilleri MJ. Clinical, etiologic, and histopathologic features of Stevens-Johnson syndrome during an 8-year period at Mayo Clinic. Mayo Clin Proc 2010;85:131–8.
56. Roujeau JC, Stern RS. Severe Adverse Cutaneous Reactions to Drugs. N Engl J Med 1994;331:1272–85.
57. Dowling JR, Anderson KL, Huang WW. Asboe-Hansen sign in toxic epidermal necrolysis. Cutis 2019;103:E6–8.
58. Schwering MS, Kayange P, Rothe C. Ocular manifestations in patients with Stevens–Johnson syndrome in Malawi—review of the literature illustrated by clinical cases. Graefes Arch Clin Exp Ophthalmol 2019;257:2343–8.
59. Bastuji-Garin S, Fouchard N, Bertocchi M, et al. SCORTEN: A Severity-of-Illness Score for Toxic Epidermal Necrolysis. J Invest Dermatol 2000;115:149–53.
60. Noe MH, Rosenbach M, Hubbard RA, et al. Development and validation of a risk prediction model for in-hospital mortality among patients with stevens-johnson

syndrome/toxic epidermal necrolysis—ABCD-10. JAMA Dermatol 2019;155: 448–54.

61. Koh HK, Fook-Chong S, Lee HY. Assessment and Comparison of Performance of ABCD-10 and SCORTEN in Prognostication of Epidermal Necrolysis. JAMA Dermatol 2020;156:1294–9.

62. Duplisea MJ, Roberson ML, Chrisco L, et al. Performance of ABCD-10 and SCORTEN mortality prediction models in a cohort of patients with Stevens-Johnson syndrome/toxic epidermal necrolysis. J Am Acad Dermatol 2021;85(4): 873–7.

63. Roujeau JC, Bioulac-Sage P, Bourseau C, et al. Acute generalized exanthematous pustulosis. Analysis of 63 cases. Arch Dermatol 1991;127:1333–8.

64. Sidoroff A, Dunant A, Viboud C, et al. Risk factors for acute generalized exanthematous pustulosis (AGEP)—results of a multinational case–control study (EuroSCAR). Br J Dermatol 2007;157:989–96.

65. Feldmeyer L, Heidemeyer K, Yawalkar N. Acute generalized exanthematous pustulosis: pathogenesis, genetic background, clinical variants and therapy. Int J Mol Sci 2016;17:1214.

66. Horwitz RI, Feinstein AR. The problem of "protopathic bias" in case-control studies. Am J Med 1980;68:255–8.

67. Sampson HA, Muñoz-Furlong A, Campbell RL, et al. Second symposium on the definition and management of anaphylaxis: summary report–second National Institute of Allergy and Infectious Disease/Food Allergy and Anaphylaxis Network symposium. Ann Emerg Med 2006;47(4):373–80.

68. Kemp SF, Lockey RF, Simons FE. World Allergy Organization ad hoc Committee on Epinephrine in A. Epinephrine: the drug of choice for anaphylaxis. A statement of the World Allergy Organization. Allergy 2008;63(8):1061–70.

69. Simons FER, Gu X, Simons KJ. Epinephrine absorption in adults: Intramuscular versus subcutaneous injection. J Allergy Clin Immunol 2001;108(5):871–3.

70. Shaker MS, Wallace DV, Golden DBK, et al. Anaphylaxis—a 2020 practice parameter update, systematic review, and Grading of Recommendations, Assessment, Development and Evaluation (GRADE) analysis. J Allergy Clin Immunol 2020;145(4):1082–123.

71. Fisher MMcD. Clinical Observations on the Pathophysiology and Treatment of Anaphylactic Cardiovascular Collapse. Anaesth Intensive Care 1986;14(1): 17–21.

72. Simons FER, Ardusso LRF, Bilò MB, et al. World allergy organization guidelines for the assessment and management of anaphylaxis. World Allergy Organ J 2011;4(2):13–37.

73. Alqurashi W, Ellis AK. Do Corticosteroids Prevent Biphasic Anaphylaxis? J Allergy Clin Immunol Pract 2017;5(5):1194–205.

74. Dodd A, Hughes A, Sargant N, et al. Evidence update for the treatment of anaphylaxis. Resuscitation 2021;163:86–96.

75. Aster RH, Bougie DW. Drug-Induced Immune Thrombocytopenia. N Engl J Med 2007;357(6):580–7.

76. Andrès E, Federici L, Weitten T, et al. Recognition and management of drug-induced blood cytopenias: the example of drug-induced acute neutropenia and agranulocytosis. Expert Opin Drug Saf 2008;7(4):481–9.

77. Lerch M, Mainetti C, Beretta-Piccoli BT, et al. Current Perspectives on Stevens-Johnson Syndrome and Toxic Epidermal Necrolysis. Clin Rev Allergy Immunol 2018;54(1):147–76.

78. Curtis JA, Christensen L-C, Paine AR, et al. Stevens-Johnson syndrome and toxic epidermal necrolysis treatments: An Internet survey. J Am Acad Dermatol 2016; 74(2):379–80.
79. Palmieri TL, Greenhalgh DG, Saffle JR, et al. A Multicenter Review of Toxic Epidermal Necrolysis Treated in U.S. Burn Centers at the End of the Twentieth Century. J Burn Care Rehabil 2002;23(2):87–96.
80. Vyles D, Antoon JW, Norton A, et al. Children with reported penicillin allergy: Public health impact and safety of delabeling. Ann Allergy Asthma Immunol 2020; 124(6):558–65.
81. Trubiano J, Phillips E. Antimicrobial stewardship's new weapon? A review of antibiotic allergy and pathways to 'de-labeling. Curr Opin Infect Dis 2013;26(6):526.
82. Macy E, Ngor EW. Safely Diagnosing Clinically Significant Penicillin Allergy Using Only Penicilloyl-Poly-Lysine, Penicillin, and Oral Amoxicillin. J Allergy Clin Immunol Pract 2013;1(3):258–63.
83. Maguire M, Hayes BD, Fuh L, et al. Beta-lactam antibiotic test doses in the emergency department. World Allergy Organ J 2020;13(1):100093.
84. Sousa-Pinto B, Blumenthal KG, Macy E, et al. Penicillin Allergy Testing Is Cost-Saving: An Economic Evaluation Study. Clin Infect Dis 2020;72(6):924–38.

Evaluation and Management of Food Allergies in the Emergency Department

Genevieve Schult Krajewski, MD[a,b,c,*], Thomas Krajewski, MD[a]

KEYWORDS

- Food allergy • Food anaphylaxis • Emergency department
- Management of food allergies

KEY POINTS

- Food allergies are a common complaint among patients evaluated in the emergency department (ED), and ED visits for food allergies are increasing.
- In someone without a previously diagnosed food allergy, diagnosis is purely clinical in the ED.
- The mainstay of therapy for those suspected of having anaphylaxis owing to a food allergy is epinephrine.
- Antihistamines and steroids are not a substitute for epinephrine in the management of anaphylaxis.
- Discharge from the ED must include education on food avoidance, follow-up with an allergist, and making sure epinephrine is readily available to the patient.

Food allergies are an important group of disorders that all emergency department (ED) providers should be comfortable treating. Their incidence is on the increase as is the frequency with which these disorders are encountered in the ED. As many as 20% of people will avoid food at some point in their life out of concern for a food allergy.[1–6] The complexity of appropriate recognition, diagnosis, and management requires a thorough understanding of the mechanisms that underlie the pathologic condition. This also means that diagnosis can be difficult. Symptoms can be broad and atypical ranging from mild to severe. It is crucial to recognize a food allergy reaction at presentation to appropriately treat and disposition patients.[7]

This article originally appeared in Emergency Medicine Clinics, Volume 40 Issue 1, February 2022.

[a] Ochsner Medical Center Emergency Department, 1514 Jefferson Highway, New Orleans, LA 70121, USA; [b] Ochsner Emergency Medicine Residency, New Orleans, LA, USA; [c] Ochsner Clinical School at the University of Queensland, New Orleans, LA, USA
* Corresponding author. 1514 Jefferson Highway, New Orleans, LA 70121.
E-mail address: Genevieve.Krajewski@Ochsner.org

Immunol Allergy Clin N Am 43 (2023) 491–501
https://doi.org/10.1016/j.iac.2022.10.003
0889-8561/23/© 2022 Elsevier Inc. All rights reserved.

Food allergies are defined as "an adverse health effect arising from a specific immune response that occur reproducibly on exposure to a given food."[7] For the emergency provider, this definitive diagnosis is particularly troublesome, as the gold standard of testing is a placebo-controlled food challenge. This obviously falls outside of the realm of an acute care visit, making the diagnosis for the acute care provider solely clinical.[8,9]

Although definitive diagnosis might not be possible at an acute care visit, the management of the most severe food allergy, anaphylaxis, is a staple of acute care medicine. The administration of epinephrine, antihistamines, and steroids is still the foundation of treatment, whereas more nuanced management and diagnosis usually fall outside of the emergency clinician's purview. Understanding these other treatments is relevant because of the disorder's widespread prevalence.

EPIDEMIOLOGY

The true incidence of ED visits for food allergy can be difficult to discern, as the diagnosis is presumptive in most cases; however, there are an estimated 203,000 emergency visits for such allergies, and of those, roughly 90,000 are anaphylactic reactions.[9,10]

The incidence of food allergy nationally is estimated to be between 3% and 4% for adults and roughly 8% for children.[11–13] Confirmatory skin testing, food challenge, and history would corroborate that 3% of adults have a true food allergy, but when patients are asked to self-report allergy, the number increases substantially. Self-reported food allergies range up to 20%, and a similar number report avoidance behavior for fear of being allergic to a specific food despite frequently lacking definitive diagnosis or true allergy.[1–5]

Although unnecessary food avoidance may not seem like a major concern, there is a genuine impact on those who do so. A study in *Allergy* found that children with peanut allergy were restricted from attending school (10%) or school trips (59%), avoided parties (68%) and restaurants (11%), and many were prevented from playing at friends' houses (14%) and attending sleepovers (26%).

There is a decade over decade increase in food allergies over the last 3 decades.[5] The increase based on confirmatory testing or serum markers is around 1.2% per decade since 1980. These seem to be most prominent in what would be described as "industrialized" countries, although there are some variances regionally and by age.[14] Although there have been attempts in Australia, the United Kingdom, and United States to determine variances based on socioeconomic divisions, there is no clear difference or pattern to be inferred, and this is a continued area of research.

Motosue and colleagues[14] analyzed pediatric anaphylaxis from food and found there to be a steadily increasing number of cases, as seen in **Fig. 1**. Previous estimates from the late 1990s had substantially underestimated the burden of this disease for the emergency system.

As recognition and investigation have increased, there has been growing interest in identifying the most at-risk cohorts as well as trying to identify risk factors or protective behavior. There are some identified risk factors, including male sex, Asian or Black race/ethnicity, and a familial history of food allergy. There are innumerable other hypotheses about risks with varying levels of evidence that range from little to no evidence, such as vitamin D deficiency, antibiotic exposure, pet exposure as well as hygiene.[15]

The leading cause in the United States of pediatric anaphylaxis is food. However, data related to ED visits and hospitalizations due to food-related anaphylaxis are limited.[14] From what is available, nut allergies are the most common, particularly peanut allergies.

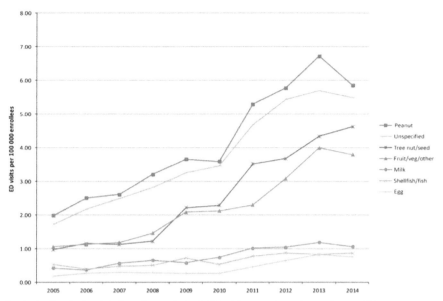

Fig, 1. Pediatric food-induced anaphylaxis ED visit rates based on trigger, 2005-2014. Veg., vegetables. (*From* Motosue et al. National trends in emergency department visits and hospitalizations for food-induced anaphylaxis in US children. Pediatr Allergy Immunol. 2018 Aug;29(5):538–544; with permission. (Figure 2 in original).)

COMMON FOOD CAUSES

The Food Allergen Labeling and Consumer Act (FALCPA) defines major food allergies as one of the 8 foods/food groups containing protein derived from milk, eggs, fish, crustacean shellfish, tree nuts, wheat, peanuts, and soybeans, as these are responsible for most food allergies.[16]

In adults, the most common of these is milk, followed by shellfish. Allergy to peanuts appears to resolve in approximately 20% of patients, but the same is not necessarily true for an allergy to tree nuts. Wheat allergies in children usually resolve by adolescence.[13,17]

An allergy to 1 food group can be predictive of a sensitivity or allergy to another group based on the cross-reactivity of the underlying immune mechanisms, as see in **Table 1** by Sicherer.[18]

For those patients who have yet to be tested definitively, these are important considerations to help avoid a repeated exposure that might precipitate another severe allergic response.

Children who have allergies to foods are likely to "outgrow them" by developing tolerance over time. Those allergic to milk or eggs have been shown likely to develop tolerance by adulthood; conversely, children allergic to fish, peanuts, or tree nuts are likely to continue to have some sensitivity or allergy into adulthood.[19,20]

TYPES OF FOOD ALLERGIES

Food allergies are an abnormal response of the immune system to a food protein. This is distinct from food intolerance, which is a nonimmune reaction. Food allergies are usually grouped into 3 categories: immunoglobulin E (IgE)-mediated, mixed IgE and non-IgE, or non-IgE-mediated. It is important for the emergency medicine physician

Table 1	
Eight major food allergies with cross-reactivity	
Primary Allergy	**Cross-Reactivity**
Cow's milk	Goat's milk, 90%, beef, 10%
Hen's eggs	Turkey, duck, and goose
Soy	Usually little cross-reactivity
Peanut	Little cross-reactivity
Fish	Very likely to be allergic to other fish
Tree nuts	Very likely to be allergic to other tree nuts
Shellfish	Likely allergic to other crustaceans and mollusks
Wheat	Little cross-reactivity

Adapted from Sicherer, Scott H. Clinical implications of cross-reactive food allergens.Journal of Allergy and Clinical Immunology, Volume 108, Issue 6, 881 - 890

to not only be aware of but also recognize the types of reactions that may fall under these subsets. They can also be divided into acute onset, which is IgE-mediated, and delayed onset, which includes IgE and/or cellular-mediated reactions.[19,21]

Traditionally, IgE-mediated reactions are the rapid onset of symptoms that are typically associated with anaphylaxis within minutes to hours. These symptoms are typical of a type I hypersensitivity reaction and include flushing, urticaria, and angioedema. These occur in more than 60% of affected children; however, isolated respiratory and gastrointestinal symptoms are possible.[21] IgE-mediated symptoms usually present within minutes to 1 to 2 hours after exposure, and the more severe the reaction, the earlier it seems to occur.[13,22] IgE-mediated are generally acute urticaria/angioedema reactions, anaphylaxis, food pollen allergy syndrome, food-associated exercise-induced anaphylaxis, and alpha-Gal mammalian meat allergy.[21,23,24]

Both IgE and non-IgE-mediated reactions are responsible for atopic dermatitis, eosinophilic esophagitis, and eosinophilic gastroenteritis.[23] Non-IgE-mediated reactions are usually delayed in onset. These include food protein-induced enterocolitis syndrome (FPIES), celiac disease, food intolerance, and contact dermatitis.[21,23–25]

Pollen-food allergy syndrome (PFAS), alternatively known as oral allergy syndrome, is a common IgE-mediated allergic disease caused by a cross-reaction among pollens and vegetables. The most common symptom is pruritus in the mouth and throat after eating raw fruit or vegetables. It is important to note these same foods are often tolerated when cooked. Systemic symptoms, such as urticaria, nausea, vomiting, and anaphylaxis, are rare but have been found in up to 1.7% of reactions. Initially, PFAS was thought to be mostly a disease of adulthood but is more prevalent in childhood than previously thought.[21,26,27]

"Alpha Gal" syndrome is secondary to a bite from the lone star tick. Diagnosis of alpha-Gal syndrome is made by a detailed history of delayed hives or anaphylaxis usually 3 to 6 hours after eating mammalian meat. Confirmatory testing for the IgE to alpha-Gal is usually not available through the ED. However, it can be done at some academic centers.[21,24,28]

Food-dependent exercise-induced anaphylaxis is the ingestion of a culprit food along with exercise. IgE to the food is crucial to the disease process. Although this is most commonly called exercise-induced anaphylaxis, other factors can precipitate a reaction when done concomitantly with ingestion of the offending food. These factors include alcohol intake or acetylsalicylic acid intake. Thus, this disease is better characterized as a type of food allergy whereby symptoms develop only in the presence of an augmenting factor.[24]

Eosinophilic gastrointestinal disorders (EGID) are mixed IgE and non-IgE-mediated with symptoms isolated to the gastrointestinal system. In patients with eosinophilic esophagitis, symptoms include long-standing dysphagia. These patients are likely to present with food impactions. Abdominal discomfort with diarrhea or constipation along with vomiting are seen in other cases of EGID. The foods most associated as triggers are milk and wheat. In most cases, patients are also treated with oral steroids, such as budesonide or fluticasone.[24]

FPIES is food protein-induced enterocolitis syndrome. It is a non-IgE-mediated food allergy seen almost exclusively in pediatric patients usually during infancy when milk and soy are introduced. Although milk and soy are the most common causes, rice, oats, and grains have also been implicated in causing reactions. True prevalence is unknown, but it is relatively rare and often seen in patients with atopic disease. The most common symptoms are emesis and nonbloody or bloody diarrhea, which can lead acutely to severe dehydration, laboratory abnormalities, and hemodynamic instability or chronic failure to thrive. There is a lack of awareness of this condition and no available confirmatory test, contributing to the diagnosis being easily missed in the ED. Treatment includes supportive care for mild reactions and intravenous (IV) corticosteroids for severe reactions. Education and avoidance of problematic foods are the definitive care.[29]

There are several mimics of food allergies that are nonimmunologic. These should be in the differential diagnosis on presentation to the ED.[30] These include scombroid poisoning caused by histamine ingestion, chemical effects caused by hot or spicy foods, Frey syndrome, and lactose intolerance, among others seen in **Box 1**.[23,30,31]

DIAGNOSIS OF FOOD ALLERGIES

The gold standard of diagnosis of food allergy is a double-blind placebo-controlled oral food challenge, but this cannot be accomplished in the ED. It is also not practical in the clinic setting, so current standard testing includes skin prick test and ssIgE (serum food allergen-specific immunoglobulin E). Some of the new diagnostic modalities under active investigation are basophil activation test, epitope analysis, and molecular allergy analysis. As exciting as this may be, none of these have application in the ED.

Box 1
Differential diagnosis for food allergy

A differential diagnosis for food allergy
- Allergic reactions to nonfood causes (eg, bee stings, medication)
- Food intolerance or sensitivity (eg, lactose intolerance, celiac disease)
- Food poisoning (eg, salmonella, staph, *Escherichia coli*)
- Food toxicity (eg, scombroid, ciguatera)
- Auriculotemporal syndrome (eg, Frey syndrome)
- Food avoidance (eg, anorexia nervosa)
- Side effects of caffeine, alcohol
- Spicy foods reaction

Adapted from Mahdavinia M. Food Allergy in Adults: Presentations, Evaluation, and Treatment. Med Clin North Am. 2020 Jan;104(1):145-155.

Therefore, the management must be guided by a history and presentation that point to a food allergy reaction.[30]

PRESENTATION

Patients with food allergies may present with a constellation of symptoms. Reactions only involving hives or angioedema not involving the posterior oropharynx or larynx are considered mild. Isolated gastrointestinal symptoms are also considered mild. Mild symptoms can be treated with antihistamines.

However, the progression to anaphylaxis with 2 body systems or respiratory or cardiovascular compromise requires escalation of treatment.[21]

Recognizing those signs and symptoms that indicate anaphylaxis is most important for guiding management in the ED and can be reviewed as in **Table 2**. Those with a history of eczema, asthma, allergic rhinitis, food allergies, and a family history of atopic disease should make suspicion for food allergy reaction even greater, as they are at higher risk of a food allergy.[30]

The National Institute of Allergy and Infectious Diseases (NIAID) and the Food Allergy and Anaphylaxis Network (FAAN) definition of anaphylaxis has been translated into clinical diagnostic criteria by Phillip Lieberman, MD in Clinical Diagnostic Criteria for Anaphylaxis, which can be seen in **Fig. 2**. Criteria include a quick onset of signs and symptoms usually within minutes but up to 2 hours and involvement of dermatologic, respiratory, cardiovascular, or gastrointestinal systems. It is important to note whether the patient has a known allergen, likely exposure, or no known allergies, as the number of criteria required to be met depends on this history. The NIAID/FAAN criteria were validated specifically in the ED, with a sensitivity of 96.7% and a specificity of 82.4%.[32] These criteria can be applied to patients in the ED and, when met, treatment with epinephrine is crucial.[33]

Some exceptions include a child with a known allergen and only cutaneous manifestations, which does not meet the diagnosis above for anaphylaxis but should be treated as such regardless.[34]

There are 3 types of anaphylactic reactions: uniphasic, biphasic, and protracted reactions. This is important to note, as some patients may need prolonged observation or extensive education at discharge even after marked improvement in ED. A uniphasic reaction is a typical anaphylactic reaction occurring within 30 minutes of exposure of the offending food allergen and resolving over the next 1 to 2 hours. A biphasic reaction has a second wave of symptoms after the initial reaction has resolved. Up to 20% of patients will experience this. The recommended observation period is 4 to 6 hours, but it is particularly important to know that reactions may occur within the next 6 to 8 hours but can occur up to 24 hours after a reaction. Protracted anaphylaxis is the most severe reaction that can last greater than 24 hours and can include shock and respiratory distress that does not improve despite aggressive therapy.[33] The treatment remains the same on recurrence in a biphasic reaction or protracted anaphylactic reactions with epinephrine, steroids, and antihistamines being the treatments of choice.

MANAGEMENT OF FOOD ALLERGIES IN THE EMERGENCY DEPARTMENT

The most important treatment for anaphylaxis is epinephrine, and it should be administered very early in the course of the allergic reaction. Patients should give themselves epinephrine at the first sign of a potential anaphylactic reaction to a food if it is available to them, and ED providers should also use epinephrine as first-line therapy. If anaphylaxis is identified and/or epinephrine administered by the patient in the out-

Table 2
System-based symptoms encountered in acute immunoglobulin E–mediated food reactions

System	Involved symptoms (usual onset within minutes to 1–2 h following food ingestion)
Cutaneous	Pruritus Flushing Urticaria Angioedema Flare of chronic eczematous rash
Ocular	Pruritus Conjunctival erythema Tearing Periorbital edema
Respiratory tract	Nasal congestion Pruritus Sneezing Laryngeal edema and hoarseness Cough Wheeze Chest tightness Dyspnea Cyanosis
Gastrointestinal	Nausea Emesis Crampy abdominal pain Oral pruritus Tongue, lip, palate, or pharyngeal angioedema
Cardiovascular	Tachycardia Bradycardia Hypotension Cardiac arrest Dizziness
Neurologic	Sense of impending doom Syncope Dizziness

From Mahdavinia M. Food Allergy in Adults: Presentations, Evaluation, and Treatment. Med Clin North Am. 2020 Jan;104(1):145-155

of-hospital setting, emergency medical services should be used to transport the patient to an ED.[35] These patients are usually monitored for 4 to 6 hours after receiving epinephrine to monitor for biphasic reactions, which occurs in 20% of cases.[21] This is not a requirement for a non-IgE-mediated reaction.[21]

Epinephrine is the most effective treatment to prevent death from anaphylaxis, and multiple doses may need to be given in the course of treatment because of its short half-life.[21,24] Despite the generally widespread knowledge of its benefit in preventing fatal anaphylaxis, epinephrine continues to be underutilized by health care providers and patients, and antihistamines are commonly overused in treating these reactions.[35]

Adjunctive treatments may also be given, but these are all second line. These include antihistamines, glucocorticoids, and inhaled beta-agonists. Histamine is produced by mast cells and basophils, which help to arrange the allergic response. Oral H1 antihistamines affect conjunctival, nasal, and cutaneous response to the allergen by decreasing the symptoms that are triggered. Onset of action of such treatment

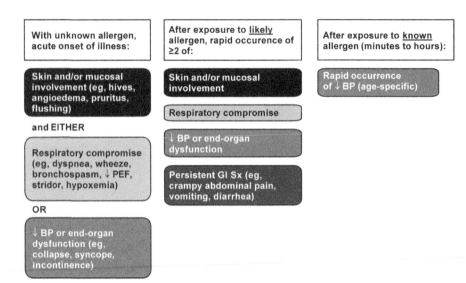

Fig. 2. Clinical diagnostic criteria for anaphylaxis. BP, blood pressure; GI Sx, gastrointestinal symptoms; PEF, peak expiratory flow. (*From* Lieberman PL. Recognition and first-line treatment of anaphylaxis. Am J Med. 2014 Jan;127(1 Suppl):S6-11; with permission (see Figure 2 in original).)

occurs within minutes to a few hours.[21] Corticosteroids have proven efficacy in the management of multiple aspects of allergic inflammation.[21] They are used to minimize the potential late-phase inflammatory response after an anaphylactic reaction, although this has yet to be proven as effective.[21] Inhaled beta-agonist medications are often given to those who present with wheezing and coughing to relieve pulmonary bronchoconstriction.[21]

To reiterate, the use of adjuvant therapy should never delay the administration of epinephrine in food-induced anaphylaxis.[21] There is some evidence that the pathophysiology of food-induced anaphylaxis differs from that of other types of anaphylaxis. In contrast to fatal venom- and drug-induced anaphylaxis, death by food-induced anaphylaxis is almost always caused by respiratory collapse. Distributive shock may be seen in cases of anaphylaxis due to rapid shifts in fluid from the intravascular space to surrounding tissues.[22] Therefore, IV fluids should be administered rapidly in patients presenting with hypotension but should not be administered in isolation.[21]

Discharge from the ED requires thorough patient education. Avoidance of the possible food allergen is the mainstay of treatment. Patients should be told to avoid any foods with ingredients to their known allergen as well as foods that have unknown ingredients. They should also be made aware that cross-contamination is possible. Although the FALCPA was passed to assist consumers with this, there are more than 160 food allergens known to cause reactions, and not all are included in the FALCPA list. In pediatrics, avoidance of food carries a different risk. Avoidance increases risk of malnutrition if it includes essential nutrients. It is especially important for pediatric patients to be closely followed up by the pediatrician[16,21] and an allergist/immunologist.[30] It is important to educate the patient on the possibility of biphasic reaction, which can occur 4 to 24 hours after the initial reaction.[22] Patients should have easy access to at least 1 epinephrine autoinjector and have an emergency action plan. The patient should be educated on when to use the epinephrine auto-injector, and that if used, he or she should seek immediate evaluation in the ED.[21,33,36]

Emergency providers may face another challenge related to food allergies. There are many medications and vaccines that use derived food products. These foods include milk, egg, fish and shellfish, soy, and gelatin.[21,37] Most patients will tolerate the medications containing the foods to which they are allergic to except for gelatin. Propofol and the flu vaccine contain egg products however, egg allergy is no longer a contraindication to receiving the flu shot. Tdap contains milk products. There is no evidence that the cohort of people allergic to eggs or milk are at an increased risk of reaction to these drugs.[37,38] The exception to this appears to be gelatin, which may be related to the larger quantity of the protein used in gelatin-containing products. This is important in the ED, as many medications have a gelatin-containing capsule. Gelatin is also used as a stabilizer in many vaccines and in IV volume expanders.[21]

CLINICS CARE POINTS

- Mild allergic symptoms like isolated urticaria, angioedema not including the larynx or posterior oropharynx, and isolated gastrointestinal symptoms can be treated with antihistamines.

- Pediatric patients with a known food allergen and isolated cutaneous manifestations are the exception to this and should be treated with epinephrine.

- Treatment of anaphylaxis owing to a food allergy is epinephrine. Anaphylaxis usually includes involvement of 2 body systems or respiratory or cardiovascular compromise.

- Treatments, such as antihistamines, glucocorticoids, and inhaled beta-agonists, are second line and are not a substitute for epinephrine in the treatment of anaphylaxis.

DISCLOSURE

The authors have nothing to disclose.

REFERENCES

1. Venter C, Pereira B, Grundy J, et al. Prevalence of sensitization reported and objectively assessed food hypersensitivity amongst six-year-old children: a population-based study. Pediatr Allergy Immunol 2006;17(5):356–63.
2. Pereira B, Venter C, Grundy J, et al. Prevalence of sensitization to food allergens, reported adverse reaction to foods, food avoidance, and food hypersensitivity among teenagers. J Allergy Clin Immunol 2005;116(4):884–92.
3. Woods RK, Thien F, Raven J, et al. Prevalence of food allergies in young adults and their relationship to asthma, nasal allergies, and eczema. Ann Allergy Asthma Immunol 2002;88(2):183–9.
4. Woods RK, Abramson M, Bailey M, et al. International prevalences of reported food allergies and intolerances. Comparisons arising from the European Community Respiratory Health Survey (ECRHS) 1991-1994. Eur J Clin Nutr 2001;55(4): 298–304.
5. Osterballe M, Hansen TK, Mortz CG, et al. The prevalence of food hypersensitivity in an unselected population of children and adults. Pediatr Allergy Immunol 2005;16(7):567–73.
6. Bock SA. Prospective appraisal of complaints of adverse reactions to foods in children during the first 3 years of life. Pediatrics 1987;79(5):683–8.
7. Boyce JA, Assa'ad A, Burks AW, et al. Guidelines for the diagnosis and management of food allergy in the United States: report of the NIAID-sponsored expert panel. J Allergy Clin Immunol 2010;126(6 Suppl):S1–58.

8. Mehta H, Groetch M, Wang J. Growth and nutritional concerns in children with food allergy. Curr Opin Allergy Clin Immunol 2013;13(3):275–9.
9. Rudders SA, Banerji A, Corel B, et al. Multicenter study of repeat epinephrine treatments for food-related anaphylaxis. Pediatrics 2010;125(4):e711–8.
10. Clark S, Bock SA, Gaeta TJ, et al. Multicenter study of emergency department visits for food allergies. J Allergy Clin Immunol 2004;113(2):347–52.
11. Jackson KD, Howie LD, Akinbami LJ. Trends in allergic conditions among children: United States, 1997-2011. NCHS Data Brief 2013;(121):1–8.
12. Gupta RS, Springston EE, Warrier MR, et al. The prevalence, severity, and distribution of childhood food allergy in the United States. Pediatrics 2011;128(1): e9–17.
13. Parrish C, Edwin K. Interventional therapies for the treatment of food allergy. Immunol Allergy Clinic N Am 2018;38(1):77–88.
14. Motosue MS, Bellolio MF, Van Houten HK, et al. National trends in emergency department visits and hospitalizations for food-induced anaphylaxis in US children. Pediatr Allergy Immunol 2018;29(5):538–44.
15. Cummings AJ, Knibb RC, King RM, et al. The psychosocial impact of food allergy and food hypersensitivity in children, adolescents and their families: a review. Allergy 2010;65:933–45.
16. Thompson T, Kane RR, Hager MH. Food Allergen Labeling and Consumer Protection Act of 2004 in effect. J Am Diet Assoc 2006;106(11):1742–4.
17. Iweala OI, Choudhary SK, Commins SP. Food allergy. Curr Gastroenterol Rep 2018;20(5):17.
18. Sicherer, SH. Clinical implications of cross-reactive food allergens J Allergy Clin Immunol 2001;108(6):881–90. doi:10.1067/mai.2001.118515.
19. Anvari S, Miller J, Yeh CY, et al. IgE-mediated food allergy. Clin Rev Allergy Immunol 2019;57(2):244–60.
20. Wood RA. The natural history of food allergy. Pediatrics 2003;111(6 Pt 3):1631–7.
21. Davis CM, Kelso JM. Food allergy management. Immunol Allergy Clin North Am 2018;38(1):53–64.
22. Keet CA, Wood RA. Food allergy and anaphylaxis. Immunol Allergy Clin North Am 2007;27(2):193–212, vi.
23. Bird JA. Food allergy point of care pearls. Immunol Allergy Clin North Am 2018; 38(2):e1–8.
24. Mahdavinia M. Food allergy in adults: presentations, evaluation, and treatment. Med Clin North Am 2020;104(1):145–55.
25. Sicherer SH, Warren CM, Dant C, et al. Food allergy from infancy through adulthood. J Allergy Clin Immunol Pract 2020;8(6):1854–64.
26. Mastrorilli C, Cardinale F, Giannetti A, et al. Pollen-food allergy syndrome: a not so rare disease in childhood. Medicina (Kaunas) 2019;55(10):641.
27. Carlson G, Coop C. Pollen food allergy syndrome (PFAS): a review of current available literature. Ann Allergy Asthma Immunol 2019;123(4):359–65.
28. Commins SP, Satinover SM, Hosen J, et al. Delayed anaphylaxis, angioedema, or urticaria after consumption of red meat in patients with IgE antibodies specific for galactose-alpha-1,3-galactose. J Allergy Clin Immunol 2009;123(2):426–33.
29. Bingemann TA, Sood P, Järvinen KM. Food protein-induced enterocolitis syndrome. Immunol Allergy Clin North Am 2018;38(1):141–52.
30. Gupta M, Cox A, Nowak-Węgrzyn A, et al. Diagnosis of food allergy. Immunol Allergy Clin North Am 2018;38(1):39–52.
31. Sampson HA, Aceves S, Bock SA, et al. Food allergy: a practice parameter update-2014. J Allergy Clin Immunol 2014;134(5):1016–25, e43.

32. Campbell RL, Hagan JB, Manivannan V, et al. Evaluation of National Institute of Allergy and Infectious Diseases/Food Allergy and Anaphylaxis Network Criteria for the diagnosis of anaphylaxis in emergency department patients. J Allergy Clin Immunol 2012;129(3):748–52.
33. Lieberman PL. Recognition and first-line treatment of anaphylaxis. Am J Med 2014;127(1 Suppl):S6–11.
34. Sampson HA, Muñoz-Furlong A, Campbell RL, et al. Second symposium on the definition and management of anaphylaxis: summary report–second National Institute of Allergy and Infectious Disease/Food Allergy and Anaphylaxis Network symposium. Ann Emerg Med 2006;47(4):373–80.
35. Jones SM, Burks AW. Food allergy. N Engl J Med 2017;377(12):1168–76.
36. Devdas JM, Mckie C, Fox AT, et al. Food allergy in children: an overview. Indian J Pediatr 2018;85(5):369–74.
37. Kelso JM. Potential food allergens in medications. J Allergy Clin Immunol 2014; 133(6):1509–18 [quiz 1519–20].
38. Kelso JM. Administering influenza vaccine to egg-allergic persons. Expert Rev Vaccin 2014;13(8):1049–57.

Allergic Acute Coronary Syndrome—Kounis Syndrome

Leen Alblaihed, MBBS, MHA, FAAEM[a],
Maite Anna Huis in 't Veld, MD[a,b],*

KEYWORDS

- Vasospastic angina • Allergic reaction • Kounis syndrome
- Acute coronary syndrome

KEY POINTS

- Acute coronary syndrome in the setting of an immune reaction is known as Kounis syndrome.
- It is an underrecognized syndrome and easily missed clinically.
- Treatment should be aimed at both the allergic component as well as the coronary vasospasm, thrombus, or plaque rupture that occurs as a result of the immune reactions.

INTRODUCTION

Kounis syndrome (KS) is defined as the occurrence of an acute coronary syndrome (ACS) associated with mast cell and platelet activation in the setting of allergic or anaphylactic reactions.[1] For many decades the association between cardiac symptoms and acute allergic reactions has been suspected. In 1950, Pfister and Plice published a case report of a 49-year-old man who presented with an acute myocardial infarction associated with the development of an urticarial rash following administration of penicillin.[2] In 1991, Kounis and Zavras introduced the terms "allergic angina" and "allergic myocardial infarction," which collectively are now better known as "Kounis Syndrome."[3] Multiple pharmacologic and environmental triggers have been identified. The proposed pathophysiological mechanism involves mast cell degranulation, resulting in inflammatory mediator release. These inflammatory mediators, including histamine, leukotriene, and prostaglandin, can induce a vasoconstrictive effect on

This article originally appeared in Emergency Medicine Clinics, Volume 40 Issue 1, February 2022.

[a] Department of Emergency Medicine, University of Maryland School of Medicine, 110 South Paca Street, 6th Floor, Suite 200, Baltimore, MD 21201, USA; [b] Department of Emergency Medicine, Diakonessenhuis Utrecht, Bosboomlaan 1, 3582 KE Utrecht, the Netherlands
* Corresponding author.
E-mail address: m.huisintveld@etz.nl
Twitter: @LeenAlblaihed (L.A.); @maiteanna (M.A.H.V.)

the coronary smooth muscle cells leading to coronary vasospasm (KS type I), cause native plaque destabilization (KS type II), or lead to stent thrombosis (KS type III).[4,5] Diagnosis is based on clinical presentation, electrocardiography, echocardiography, and angiography. The treatment of KS is challenging as there are limited data available on therapeutic options. Many physicians are not aware of KS; therefore, it is underrecognized and underreported. It is imperative for the emergency physician to be aware of this disease in order to promptly diagnose and manage patients who present with KS in the emergency department. This article discusses KS, its underlying pathophysiologic mechanism, diagnosis, and treatment.

DISCUSSION
Pathophysiology

The exact pathophysiologic mechanism of KS remains elusive, as most of the literature pertaining to KS consists of case reports or case series. The main proposed pathophysiological mechanism is thought to be vasospasm, plaque rupture, and thrombosis due to the rapid release of inflammatory mediators during a hypersensitivity reaction.

Mast cells play an essential role in the development of allergic reactions. During allergic reactions mast cells are activated through the cross-linking of immunoglobulin E (IgE) bound to antigen at high-affinity receptors, FcεRIs. Mast-cell activation can also occur in the presence of anaphylatoxins such as C3a and C5a, adenosine, or other stimuli.[6] Activation leads to release of multiple preformed inflammatory mediators such as histamine, tryptase, and chymase, as well as de novo produced arachidonic acid–derived mediators, cytokines, and chemokines.[7] Mast cells are omnipresent in cardiac tissue and are preferentially located at sites of coronary plaques.[8–10] Mast cells can infiltrate areas of plaque erosion or rupture and act on the underlying smooth muscle cells. The cardiac mast cell load of patients with coronary plaques is up to 200-fold higher than in coronary arteries of healthy people.[11]

Mast cell–induced release of mediators has many effects on the coronary arteries including vasospasm, plaque rupture, and thrombosis. Histamine release can lead to coronary vasoconstriction, decreased diastolic blood pressure, and increased intimal thickening; this may contribute to coronary plaque rupture and subsequent coronary artery thrombosis.[3,12] Histamine can also initiate platelet activation and aggregation. The presence of mast cells in and around thrombi has been thought to lead to heparin- and tryptase-induced degradation of fibrinogen, which contributes to destabilization and maturation of thrombi.[11,13] Leukotrienes are potent vasoconstrictors, and chymase and cathepsin-D might act to convert angiotensin I to angiotensin II, a potent vasoconstrictor.[1]

Even in patients with nonallergic ACS, increased levels of serum inflammatory mediators are found, including tryptase, chymase, and arachidonic acid products such as thromboxane and leukotrienes.[14] The mast cell activation in acute coronary syndrome has been thought to be a primary event, not the result from the coronary artery spasm, and this has been supported by evidence that tryptase levels in peripheral blood increases during spontaneous myocardial ischemia but not during pharmacologically induced coronary spasms.[12]

Multiple causes have been identified to trigger KS (**Table 1**). Among these are many well-known triggers of typical allergic reactions and anaphylaxis. In one review by Abdelghany and colleagues of 175 previously reported cases of KS, the most common triggers were antibiotics (27.4%) and insect bites (23.4%).[13]

Table 1
Known causes of Kounis syndrome

Drugs	Foods	Environmental Exposures
Analgesics (aspirin, dipyrone, tramadol)	Canned food	Bee stings
Anesthetics (etomidate, isoflurane, midazolam, propofol, remifentanil, rocuronium bromide, succinylcholine, suxamethonium, trimethaphan)	Fish	Black widow spider bite
Antibiotics (penicillins, cephalosporins, amikacin, cinoxacin, ciprofloxacin, clindamycin, lincomycin, metronidazole trimethoprim sulfamethoxazole, vancomycin)	Kiwi	Dialysate
Antifungals (fluconazole)	Mushrooms (Coprinopsis atramentaria)	Grass
Anticoagulants (heparin, lepirudin)	Shellfish	Hymenoptera stings
Antineoplastics (5-fluorouracil, capecitabine, carboplatin, denileukin, interferons, paclitaxel, vinca alkaloids)	Tomato	Jellyfish stings
Antivirals (brivudine, oseltamivir)	Vegetables	Latex
Contrast media (iohexol, ioxaglate, meglumine diatrizoate, sodium indigotindisulfonate)		Scorpion stings
Glucocorticoids (betamethasone, hydrocortisone)		
Nonsteroidal antiinflammatory drugs (alclofenac, diclofenac, naproxen)		Wasp stings
Proton pump inhibitors (lansoprazole)		
Skin disinfectants (chlorhexidine, povidone iodine)		
Thrombolytics (streptokinase, tissue plasminogen activator, urokinase)		
Others (allopurinol, bupropion, clopidogrel, dextran, enalapril, esmolol, fructose, gelofusine, insulin, iodine, iron, losartan, protamine, tetanus antitoxin, glafenine, mesalamine)		

Disease Presentation

Patients with KS will present with signs and symptoms of an acute coronary syndrome while simultaneously demonstrating evidence of an acute hypersensitivity reaction. Signs and symptoms can be waxing and waning. Cardiac symptoms may include chest pain, chest discomfort, palpitations, dyspnea, nausea, vomiting, lightheadedness, pallor, diaphoresis, and bradycardia.[14] The signs and symptoms of an allergic reaction may include skin rash, pruritus, hives, nausea, vomiting, wheezing, and angioedema. Both cardiac and allergic components can lead to hypotension, shock, and cardiac arrest. Abdelghany and colleagues found that in 80% of cases, the cardiac symptoms will occur within the first hour of trigger exposure.[13]

Risk Factors

Risk factors for KS include a history of a previous allergy, hypertension, smoking, diabetes, and hyperlipidemia. Twenty five percent of patients with KS will have a known history of allergy. KS can occur at any age, but it is most commonly seen in patients aged 40 to 70 years.[13]

Definitions

Kounis and Zavras described the "allergic angina syndrome" that progresses to allergic acute myocardial infarction due to histamine-mediated vasospasm of the coronary arteries when triggered by certain antigens.[3] It is defined as the "concurrence of acute coronary syndromes associated with mast cell and platelet activation in the setting of allergic or anaphylactic insults."[14] There are 3 known variants to KS based on the mechanism of coronary artery obstruction; however, they all have a common initial mechanism of an allergic response that induces mast cell–mediated inflammatory cascade that leads to compromise of the coronary circulation:[4,14]

- Type I: this is the most common variant of KS, occurring in 72.6% of cases.[14] This occurs in younger people without underlying native atherosclerotic artery disease who have ACS due to an allergic insult. The allergic reaction causes *coronary artery spasm* usually without an increase in troponin or other cardiac biomarkers. However, if this spasm results in myocardial infarction, troponin levels might be elevated. This variant is one of the causes of myocardial infarction with nonobstructive coronary arteries and represents microvascular angina or endothelial dysfunction.[15]
- Type II: occurs in 22.3% of cases. This variant occurs in those with preexisting atheromatous disease in whom the acute release of inflammatory mediators can cause coronary artery spasm, in addition to *plaque erosion or rupture*, thus presenting as acute myocardial infarction.[14]
- Type III: this is the least common variant, accounting for 5.1% of cases. This variant was further subdivided into *stent thrombosis* (subtype a) and *stent restenosis* (subtype b) that occur due to allergic inflammation.[16] Coronary stents that contain nickel have been implicated as a trigger of KS.[17] The aspirated thrombus, when stained with hematoxylin-eosin and Giemsa, demonstrates the presence of eosinophils and mast cells, respectively.[18] Furthermore, both subtypes have been diagnosed post mortem in patients with stent implantation who died suddenly. The histologic examination of the coronary intima, media, and adventitia adjacent to stent deployment showed infiltration of eosinophils and mast cells.[16]

Diagnosis

KS is not a rare disease, but it is likely underdiagnosed in the clinical setting and can be easily overlooked or missed. It is important to keep this entity in mind when evaluating patients who come in with chest pain or even myocardial infarction in the setting of symptoms of an allergic reaction. It is important to focus on the duration of time between exposure to the trigger and the onset of symptoms. Most of the patients will have an interval of less than 1 hour but almost 10% were reported more than 6 hours after exposure.[19]

The diagnosis of KS is made based on clinical signs and symptoms, history of previous allergies, and the results of laboratory tests, electrocardiogram (ECG), echocardiogram, angiogram, and MRI.

- Clinical signs and symptoms
  - Cardiac component: 86.6% of patients will present with chest pain; it is the most common presentation. Similar to ACS pain, it is described as crushing or constrictive, and it may radiate to the neck, jaw, or arms. It may also be associated with diaphoresis, pallor, nausea, vomiting, palpitations, and shortness of breath.
  - Allergic manifestations: ranges from mild and localized to widespread and life-threatening. Some common findings include hives, rash, mucous membrane involvement, edema of the face or tongue, wheezing, hypotension, and shock.
- History
  - 25% of patients have a known history of allergies or have experienced an allergic reaction in the past. It is imperative to obtain a medication history in the patient and review medication allergies, including allergy to iodinated contrast media.
- Laboratory tests
  - There is no laboratory test that will definitely diagnose KS; however, obtaining a complete blood count, particularly looking at eosinophils, cardiac biomarkers (CK, CK-MB) and troponin I or T, C-reactive protein (high sensitivity), total and specific immunoglobulin E (IgE), histamine, chymase, and serum tryptase levels can all aid in the diagnosis of KS in the right clinical setting. Note that histamine has a very short half-life of approximately 8 minutes; therefore, a low level does not exclude the diagnosis. Other laboratories that might be helpful include levels of arachidonic acid products (thromboxane, leukotrienes, prostaglandins), tumor necrosis factor, interferon, and interleukin-6.[13]
- ECG
  - ECG changes are usually transient and occur during an episode of pain. ST elevation myocardial infarction (usually involving the inferior leads) is the most common ECG change seen with KS.[19] There are no specific changes to distinguish KS from a nonallergic form of ACS. ST-T changes suggesting ischemia (ST segment depression and T wave inversion), sinus tachycardia or bradycardia, heart blocks, atrial fibrillation, ventricular fibrillation, ectopic beats, QRS and QT prolongation, and findings similar to digoxin toxicity have all been reported in KS.[14,19]
- Echocardiogram
  - In KS, echocardiogram studies might reveal regional wall motion abnormality in the distribution of the affected artery.[1,20] The subendocardial layer of the myocardium is affected in that coronary territory in contrast to acute myocarditis where heterogeneous and subepicardial involvement is detected.[21]

- Coronary artery angiogram may show coronary vasospasm or stenosis. The right coronary artery is the culprit lesion in more than half the cases.[13]
- Thallium-201 single-photon emission computed tomography (SPECT) and 125I-15-(p-iodophenyl)-3-(R,S) methyl pentadecanoic acid SPECT demonstrated severe myocardial ischemia in a 66-year-old who developed KS after local anesthetic infiltration for a dental procedure. The patient underwent coronary angiography, which demonstrated normal coronary arteries consistent with KS type I.[22]
- Cardiac MRI has demonstrated normal washout in the subendocardial lesion area with delayed contrast-enhanced images.[23]

Differential Diagnoses

- Obstructive coronary artery disease (CAD)
- Unstable angina
- Stress-induced cardiomyopathy (Takotsubo) is one of the major differential diagnoses to consider when diagnosing KS. Furthermore, those 2 entities can also coexist and present in the same patient.[24]
- Hypersensitivity myocarditis
- Acute pericarditis
- Prinzmetal angina
- Eosinophilic coronary periarteritis
- Coronary allograft vasculopathy
- Esophageal spasm

Management

Revascularization of the myocardium while simultaneously managing the allergic reaction is the mainstay of treatment of KS. When patients present with acute coronary syndrome, they should be managed according to the ACS guidelines.[12] Unfortunately, these guidelines lack in specific details regarding the management of ACS due to KS. Most data come from case reports or case series. What complicates matters further is some drugs administered to treat cardiac manifestations of KS can worsen the allergic component, and other drugs given for the allergic symptoms can aggravate the cardiac dysfunction.[16]

Treating the allergic reaction in the type I variant usually resolves the cardiac manifestation:

- Corticosteroids (hydrocortisone 1–2 mg/kg/d) suppress the arterial hyperreactivity and relieves inflammation.[25] Prevention of biphasic reactions has not been demonstrated.[26]
- H1 and H2 blockers (diphenhydramine 1–2 mg/kg and ranitidine 1 mg/kg) can also decrease the allergic manifestations.[27] These should be administered as a slow intravenous push because they may induce hypotension and worsen coronary perfusion.[16]
- Calcium channel blockers (CCB) and nitrates can help abolish the vasospasm induced by hypersensitivity and should be used if the blood pressure is satisfactory.[16,28] However, caution must be taken with nitroglycerin because it may cause hypotension and tachycardia and further complicate the allergic reaction.[1]
- Because epinephrine can worsen myocardial ischemia and induce coronary vasospasm and arrhythmias it should be used with caution in KS.[11] However, if the patient presents with anaphylaxis, the risks of untreated anaphylaxis outweighs the risk of possible worsening myocardial ischemia.[29]

In patients with type II variant of KS, the management is similar to that of ACS with additional treatment with antihistamines and steroids.[14] Vasodilators such as nitrates and CCBs may be used as necessary.[16] Beware that using β-blockers can exaggerate coronary vasospasm due to unopposed α-adrenergic receptors action. Epinephrine can aggravate ischemia and worsen coronary vasospasm. Using a sulfite-free epinephrine is preferable (dose of 0.2–0.5 mg of the 1:1000 concentration intramuscularly [IM]).[30] Epinephrine may be ineffective in patients already on β-blockers. In those patients administer glucagon 1 to 5 mg intravenously (IV) followed by infusion at 0.05 to 0.1 mg/kg/h if needed.

Treatment in type III variant KS should also follow the ACS guidelines. Per guidelines, when indicated, aspiration of the in-stent thrombus is of crucial importance in histologic analysis and staining of the thrombus for eosinophils and mast cells. These can suggest an allergic reaction, which can alter management.[14] In addition, if a patient develops an allergic reaction following coronary stent placement, steroids, antihistamines, and mast cell stabilizers (eg, sodium cromoglycate) can help relieve the allergic manifestations. Identifying the culprit cause via patch or skin test followed by desensitization might be indicated especially if these measures fail.[14] If allergy to nickel-titanium alloy is confirmed by patch test, with failed desensitization, removal of the implanted stent might be necessary.[31]

Management of Kounis Syndrome in the Emergency Department

Diagnosing KS in the ED is challenging. The allergic component of the presentation can easily be missed (eg, if a patient has underlying asthma and presents with wheezing and chest pain).

The following are steps that can you take to help manage a patient with suspected KS (**Fig. 1**):

- Ask about exposure to known allergens and when the exposure occurred. Most patients will present less than an hour postexposure.

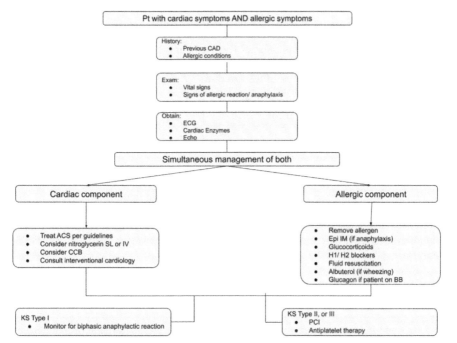

Fig. 1. Algorithm for management of patients suspected to have Kounis syndrome in the emergency department.

- Ask about prior similar presentations, especially if they were previously evaluated with coronary angiography studies or MRI.
- Ask about previously diagnosed CAD:
  - No history of CAD: this presentation can be KS type I or new ACS.
  - History of CAD: this can be KS type II, III, or ACS—all of these are managed according to ACS guidelines.
- On examination, look for signs of allergic reaction.
- Manage the cardiac and allergic components of KS simultaneously.
  - Nitroglycerine (if BP acceptable)
  - Calcium channel blockers
  - IM epinephrine if anaphylaxis is present
  - Glucocorticoids, H1 and H2 blockers
  - Consult interventional cardiology if cardiac ischemia is suspected by ECG, elevated troponin level, or based on clinical picture.

Drugs to Avoid

- Nonselective β-blockers can exacerbate vasospasm.
- Opioids (eg, morphine, codeine and meperidine) may induce massive mast cell degranulation and aggravate allergic reaction.[1] Fentanyl and its derivatives are weak mast cell triggers and therefore are preferable.[1]
- Acetaminophen (especially IV) has been associated with the development of severe hypotension due to a reduction in cardiac output.[32]
- High-dose aspirin because it inhibits prostacyclin production.
- Oral sumatriptan can cause coronary vasospasm and myocardial infarction.
- 5-Fluorouracil has been reported to induce coronary artery spasm.

Prognosis

With appropriate treatment, KS generally has a good prognosis with complete recovery in most patients. Type I variant of KS is the most prevalent and most common of all variants. In this type, early identification and hence treatment is possible because of early appearance of allergic manifestations. The resultant coronary vasospasm can be reversed with vasodilators, and based on previous reports it also has good prognosis.[33]

Overall, serious complications of KS are rare:

- Cardiogenic shock occurs in 2.3%.
- Cardiac arrest occurs in 6.3%.
- Mortality is 2.9%.

SUMMARY

ACS in the setting of an allergic/immunologic reaction is known as KS. It is an underdiagnosed and underrecognized disease entity. One must keep a high index of suspicions when managing a patient presenting with cardiac as well as allergic symptoms. There are 3 main variants to the syndrome. Treating the allergic reaction may alleviate the pain; however, ACS guidelines should be followed if cardiac ischemia is present.

CLINICS CARE POINTS

- Keep a high index of suspicion for the possibility of KS when treating patients with chest pain or ACS-like picture.

- When treating patients with anaphylaxis, obtain ECG and troponins to rule out KS.
- Treat the allergic as well as the cardiac components simultaneously.
- Epinephrine, although a life-saving necessity for anaphylaxis treatment, may worsen cardiac ischemia. The risk of untreated (true) anaphylaxis usually outweighs the risk of worsening ischemia.
- Avoid β-blockers, as they can worsen vasospasm.

DISCLOSURE

There are no commercial or financial conflicts of interest.

REFERENCES

1. Kounis NG. Coronary hypersensitivity disorder: the kounis syndrome. Clin Ther 2013;35(5):563–71.
2. Pfister CW, Plice SG. Acute myocardial infarction during a prolonged allergic reaction to penicillin. Am Heart J 1950;40(6):945–7.
3. Kounis NG, Zavras GM. Histamine-induced coronary artery spasm: the concept of allergic angina. Br J Clin Pract 1991;45(2):121–8.
4. Ferreira RM, Villela PB, Almeida JCG, et al. Allergic recurrent coronary stent thrombosis: A mini-review of Kounis syndrome. Cardiovasc Revasc Med 2018; 19(7 pt B):890–5.
5. Lanza GA, Careri G, Crea F. Mechanisms of coronary artery spasm. Circulation 2011;124(16):1774–82.
6. Gilfillan AM, Tkaczyk C. Integrated signalling pathways for mast-cell activation. Nat Rev Immunol 2006;6(3):218–30.
7. Moon TC, Dean Befus A, Kulka M. Mast cell mediators: Their differential release and the secretory pathways involved. Front Immunol 2014;5(NOV):1–18.
8. Brown SGA. Cardiovascular aspects of anaphylaxis: implications for treatment and diagnosis. Curr Opin Allergy Clin Immunol 2005;5(4):359–64.
9. Jeziorska M, McCollum C, Woolley DE. Mast cell distribution, activation, and phenotype in atherosclerotic lesions of human carotid arteries. J Pathol 1997; 182(1):115–22.
10. Marone G, de Crescenzo G, Adt M, et al. Immunological characterization and functional importance of human heart mast cells. Immunopharmacology 1995; 31(1):1–18.
11. Fassio F, Losappio L, Antolin-Amerigo D, et al. Kounis syndrome: A concise review with focus on management. Eur J Intern Med 2016;30:7–10.
12. Fassio F, Almerigogna F. Kounis syndrome (allergic acute coronary syndrome): different views in allergologic and cardiologic literature. Intern Emerg Med 2012;7(6):489–95.
13. Abdelghany M, Subedi R, Shah S, et al. Kounis syndrome: A review article on epidemiology, diagnostic findings, management and complications of allergic acute coronary syndrome. Int J Cardiol 2017;232:1–4.
14. Kounis NG. Kounis syndrome: an update on epidemiology, pathogenesis, diagnosis and therapeutic management. Clin Chem Lab Med 2016;54(10):1545–59.
15. Kounis NG, Koniari I, Soufras GD, et al. The humble relation of Kounis Syndrome, MINOCA (Myocardial Infarction With Nonobstructive Coronary Arteries) and MACE (Major Adverse Cardiac Events). Can J Cardiol 2018;34(8):1089, e7.

16. Kounis NG, Koniari I, Velissaris D, et al. Kounis Syndrome-not a Single-organ Arterial Disorder but a Multisystem and Multidisciplinary Disease. Balk Med J 2019;36(4):212–21.

17. Köster R, Vieluf D, Kiehn M, et al. Nickel and molybdenum contact allergies in patients with coronary in-stent restenosis. Lancet 2000;356:1895–7.

18. Gangadharan V, Bhatheja S, Al Balbissi K. Kounis syndrome - an atopic monster for the heart. Cardiovasc Diagn Ther 2013;3(1):47–51.

19. Giovannini M, Koniari I, Mori F, et al. Kounis syndrome: a clinical entity penetrating from pediatrics to geriatrics. J Geriatr Cardiol 2020;17(5):294–9.

20. Biteker M, Duran NE, Biteker FS, et al. Kounis syndrome secondary to amoxicillin/clavulanic acid use in a child. Int J Cardiol 2009;136(1):e3–5.

21. Almpanis GC, Mazarakis A, Dimopoulos DA, et al. The conundrum of hypersensitivity cardiac disease: hypersensitivity myocarditis, acute hypersensitivity coronary syndrome (Kounis syndrome) or both? Int J Cardiol 2011;148:237–40.

22. Goto K, Kasama S, Sato M, et al. Myocardial scintigraphic evidence of Kounis syndrome: what is the aetiology of acute coronary syndrome? Eur Heart J 2016;37(14):1157.

23. Okur A, Kantarci M, Karaca L, et al. The utility of cardiac magnetic resonance imaging in Kounis syndrome. Postep Kardiol Inter 2015;11(3):218–23.

24. Yanagawa Y, Nishi K, Tomiharu N, et al. A case of takotsubo cardiomyopathy associated with Kounis syndrome. Int J Cardiol 2009;123(2):e65–7.

25. Takagi S, Goto Y, Hirose E, et al. Successful treatment of refractory vasospastic angina with corticosteroids: coronary arterial hyperactivity caused by local inflammation? Circ J 2004;68(1):17–22.

26. Alqurashi W, Ellis AK. Do Corticosteroids Prevent Biphasic Anaphylaxis? J Allergy Clin Immunol Pract 2017;5(5):1194–205.

27. Ioannidis TI, Mazarakis A, Notaras SP, et al. Hymenoptera sting-induced Kounis syndrome: effects of aspirin and beta-blocker administration. Int J Cardiol 2007; 121(1):105–8.

28. Terlemez S, Eryilmaz U, Tokgoz Y, et al. Kounis syndrome caused by metronidazole–a case of 14 year-old boy. Int J Cardiol 2015;179:222–4.

29. Singer E, Zodda D. Allergy And Anaphylaxis: Principles Of Acute Emergency Management. Emerg Med Pr 2015;17(8):1–19, quiz: 20]. Available at: https://pubmed.ncbi.nlm.nih.gov/26237051/.

30. Kounis NG, Mazarakis A, Almpanis G, et al. The more allergens an atopic patient is exposed to, the easier and quicker anaphylactic shock and Kounis syndrome appear: Clinical and therapeutic paradoxes. J Nat Sci Biol Med 2014;5(2):240–4.

31. Dasika UK, Kanter KR, Vincent R. Nickel allergy to the percutaneous patent foramen ovale occluder and subsequent systemic nickel allergy. J Thorac Cardiovasc Surg 2003;126(6):2112.

32. Cantais A, Schnell D, Vincent F, et al. Acetaminophen-induced changes in systemic blood pressure in critically ill patients. Crit Care Med 2016;44(12):2192–8.

33. Bory M, Pierron F, Panagides D. Coronary artery spasm in patients with normal or near normal coronary arteries. Long-term follow-up of 277 patients. Eur Heart J 1996;17(7):1015–21.

Angiotensin-Converting Enzyme Inhibitor–Induced Angioedema

R. Gentry Wilkerson, MD*, Michael E. Winters, MD, MBA

KEYWORDS

- ACE inhibitor–induced angioedema • C1-inhibitor • Bradykinin • Quincke disease
- Difficult airway

KEY POINTS

- Inhibition of ACE prevents the conversion of angiotensin I to angiotensin II but it also inhibits the other function of ACE, which is the metabolism of bradykinin.
- There are no laboratory biomarkers that confirm the diagnosis of ACEi-induced angioedema, but some laboratories may be useful when considering other diagnoses such as infections and allergic reactions.
- Use of fiberoptic nasopharyngoscopy allows for visualization of deeper airway structures to determine extent of the swelling and the need to secure the airway.
- No medication has sufficient evidence from clinical trials to support its use in cases of ACEi-induced angioedema.
- Clinical findings associated with need for definitive airway management include voice change, hoarseness, stridor, and dyspnea.

INTRODUCTION

Angioedema is a well-recognized and potentially lethal complication of angiotensin-converting enzyme inhibitor (ACEi) therapy. Similar to cases of hereditary angioedema (HAE), ACEi-induced angioedema occurs as a result of the accumulation of the vasoactive peptide bradykinin. In most cases of HAE there is increased production of bradykinin due to decreased amount or function of C1-esterase inhibitor (C1-INH), which normally inhibits bradykinin formation through the inhibition of multiple steps of the complement, fibrinolytic, and contact activating systems. However, in ACEi-induced

This article originally appeared in Emergency Medicine Clinics, Volume 40 Issue 1, February 2022.

Department of Emergency Medicine, University of Maryland School of Medicine, 110 South Paca Street, 6th Floor, Suite 200, Baltimore, MD 21201, USA

* Corresponding author.

E-mail address: gwilkerson@som.umaryland.edu

Twitter: @gentrywmd (R.G.W.); @critcareguys (M.E.W.)

Immunol Allergy Clin N Am 43 (2023) 513–532
https://doi.org/10.1016/j.iac.2022.10.013

angioedema, bradykinin accumulates due to a decrease in its metabolism by ACE, the enzyme that is primarily responsible for this function. The action of bradykinin at bradykinin type 2 receptors (B2R) leads to increased vascular permeability and the accumulation of fluid in the subcutaneous and submucosal space. Patients with ACEi-induced angioedema are at risk for airway compromise because of the tendency for the face, lips, tongue, and airway structures to be affected. To date, there have been no medications proved to treat ACEi-induced angioedema. The emergency physician should focus on airway evaluation and management when treating patients with ACEi-induced angioedema.

BACKGROUND

ACEi medications were developed after it was noted that people bitten by the Brazilian pit viper *Bothrops jararaca* developed profound hypotension and frequently died from shock. Peptides in the pit viper venom were identified as Bradykinin Potentiating Factors (BPFs).[1] When studied further, these BPFs were determined to inhibit ACE, the enzyme responsible for the conversion of angiotensin I to angiotensin II.[2] At the time BPFs were discovered, ACE was thought to play a minor role in hypertension. Further research clarified the role that the renin-angiotensin-aldosterone system has in blood pressure and led to the development of captopril, the first oral ACEi approved to treat hypertension.[3,4]

The first reports of angioedema associated with ACEi occurred in 1980, just months before captopril being approved by the US Food and Drug Administration (FDA). In the first report of ACEi-induced angioedema, Wilkin and colleagues described 7 new cases of cutaneous reactions due to captopril therapy. In 2 of these cases, the reactions were described as "angioedematous." The investigators recognized that the reactions were likely due to the potentiation of kinins.[5] Angioedema is now a well-recognized complication of ACEi therapy, but despite this the FDA has not required a boxed warning to be added to the label for this class of medications.

EPIDEMIOLOGY

In the United States, there are more than 100,000 annual emergency department (ED) visits for angioedema.[6] ACEi-induced angioedema accounts for 30% to 50% of all cases of angioedema seen in the ED.[7,8] The incidence of ACEi-induced angioedema has been reported to be between 0.1% and 0.7% of patients taking an ACEi.[9,10] Despite the relatively low overall incidence, ACEi-induced angioedema is a fairly common presentation in the ED because of how frequently ACEi medications are prescribed to treat hypertension. Among patients prescribed a medication for hypertension, 28.5% were prescribed an ACEi, making it the most frequently prescribed class of antihypertensives.[11] In the United States, lisinopril is the most frequently prescribed ACEi and the second most frequently prescribed medication overall, with more than 100 million prescriptions written in 2015.[12] Black patients taking an ACEi have a much higher risk of developing angioedema (5%) than do white patients (0.7%).[13] The data are inconsistent regarding sex as a risk factor. Some studies have found no statistical difference in the incidence between men and women.[2] Other studies have found a slightly higher incidence among women taking an ACEi.[14–16] A history of smoking is associated with an increased risk of developing ACEi-induced angioedema.[15,17] Patients with ACEi-induced angioedema tend to be older, likely reflective of the increased incidence of hypertension with age. In a single-center retrospective case series involving 88 patients with ACEi-induced angioedema, the average age of diagnosis was 59.3 years, with a range of 33 to 89 years.[18]

Another common side effect of ACEi use is development of a persistent dry cough. This side effect has been reported to occur in 5% to 35% of patients taking an ACEi. The mechanism for development of cough is not clear but is thought to be similar to the mechanism for ACEi-induced angioedema—accumulation of bradykinin and substance P due to inhibition of the ACE enzyme.[19] It is also uncertain why some patients will develop cough, whereas others go on to develop angioedema. One study found that women had a 3-fold higher risk of developing ACEi-induced cough compared with men.[20] Other demographic factors associated with ACEi-induced cough include age greater than 60 years and being of East Asian descent.[15] The only effective treatment is discontinuation of the ACEi.

PATHOPHYSIOLOGY

Development of angioedema is a potential class effect of ACEi medications. Inhibition of ACE, which is also known as kininase II, interferes with the conversion of angiotensin I to angiotensin II. This is the mechanism by which ACEi medications exert their desirable blood pressure–lowering effects. ACE is also the enzyme that is primarily responsible for the degradation of bradykinin. Bradykinin is a nonapeptide that acts as a potent vasodilator and increases capillary wall permeability. In humans, bradykinin is formed through plasma kallikrein–mediated cleavage of high-molecular-weight kininogen (HMWK) or through the conversion of kallidin (lys-bradykinin) by the enzyme aminopeptidase. Kallidin is created by tissue kallikrein-mediated cleavage of low-molecular-weight kininogen (LMWK).[21] The half-life of bradykinin in normal human plasma is very short (~34 seconds). In the presence of ACEi medications the plasma half-life duration is increased 5- to 12-fold leading to higher overall plasma concentration of bradykinin.[22]

Bradykinin is normally metabolized by the action of several enzymes that are collectively known as kininases. The cleavage sites and resultant metabolites differ for each kininase (**Fig. 1**). ACE is the primary enzyme responsible for the breakdown of bradykinin. Other major enzymes involved in bradykinin metabolism include aminopeptidase P (APP) and dipeptidyl peptidase IV (DPP-IV). Kininase I, a collective term for different carboxypeptidases, metabolizes bradykinin into des-Arg^9-bradykinin. Under normal conditions this is a minor pathway, but when ACE is inhibited, carboxypeptidase-mediated metabolism becomes a major metabolic pathway. Des-Arg^9-bradykinin is further degraded by APP into inactive metabolites.[23] Various genetic polymorphisms of the enzymes capable of metabolizing bradykinin have been

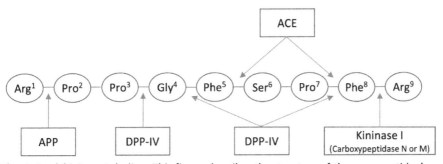

Fig. 1. Bradykinin metabolism. This figure describes the structure of the nonapeptide, bradykinin, and the sites of cleavage by the various enzymes involved in bradykinin degradation.

described with varying degrees of association with the risk of developing ACEi-induced angioedema.[12] During episodes of ACEi-induced angioedema, the levels of plasma bradykinin have been shown to be elevated, whereas the levels of its precursor HMWK are not.[24] In addition, the ratio of bradykinin to its degradation products is elevated,[25] and this suggests that impaired degradation of bradykinin rather than increased production is associated with the development of ACEi-induced angioedema.

The 2 members of the bradykinin receptor family are G protein–coupled receptors. The bradykinin type 1 receptor (B1R) is normally not present in tissue but can be rapidly induced during periods of inflammation.[26] Bradykinin has no specific affinity for B1R, whereas the metabolite lys-des-Arg^9-bradykinin is the most potent agonist.[27] B2R is expressed throughout the human body, and activation through the binding of its ligand, bradykinin, leads to vasodilatation and increased capillary leakage into surrounding tissue.

Substance P is another vasoactive peptide consisting of 11 amino acids that has been hypothesized to be involved in the development of ACEi-induced angioedema. Substance P exerts its activity through association with the high-affinity neurokinin 1 receptor, resulting in increased vascular permeability. Substance P is also degraded by ACE but during ACE inhibition it is metabolized primarily by DPP-IV.[28] Contribution of substance P in addition to bradykinin for the development of ACEi-induced angioedema is supported by the fact that patients taking a DPP-IV inhibitor for glycemic control in type 2 diabetes mellitus are at increased risk of developing ACEi-induced angioedema.[29,30]

In contrast to the pathophysiology of ACEi-induced angioedema, nonsteroidal anti-inflammatory drug (NSAID)-induced angioedema can be due to a type 1 hypersensitivity reaction, leading to release of preformed mediators such as histamine from mast cells and basophils. Alternatively, NSAID-induced angioedema may also be the result of inhibition of cyclooxygenase-1 enzymes, which causes a shift of arachidonic acid metabolism from the COX pathway to the leukotriene pathway, and this results in accumulation of cysteinyl leukotrienes, potent proinflammatory mediators.[31]

CLINICAL PRESENTATION

Angioedema is characterized by asymmetric, nonpitting swelling of the subcutaneous layer of the skin and submucosal tissue of the respiratory and gastrointestinal tracts.[32] Urticaria with accompanying pruritus is not typically present in ACEi-induced angioedema because the primary mediator is bradykinin rather than histamine. The presence of urticaria and pruritus with angioedema suggests a different cause and pathophysiology.

The head and neck are the predominant areas affected in ACEi-induced angioedema with involvement of the tongue, lips, face, and laryngeal structures. Chan and Soliman performed a retrospective analysis of cases of ACEi-induced angioedema that presented to a single, urban, academic hospital in the United States. The most common site affected was the lips (60.2%), followed by tongue (39.7%), larynx (29.5%), soft palate and uvula (17.0%), face (12.5%), and floor of mouth (6.8%). Less than half the patients included in this study had fiberoptic nasopharyngoscopy performed, which may have led to underreporting of laryngeal involvement.[18] A report by Javaud and colleagues included cases of ACEi-induced angioedema seen at 4 French hospitals. The larynx was involved in 15 of 62 cases (24%).[33]

Visceral angioedema leading to abdominal pain, diarrhea, and occasionally obstruction is less frequently described although it is likely underreported due to the diagnosis not being considered;[34,35] this is in contrast to HAE, where abdominal pain due to swelling of the intestinal tract is a prominent feature—in fact the most common presenting complaint.[36] The severity of symptoms when the intestines are involved can be such that it mimics an acute abdomen leading to unnecessary surgical intervention.[37,38]

The interval between the initiation of therapy with an ACEi and the development is variable. Some reports have suggested that most cases of ACEi-induced angioedema occur within the first weeks to months of therapy.[39,40] A retrospective, single-center study based in Romania found that only 10% of included patients developed angioedema during the first year of treatment.[41] In a study by Banerji and colleagues, there were 888 cases of angioedema that developed in the first 5 years of therapy with an ACEi. Ten percent of the cases developed in the first month and 35% in the first year. During each of the subsequent 4 years, an additional 15% to 17% of the cases occurred.[10] In a study by Sandefur and colleagues, angioedema developed after more than 1 year of ACEi therapy in 74% of patients. Only 6% of this study's population were Black, which may limit the generalizability of the findings.[42] ACEi-induced angioedema has been reported as late as 23 years after the initiation of treatment.[43]

DIAGNOSTIC EVALUATION
Laboratory Testing

There are no laboratory biomarkers that confirm the diagnosis of ACEi-induced angioedema. The diagnosis is made based on the presence of angioedema in the setting of ACEi treatment regardless of timing of initiation and the absence of signs and symptoms associated with histaminergic causes (eg, urticarial, pruritus, lack of history of HAE or acquired C1-INH deficiency). The complement component 4 (C4) level is a cost-effective screening test for HAE.[44] The ideal time to screen for HAE and acquired angioedema (AAE) is during an acute attack. During periods between HAE attacks, the sensitivity of C4 for diagnosis is decreased to 81% to 96%.[45–47] Quantitative and functional measurements of C1-INH antigen can be reserved for follow-up evaluation in patients who have a positive screen with C4. These are used to confirm or exclude the diagnosis of HAE and to differentiate HAE-C1-INH type 1 from type 2. Quantitative and functional levels are less than 50% of normal in HAE-C1-INH type 1, whereas in type 2 the quantitative levels are normal but the function is decreased. Diagnosis of HAE with normal levels of C1-INH (HAE-nl-C1-INH) requires special genetic testing. Most cases of HAE-nl-C1-INH are due to mutations in the genes for plasminogen, high- and low-molecular-weight kininogen, or angiopoietin-1.[48] Patients who develop an acquired deficiency of C1-INH (AAE) will have decreased levels of C4 as well as decreased quantitative and functional C1-INH levels.[49] Testing for CH50, which measures overall complement activity, and for complement component 3 (C3) is not helpful to aid with the diagnosis of HAE.[50] In ACEi-induced angioedema, C4 levels and C1-INH studies will be normal.

Additional laboratory testing should be obtained to evaluate for other conditions that are being considered as causes for the patient's presentation. Although the result may not be available during a patient's stay in the ED, a tryptase level can be used for the evaluation of anaphylaxis or other mast cell disorders. A C-reactive protein (CRP) level may be sent to evaluate for infection (eg, lip abscess). However, one study of 25 patients with ACEi-induced angioedema demonstrated a greater than 7-fold increase in CRP. An elevation in white blood cell counts was not seen in this study.[51] Importantly, marked leukocytosis has been reported in cases of

ACEi-induced angioedema, especially those with abdominal symptoms as opposed to head and neck swelling.[52,53]

Radiographic Testing

Imaging studies are often obtained to evaluate for alternative diagnoses and causes of the patient's symptoms. Imaging can help establish angioedema as the cause of a patient's presenting complaint, but it cannot distinguish between the different causes of angioedema. Soft tissue neck radiographs and computed tomography (CT) of the neck may be obtained to evaluate for angioedema mimics, such as infections and malignancies. For patients with abdominal symptoms, a contrast-enhanced CT of the abdomen and pelvis is the study of choice. Findings may include thickening of the small bowel wall with submucosal and subserosal enhancement without adjacent fat stranding. This pattern seen on cross-sectional view has been called the "halo" sign, which is also seen in nonocclusive mesenteric ischemia.[54] In one retrospective case series of 20 patients, the mean diameter of the small bowel wall was 1.3 cm.[55] Normally, the small bowel wall thickness is 1 to 2 mm when the lumen is distended and 3 to 4 mm when the lumen is collapsed.[56] Fluid extravasation into the areas adjacent to swollen segments of intestine due to angioedema leads to the development of ascites, which is frequently found on CT imaging.[38] Abdominal ultrasound can also demonstrate bowel wall thickening and the presence of ascites.[57] Ultrasound can be repeated to assess for response to treatment, thereby avoiding repeated exposure to radiation.[58] Point-of-care ultrasound in the ED has been used to identify upper airway edema.[59] Further research is needed to determine if this noninvasive approach provides adequate sensitivity and specificity to be used in the place of direct visualization.

Fiberoptic Nasopharyngoscopy

Direct visualization can identify patients who have angioedema of the tongue, soft palate, or floor of the mouth and are at risk for involvement of deeper airway structures that increase the risk of asphyxiation due to airway obstruction. Fiberoptic nasopharyngoscopy to identify the presence of swelling of the deeper upper airway structures is recommended in consensus guidelines endorsed by the American College of Allergy, Asthma and Immunology and the Society for Academic Emergency Medicine.[60] A clinical practice guideline endorsed by the American Academy of Emergency Medicine (AAEM) also recommends the use of nasopharygoscopy to evaluate patients with angioedema who have signs or symptoms of upper airway involvement including odynophagia, dyspnea, dysphonia, hoarseness, or dysphagia.[61] In patients with angioedema due to any underlying cause, minor trauma, including nasopharyngoscopy, can result in increased swelling. The patient and treatment area should be fully prepped to perform an intubation before performing any evaluation of the deeper upper airway structures. If possible, an endotracheal tube should be preloaded on the nasopharyngoscope and airway medications made available so that the tube can be passed if severe swelling is noted or the patient develops distress.[60] Visualization of laryngeal structures seen on nasopharyngoscopic examination is used to categorize a patient according the Ishoo staging system (see Section VIII. Airway Management).[62]

PHARMACOLOGIC TREATMENT

Since 2008, multiple medications have been developed and approved by the FDA for the treatment of HAE. Unfortunately, no medication has sufficient evidence from clinical trials to support its use in cases of ACEi-induced angioedema.[63] When there remains clinical concern that the underlying cause of angioedema may be due to an allergic or immunologic process, the patient should be treated with medications targeting this process. In cases of anaphylaxis, epinephrine is the first-line medication and should be given as an intramuscular injection in the anterolateral thigh for best absorption.[64–66] Additional information on the emergency management of allergic reactions and anaphylaxis can be found in the accompanying article in this issue: Anaphylaxis: Emergency Department Treatment. The treatment of HAE is based on interrupting the action of bradykinin at the B2 receptor expressed in subcutaneous and submucosal tissue—either through direct antagonism of the receptor or through limiting the production of bradykinin.

Fresh Frozen Plasma

Fresh frozen plasma (FFP) is produced by the separation of plasma from whole blood, which is then frozen at -30°C. FFP contains C1-INH and has been used as a treatment of patients with C1-INH deficiency since Pickering and colleagues first described its use for 2 patients in 1969.[67] FFP also contains components used to generate additional bradykinin such as HMWK, prekallikrein, and FXII as well as ACE, which would metabolize the bradykinin that has accumulated. The clinical outcome that results from the balance of additional inhibition by C1-INH, metabolism by ACE, and the possibility of increased production of bradykinin has never been assessed in a controlled clinical trial. Despite decades of use in HAE, data regarding its efficacy are limited to fewer than several hundred cases.[68–71] The theoretic concern that FFP could worsen swelling has not been established in these reports. Winnewisser and colleagues reported successful treatment of 30 patients with HAE in 1997.[67] In a 2007 retrospective report by Prematta and colleagues, 11 patients with HAE were given FFP to treat acute symptoms. Two patients in that case series had worsening abdominal pain during or shortly after the start of treatment; this was thought to be due to progression of illness rather than the FFP.[69] The US HAEA Medical Advisory Board 2020 Guidelines suggest that FFP can be considered for treatment of acute attacks of HAE in the absence of other approved therapeutics "as long as precautions are taken to protect the patient's airway."[72]

FFP has been used in cases of ACEi-induced angioedema owing to the presence of ACE in this treatment. As with HAE, no prospective clinical trial has been performed to determine effectiveness and safety. A retrospective analysis performed by Saeb and colleagues included 128 patients with non-HAE angioedema, 86% of whom were taking an ACEi. Of these 128 patients, 20 (15.6%) received FFP. In comparison to patients who did not receive FFP, those who did receive had shorter duration of intensive care unit (ICU) stay (3.5 days vs 1.5 days; $P < .001$). The rate of intubation for the FFP group was 35% compared with 60% for the no-FFP group ($P = .05$). The degree of swelling was not reported for the 2 groups, so it is unlikely that the groups were balanced making this comparison of questionable value.[73] There has also been one case report of the successful use of 4-factor prothrombin complex concentrate for a patient on an ACEi as well as a DPP-IV inhibitor.[74] There are reports of ACEi-induced angioedema that is refractory to FFP treatment[75] and one report of worsening symptoms after FFP administration.[76] Chen and colleagues demonstrated that there can be as much as a 20-fold difference in ACE activity between different donors. They suggest that this variation may account for why FFP may have varying degrees of effectiveness.[77] FFP for ACEi-induced angioedema continues to be controversial.[78,79] The AAEM Clinical Practice Guideline states that there is insufficient evidence to support its use.[63]

C1-Esterase Inhibitor Concentrate

Donaldson and Evans first identified that cases of HAE were due to deficiency of C1-INH in 1963.[80] A decade later the first case of administration of a partially purified concentrate was published.[81] Three groups independently worked to purify concentrates of C1-INH from plasma: the American Red Cross, the Dutch Red Cross, and the Behring Company in Germany. Bork and Witzke working for the Behring Company were the first to publish successful use of C1-INH concentrate.[82] The following year, Gadek and colleagues working with the American Red Cross and Agostoni and colleagues collaborating with the Dutch Red Cross independently published reports of successful purification and administration of C1-INH concentrate in patients with acute exacerbations of HAE.[83,84] The American effort was abandoned in the 1980s when the American Red Cross turned its attention to the issue of transfusion-related HIV transmission.[85] The remaining preparations were available but not to the United States; this continued until 2009, when the FDA gave approval to the CSL Behring plasma-derived C1-INH product Berinert (CSL Behring, Marburg, Germany) based on the success of the IMPACT studies that demonstrated its effectiveness in treating acute attacks of HAE.[86,87] Another preparation, Cinryze (Takeda, Lexington, MA, USA), is now approved for use as prophylaxis for HAE. A recombinant form of C1-INH produced in the milk of transgenic rabbits, rhC1-INH, was approved by the FDA in 2014 for the treatment of adults and adolescents with acute HAE attacks excluding laryngeal involvement. Recombinant C1-INH has the same amino acid structure as naturally produced C1-INH but is more highly glycosylated, leading to much faster clearance from the plasma.[88]

C1-INH concentrates have been used in ACEi-induced angioedema. In 2017, Riha and colleagues published a review in which they found 8 publications detailing C1-INH concentrate treatment in 27 patients with ACEi-induced angioedema. Since that publication, Perza and colleagues published a case series of an additional 7 patients who had a range of responses but led the investigators to conclude that C1-INH should not be routinely used for ACEi-induced angioedema.[89] Kovaltchouk and colleagues, published a series of 9 patients in 2021 who were treated with C1-INH concentrate after developing ACEi-induced angioedema. Seven of the 9 patients were intubated before receiving the C1-INH, limiting the potential benefit of this treatment.[90] A randomized, blinded, phase III study of Berinert for the treatment of ACEi-induced angioedema (NCT01843530) completed enrollment in 2019 but the results have not been published.[91] Use of C1-INH concentrate is not currently recommended for ACEi-induced angioedema.[63]

Inhibition of Kallikrein

As noted, plasma kallikrein is the enzyme responsible for the release of bradykinin from HMWK, and tissue kallikrein mediates the release of kallidin from LMWK, which is then converted to bradykinin by APP. Ecallantide is a novel recombinant 60-amino acid protein expressed in the yeast *Pichia pastoris*, which is a potent, specific, and reversible inhibitor of plasma kallikrein that leads to decreased levels of plasma bradykinin. The degree of inhibition is similar to that provided by C1-INH, but the inhibition by C1-INH is not reversible, as it forms covalent bonds with the enzymes it inhibits.[92] Ecallantide, administered as a 30 mg dose given subcutaneously, demonstrated improved time to symptom resolution in 2 randomized, double-blind, placebo-controlled trials.[93,94] Based on the results of these studies the FDA approved ecallantide for the treatment of acute attacks of HAE in patients 12 years of age and older. The risk of anaphylaxis after the administration was 3% to 4% in the early studies, so the FDA applied a black box warning that ecallantide could only be administered by a health care professional equipped to treat anaphylaxis.[95,96]

Bernstein and colleagues performed a randomized, triple-blind, controlled phase 2 trial with rescue crossover design to estimate the degree of efficacy and monitor for safety of use of ecallantide for the treatment of ACEi-induced angioedema. More than half of the subjects enrolled in this study were Ishoo stage I in which the swelling is isolated to the face or lips. Improvement to meeting discharge criteria within 4 hours, the primary outcome of interest, was achieved in 31% of subjects randomized to the ecallantide and 21% randomized to placebo.[97] The results of this study were used to design a second multicenter, randomized, controlled trial of ecallantide at doses of 10 mg, 30 mg, and 60 mg as compared with placebo. The primary outcome of interest was the proportion of patients meeting discharge criteria within 6 hours. An unplanned interim analysis revealed that the study was underpowered to detect a difference in the primary outcome due to a higher-than-expected rate of subjects in the placebo arm meeting the primary endpoint and the study was halted early. Data collected before study termination were analyzed and found that 88% of subjects in the ecallantide group met discharge criteria by 6 hours as compared with 72% in the placebo group (difference vs placebo 16%; 95% confidence interval [CI]: 11%–41%). As with the first study, this trial enrolled very few patients with severe angioedema. Only 7.9% of the subjects had Ishoo stage IV edema where laryngeal structures are involved, whereas 44.8% had Ishoo stage I edema.[98] Based on the failure of these 2 trials to demonstrate effectiveness, ecallantide is not recommended for the treatment of ACEi-induced angioedema.[63]

Antagonism of the Bradykinin B2 Receptor

The selective, competitive B2R inhibitor, icatibant, is a synthetic decapeptide with a similar structure to bradykinin but containing 5 nonproteinogenic amino acids. Icatibant is resistant to metabolism by ACE and carboxypeptidase, enzymes that normally degrade bradykinin.[99] It has a similar affinity to the B2R as bradykinin does. After subcutaneous absorption, icatibant has approximately 97% bioavailability and reaches maximum concentration within 30 minutes.[100]Efficacy of icatibant for the treatment of acute attacks of HAE was demonstrated in 3 randomized, multicenter, double-blind clinical trials—For Angioedema Subcutaneous Treatment (FAST) 1 through 3.[101,102] The FDA granted approval of icatibant for the treatment of acute attacks of HAE in adult patients in 2011. It is supplied at a concentration of 10 mg/mL, and a single dose is given as a subcutaneous injection of 30 mg. Repeat dosing can occur after 6 hours when there is inadequate response. No more than 3 doses should be given in a 24-hour period. In early clinical trials, greater than 97% of patients receiving icatibant had an injection site reaction. This reaction was shown in a population of healthy volunteers to be mediated by release of the preformed mast cell mediators, histamine, and tryptase. The severity of reaction could be attenuated by prophylactic administration of an H_1-receptor antagonist such as cetirizine.[103] The patent on icatibant expired in 2019, and multiple generic versions are now available.

The understanding that ACEi-induced angioedema was caused by excess bradykinin that resulted from inhibition of the ACE enzyme was supported by reports that administration of icatibant led to improvement of symptoms[104,105]; this was further supported by the AMACE study, a multicenter, double-blind, randomized, phase 2 study performed at 4 sites in Germany comparing icatibant with standard treatment consisting of prednisolone and a first-generation antihistamine, clemastine. This study included 27 subjects for analysis and demonstrated a shorter time to complete resolution of edema for subjects who were randomized to receive icatibant as compared with those who only received standard treatment (8.0 vs 27.1 hours; $P = .002$). A shorter time to onset of symptom relief was also noted in the icatibant group (2.0 vs 11.7 hours; $P = .03$).[106] A phase 3 double-blind, placebo-controlled study was performed comparing icatibant to placebo. The study enrolled 33 subjects, 32 of whom were enrolled at the primary study site and treated at a Clinical Research Center rather than in the ED. The study failed to demonstrate a statistically significant difference between the 2 groups regarding the primary efficacy outcome of mean time to resolution for icatibant-treated subjects 35.3 ± 5.25 hours versus 27.2 ± 4.8 hours for placebo (N. Brown, personal communication August 31, 2021).[107] The CAMEO study, a multinational, multicenter, randomized, double-blind, placebo-controlled phase 3 clinical trial, was subsequently performed. This study included 121 subjects in the intention-to-treat analysis and found no difference between the groups for the primary efficacy endpoint of median time to meeting discharge criteria (4.0 hours vs 4.0 hours; P = .63). In addition, there were no differences in any of the secondary endpoints of interest.[108] Possible reasons why the subsequent phase 3 studies were unable to confirm the efficacy of icatibant for the treatment of ACEi-induced angioedema include the differences in race in the study population and time to study drug administration. In the AMACE study, all the subjects were white, and the time to study drug administration was 6.1 hours in the icatibant group and 5.1 hours in the control group.[106] In the Straka and colleagues study, two-thirds of the subjects enrolled were Black, and the time to study drug administration was 10.3 hours in the icatibant group and 12.7 hours for the placebo group.[107] In the CAMEO trial, 69.4% of the subjects were Black and the overall median time to study drug administration was 7.8 hours.[108] The recent AAEM guidelines also do not support the use of icatibant for the treatment of ACEi-induced angioedema.[63]

AIRWAY MANAGEMENT

The major focus of an emergency physician's care of a patient presenting with angioedema is on ensuring airway patency. In a retrospective review of 311 patients with ACEi-induced angioedema who were evaluated with nasopharyngoscopy by an otolaryngologist in the ED, Kieu and colleagues found that 16% required intubation and 1% had a tracheostomy performed. They found that patients presenting within 4 hours of symptom onset, those reporting dysphagia, dysphonia, and globus sensation, and those with drooling or respiratory distress were most likely to require airway intervention.[109] McCormick and colleagues performed a retrospective analysis of 133 patients with angioedema to assess the relationship of the sites involved and the need for airway intervention. Two-thirds of the patients included in this study were on an ACEi. There was a statistically significant increase in the likelihood of intubation or surgical airway when the anterior tongue, the base of the tongue, or the larynx was involved. When the base of the tongue or larynx was involved, 38% of cases required airway intervention, whereas when these structures were not involved only 7% did.[110]

Based on a retrospective analysis, Ishoo and colleagues proposed a 4-tiered system to help predict the site of disposition as well as the need for airway intervention based on the location of swelling (**Table 1**). The term "stage" was used but the swelling of angioedema does not follow a typical pattern, and therefore, the different groupings should not be considered sequential. ACEi medications were involved in 39% of the episodes included in this analysis. Stridor, voice change, hoarseness, and dyspnea were associated with a need for airway intervention and admission to an ICU. All patients with either stage I (face, lip) or stage II (soft palate) angioedema were managed as outpatients or hospitalized outside of the ICU. Most (67%) patients with stage III (tongue) angioedema were managed in the ICU; however, 26% were managed as outpatients. When the swelling involved the larynx (Stage IV), all were treated in an ICU setting. Seven percent of patients with stage III and 24% of patients with stage IV angioedema required an airway intervention. This staging system is useful to describe

Table 1
Ishoo staging of angioedema[62]

Stage	Site	Episodes (%)	Outpatient (%)	Floor (%)	ICU (%)	Intervention (%)
I	Facial, lip	31	48	52	0	0
II	Soft palate	5	60	40	0	0
III	Tongue	32	26	7	67	7
IV	Laryngeal	31	0	0	100	24

the location of angioedema and to get a general sense of likely disposition and need to have an airway established; however, it has not been prospectively validated.[62]

Using retrospective data from 108 patients who presented to 2 tertiary hospitals during a 7-year period with angioedema due to any cause, Chiu and colleagues described a different 3-tiered classification system to describe cases based on the initial physical examination findings (**Table 2**). In this study, ACEi medications were involved in 68.5% of the cases. Cases were classified as type 1 when angioedema was limited to the face and oral cavity excluding the floor of the mouth. Type 2 cases involved the floor of the mouth and oropharyngeal structures such as the uvula, base of the tongue, and soft palate. In type 3, there was involvement of oropharyngeal structures with extension to supraglottic and glottic structures. Half the patients with type 3 required admission to the ICU. No patients with type 1 angioedema where the swelling was limited to the face and oral cavity excluding the floor of the mouth required airway management. Rates of intubation for types 2 and 3 were 21.4% and 33.3%, respectively. Only 2 patients in the entire study required a surgical airway—both were type 2.[111]

The prediction of a "difficult" airway in an otherwise anatomically normal patient is challenging even when using bedside screening tests such as the Mallampati classification and thyromental distance.[112] Any patient with angioedema of the head and neck should immediately be considered to have a "difficult" airway. Failure to recognize the difficult nature of the airway leading to suboptimal management can result in devastating outcomes. If the patient with angioedema is not in extremis requiring immediate control of the airway, the emergency physician should take the time to prepare to ensure optimal conditions to successfully intubate the patient. Because physical manipulation of the airway can worsen the degree of swelling, first pass

Table 2
Chiu classification of angioedema based on anatomic location[65]

Type	Site	Episodes (%)	Discharged from ED (%)	Floor (%)	ICU (%)	Intubated (%)	Surgical Airway (%)
I	Facial, oral cavity excluding floor of mouth	57.4	69.4	22.6	8.0	0.0	0.0
II	Floor of mouth, oropharyngeal structures (uvula, base of the tongue, and soft palate)	25.9	10.7	28.6	32.1	21.4	7.1
III	Oropharyngeal structures with extension to supraglottic and glottic structures	16.7	5.6	11.1	50.0	33.3	0.0

success is critical to increase the likelihood of success. For this reason, the most experienced person in airway management should perform the intubation. Supraglottic airway devices such as a laryngeal mask airway cannot be used as a temporizing measure in cases of angioedema because these are placed above the site of obstruction.[60,113] Positive pressure ventilation with bilevel positive airway pressure or continuous airway pressure also should not be used, as these modalities do nothing to fix the underlying problem and the barotrauma associated with them may worsen the swelling. Successful preparation includes delineating roles for care team members, ensuring proper equipment including suction and rescue devices are present, having appropriate medications, and developing a backup plan in the case of failure to intubate. Before intubation, glycopyrrolate (0.1–0.2 mg intravenously) can be given to reduce oral secretions to aid in visualization. The onset of action is 3 to 5 minutes and will continue to work for 30 to 60 minutes.[114] The patient should also be preoxygenated using a nonrebreather mask.

Rapid sequence intubation (RSI) uses a hypnotic to provide sedation and a neuromuscular blocker as a paralytic agent and in most cases of emergent intubation improves conditions for intubation and leads to improved first pass success rate. RSI is not recommended by many experts in cases of angioedema as this may lead to a situation where the patient cannot be intubated and cannot be oxygenated. Using the technique of awake intubation allows for vocal cord visualization without preventing the patient from spontaneous breathing. Before performing an awake intubation, the airway should have a local anesthetic applied to provide patient comfort and lessen the risk of coughing or gagging. A recent trial demonstrated that use of lidocaine spray was superior to nebulized lidocaine for topical anesthesia during diagnostic flexible bronchoscopy.[115] Use of vasoconstrictors such as oxymetazoline (0.5% nasal spray) or phenylephrine (0.5% nasal spray) decreases mucosal edema of the nasal passageway, allowing for better passage of the endotracheal tube and reducing the likelihood of iatrogenic epistaxis.

In practice, multiple methods of airway management are used for patients with angioedema. In a retrospective, single-center analysis, Driver and McGill reviewed the method of intubation for 45 patients with angioedema. Fiberoptic nasotracheal intubation was the most commonly used initial technique (51.1%) followed by blind nasotracheal intubation (22.2%). Other techniques used were video laryngoscopy (15.6%), fiberoptic oral (6.7%), and direct laryngoscopy (4.4%). The overall first pass success rate was 60%. A tracheal tube introducer (Bougie) was used in all cases where direct and video-assisted laryngoscopy methods were used.[116] Regardless of the method chosen, it is important to remember that physical manipulation of the airway can cause sudden and severe worsening of the swelling. Prepping the patient for a surgical airway—a double setup—before any attempt to evaluate or manage the airway has been recommended.[32]

DISPOSITION

The disposition of patients with ACEi-induced angioedema is determined by the location of swelling and the severity of symptoms. The aforementioned Ishoo staging and Chiu classification provides some information about the disposition of patients based on anatomic location. Most would consider a minimum period of observation in the ED of 4 to 6 hours for patients with only mild symptoms that only involve the face and lips; this allows for monitoring of the patient for progression of symptoms. When oropharyngeal and laryngeal structures are involved longer periods of observation are required. If there is substantial concern that the patient may progress to the point of needing airway intervention, the patient should be placed in an area where there is close monitoring and where there are supplies and providers with airway expertise. Patients who are intubated or who have a surgical airway performed will need to be admitted to an ICU. All patients should have their ACEi medication discontinued. The patient should be educated that this reaction is a class effect and that use of any form of ACEi carries a high likelihood of recurrence of angioedema. The use of an angiotensin receptor blocker (ARB) after an episode of ACEi-induced angioedema is controversial. Patients taking ARBs have been reported to develop angioedema although studies have shown that the risk is not higher than for patients taking other antihypertensives such as β-blockers.[117,118] Despite the fact that ARBs do not seem themselves associated with a high incidence of developing angioedema, one metanalysis found that the risk of developing angioedema on an ARB was 3.5% for cases of confirmed ACEi-induced angioedema and 9.4% for possible cases.[119]

CONCLUSION

Angioedema that develops as a result of treatment with an ACEi is a potentially life-threatening complication that requires prompt evaluation by a physician trained in emergency stabilization and airway management. Although the entire pathophysiologic processes for why this complication develops is not entirely clear, it is thought to be largely driven by the accumulation of bradykinin with some possible role for substance P. Importantly, ACEi-induced angioedema is not a type I hypersensitivity reaction that results in the release of preformed mediators such as histamine from mast cells and basophils. There are no medications that have proved efficacy in the treatment of ACEi-induced angioedema. Given the relative frequency that this is seen in the ED, this is an important area for future research. The most important role that the emergency physician has is to evaluate and manage the airway based on the location of swelling and the severity of symptoms. Classification systems have been developed to describe the location of angioedema and provide some information on disposition and need for airway intervention. The emergency physician can use the systems to provide some context; however, the management of each patient should be individualized based on the global assessment performed by the treating physician.

CLINICS CARE POINTS

- Patients may present with ACEi-induced angioedema despite being on an ACEi for multiple years.
- There are no tests that can definitively rule in that angioedema is due to use of an ACEi. If there is concern of an alternative cause, such as an allergic reaction, then treatment focused on allergic reactions should be given.
- A C4 level is useful to screen for cases of HAE that may have been previously undiagnosed.
- ACEi-induced angioedema may affect the gastrointestinal tract, so this diagnosis should be considered in any patient on an ACEi presenting with abdominal pain.
- Patients with voice change, hoarseness, stridor, and dyspnea are at high risk for needing an airway.
- It is recommended to perform fiberoptic nasopharyngoscopy on patients who may be at risk for airway obstruction. The patient should be prepared for intubation, as performing nasopharyngoscopy may result in worsening of the swelling encountered.
- The Ishoo staging system and the Chiu classification provide some guidance as to which patients will need a higher level of care and an airway intervention based on the anatomic site of swelling.

- Patients with ACEi-induced angioedema should be counseled to avoid ACEi medications. The use of an ARB after an episode of ACEi-induced angioedema is controversial.

DISCLOSURE

The authors have nothing to disclose.

REFERENCES

1. Ferreira SH. A Bradykinin-Potentiating Factor (BPF) Present int eh Venom of Bothrops Jararaca. Br J Pharm Chemoth 1965;24(1):163–9.
2. Skeggs LT, Lentz KE, Kahn JR, et al. THE amino acid sequence of hypertensin II. J Exp Med 1956;104(2):193–7.
3. Cushman DW, Ondetti MA. History of the design of captopril and related inhibitors of angiotensin converting enzyme. Hypertension 2018;17(4):589–92.
4. Kostis WJ, Kostis JB. ACE inhibitor-induced angioedema: a review. Curr Hypertens Rep 2018;20(7):55.
5. Wilkin JK, Hammond JJ, Kirkendall WM. The captopril-induced eruption. A possible mechanism: cutaneous kinin potentiation. Arch Dermatol 1980; 116(8):902–5.
6. Kelly M, Donnelly JP, McAnnally J-R, et al. National estimates of emergency department visits for angioedema and allergic reactions in the United States. Allergy asthma Proc 2013;34(2):150–4.
7. Banerji A, Clark S, Blanda M, et al. Multicenter study of patients with angiotensin-converting enzyme inhibitor-induced angioedema who present to the emergency department. Ann Allergy Asthma Immunol 2008;100(4): 327–32.
8. Weisman DS, Arnouk N, Asghar MB, et al. ACE inhibitor angioedema: characterization and treatment versus non-ACE angioedema in acute hospitalized patients. J Community Hosp Intern Med Perspect 2020;10(1):16–8.
9. Slater EE, Merrill DD, Guess HA, et al. Clinical profile of angioedema associated with angiotensin converting-enzyme inhibition. JAMA 1988;260(7):967–70.
10. Banerji A, Blumenthal KG, Lai KH, et al. Epidemiology of ACE Inhibitor Angioedema Utilizing a Large Electronic Health Record. J Allergy Clin Immunol Pract 2017;5(3):744–9.
11. Shah SJ, Stafford RS. Current trends of hypertension treatment in the United States. Am J Hypertens 2017;30(10):1008–14.
12. Liau Y, Chua I, Kennedy MA, et al. Pharmacogenetics of angiotensin-converting enzyme inhibitor-induced angioedema. Clin Exp Allergy 2019;49(2):142–54.
13. Asad H, Gohar A. Incidence of angiotensin-converting enzyme-associated angioedema among African Americans compared to other races. Presented at: CHEST Annual Meeting 2020; October 18–21, 2020. Presentation 1123A.
14. Kostis JB, Kim HJ, Rusnak J, et al. Incidence and characteristics of angioedema associated with enalapril. Arch Intern Med 2005;165(14):1637–42.
15. Do TP, Seetasith A, Belleli R, et al. A database cohort study to assess the risk of angioedema among patients with heart failure initiating angiotensin-converting enzyme inhibitors in the USA. Am J Cardiovasc Drugs 2018;18(3):205–11.
16. Pall AH, Lomholt AF, Buchwald C von, et al. Clinical features and disease course of primary angioedema patients in a tertiary care hospital. J asthma Allergy 2020;13:225–36.

17. Morimoto T, Gandhi TK, Fiskio JM, et al. Development and validation of a Clinical prediction rule for angiotensin-converting enzyme inhibitor-induced cough. J Gen Intern Med 2004;19(6):684–91.

18. Chan NJ, Soliman AMS. Angiotensin converting enzyme inhibitor-related angioedema: onset, presentation, and management. Ann Otology Rhinology Laryngol 2015;124(2):89–96.

19. Dicpinigaitis PV. Angiotensin-Converting Enzyme Inhibitor-Induced Cough ACCP Evidence-Based Clinical Practice Guidelines. Chest 2006;129(1): 169S–73S.

20. Os I, Bratland B, Dahlöf B, et al. Female preponderance for lisinopril-induced cough in hypertension. Am J Hypertens 1994;7(11):1012–5.

21. Campbell DJ. Towards understanding the kallikrein-kinin system: insights from measurement of kinin peptides. Braz J Med Biol Res 2000;33(6):665–77.

22. Marceau F, Rivard GE, Gauthier JM, et al. Measurement of Bradykinin Formation and Degradation in Blood Plasma: Relevance for Acquired Angioedema Associated With Angiotensin Converting Enzyme Inhibition and for Hereditary Angioedema Due to Factor XII or Plasminogen Gene Variants. Front Med 2020; 7:358.

23. Cyr M, Lepage Y, Blais C, et al. Bradykinin and des-Arg9-bradykinin metabolic pathways and kinetics of activation of human plasma. Am J Physiol-heart C 2001;281(1):H275–83.

24. Cugno M, Nussberger J, Cicardi M, et al. Bradykinin and the pathophysiology of angioedema. Int Immunopharmacology 2003;3(3):311–7.

25. Hubers SA, Kohm K, Wei S, et al. Endogenous bradykinin and B1-B5 during angiotensin-converting enzyme inhibitor-associated angioedema. J Allergy Clin Immunol 2018;142(5):1636–9, e5.

26. Campos MM, Mata LV, Callxto JB. Expression of B1 kinin receptors mediating paw edema and Formalin-induced nociception. Modulation by glucocorticoids. Can J Physiol Pharm 1995;73(7):812–9.

27. Hoover T, Lippmann M, Grouzmann E, et al. Angiotensin converting enzyme inhibitor induced angio-oedema: a review of the pathophysiology and risk factors. Clin Exp Allergy 2010;40(1):50–61.

28. Byrd JB, Woodard-Grice A, Stone E, et al. Association of angiotensin-converting enzyme inhibitor-associated angioedema with transplant and immunosuppressant use. Allergy Published Online June 2010;19.

29. Byrd JB, Touzin KK, Sile SS, et al. Dipeptidyl peptidase IV in angiotensin-converting enzyme inhibitor associated angioedema. Hypertension 2008; 51(1):141–7.

30. Brown NJ, Byiers S, Carr D, et al. Dipeptidyl peptidase-IV inhibitor use associated with increased risk of ACE inhibitor-associated angioedema. Hypertension 2009;54(3):516–23.

31. Giavina-Bianchi P, Aun MV, Jares EJ, et al. Angioedema associated with nonsteroidal anti-inflammatory drugs. Curr Opin Allergy Clin Immunol 2016;16(4): 323–32.

32. Wilkerson RG. Angioedema in the emergency department: an evidence-based review. Emerg Med Pract 2012;14(11):1–21.

33. Javaud N, Achamlal J, Reuter P-G, et al. Angioedema related to angiotensin-converting enzyme inhibitors: attack severity, treatment, and hospital admission in a prospective multicenter study. Medicine 2015;94(45):e1939.

34. Farraye FA, Peppercorn MA, Steer ML, et al. Acute small-bowel mucosal edema following enalapril use. Jama 1988;259(21):3131.

35. Byrne TJ, Douglas DD, Landis ME, et al. Isolated visceral angioedema: an underdiagnosed complication of ACE inhibitors? Mayo Clinic Proc Mayo Clinic 2000;75(11):1201–4.

36. Javaud N, Altar A, Fain O, et al. Hereditary angioedema, emergency management of attacks by a call center. Eur J Intern Med 2019;67:42–6.

37. Parreira R, Amaral R, Amaral L, et al. ACE inhibitor-induced small bowel angioedema, mimicking an acute abdomen. J Surg Case Rep 2020;2020(10):rjaa348.

38. Bloom AS, Schranz C. Angiotensin-converting enzyme inhibitor–induced angioedema of the small bowel—a surgical abdomen mimic. J Emerg Med 2015;48(6):e127–9.

39. Prisant LM. Angioneurotic edema. J Clin Hypertens (Greenwich, Conn) 2001; 3(4):262–3.

40. Agah R, Bandi V, Guntupalli KK. Angioedema: the role of ACE inhibitors and factors associated with poor clinical outcome. Intensive Care Med 1997;23(7): 793–6.

41. Leru PM, Anton VF, Bocsan C, et al. Acquired angioedema induced by angiotensin-converting enzyme inhibitors - experience of a hospital-based allergy center. Exp Ther Med 2020;20(1):68–72.

42. Sandefur B, Silva LOJ e, Lohse C, et al. Clinical features and outcomes associated with angioedema in the emergency department. West J Emerg Med 2019; 20(5):760–9.

43. Howarth D. ACE inhibitor angioedema - a very late presentation. Aust Fam Physician 2013;42(12):860–2.

44. Manning ME. Hereditary angioedema: differential diagnosis, diagnostic tests, and family screening. Allergy Asthma Proc 2020;41(6):S22–5.

45. Tarzi MD, Hickey A, Förster T, et al. An evaluation of tests used for the diagnosis and monitoring of C1 inhibitor deficiency: normal serum C4 does not exclude hereditary angio-oedema. Clin Exp Immunol 2007;149(3):513–6.

46. Ohsawa I, Honda D, Nagamachi S, et al. Clinical and laboratory characteristics that differentiate hereditary angioedema in 72 patients with angioedema. Allergol Int 2014;63(4):595–602.

47. Zanichelli A, Arcoleo F, Barca MP, et al. A nationwide survey of hereditary angioedema due to C1 inhibitor deficiency in Italy. Orphanet J Rare Dis 2015; 10(1):11–6.

48. Santacroce R, D'Andrea G, Maffione AB, et al. The genetics of hereditary angioedema: a review. J Clin Med 2021;10(9):2023.

49. Patel G, Pongracic JA. Hereditary and acquired angioedema. Allergy asthma Proc 2019;40(6):441–5.

50. Bowen T, Cicardi M, Farkas H, et al. 2010 International consensus algorithm for the diagnosis, therapy and management of hereditary angioedema. Allergy asthma, Clin Immunol 2010;6(1):24.

51. Bas M, Hoffmann TK, Bier H, et al. Increased C-reactive protein in ACE-inhibitor-induced angioedema. Br J Clin Pharmacol 2005;59(2):233–8.

52. Ferreira TA, Alves MR, Oliveira AMP, et al. A rare cause of abdominal pain: intestinal angioedema. J Med Cases 2021;12(4):138–40.

53. Wilin KL, Czupryn MJ, Mui R, et al. ACE inhibitor-induced angioedema of the small bowel: a case report and review of the literature. J Pharm Pract 2018; 31(1):99–103.

54. Ishigami K, Averill SL, Pollard JH, et al. Radiologic manifestations of angioedema. Insights into Imaging 2014;5(3):365–74.

55. Scheirey CD, Scholz FJ, Shortsleeve MJ, et al. Angiotensin-converting enzyme inhibitor-induced small-bowel angioedema: clinical and imaging findings in 20 patients. AJR Am J roentgenology 2011;197(2):393–8.
56. Wittenberg J, Harisinghani MG, Jhaveri K, et al. Algorithmic Approach to CT Diagnosis of the Abnormal Bowel Wall. Radiographics 2002;22(5):1093–107.
57. Sofia S, Casali A, Bolondi L. Sonographic findings in abdominal hereditary angioedema. J Clin Ultrasound 1999;27(9):537–40.
58. Riguzzi C, Losonczy L, Teismann N, et al. Gastrointestinal manifestations of hereditary angioedema diagnosed by ultrasound in the emergency department. The West J Emerg Med 2014;15(7):816–8.
59. Schick M, Grether-Jones K. Point-of-care sonographic findings in acute upper airway edema 2016;17(6):822–6.
60. Moellman JJ, Bernstein JA, Lindsell C, et al. A consensus parameter for the evaluation and management of angioedema in the emergency department. Goldstein JN. Acad Emerg Med 2014;21(4):469–84.
61. Winters ME, Rosenbaum S, Vilke GM, et al. Emergency department management of patients with ace-inhibitor angioedema. J Emerg Med 2013;45(5):775–80.
62. Ishoo E, Shah UK, Grillone GA, et al. Predicting airway risk in angioedema: staging system based on presentation. Otolaryngology–head neck Surg 1999;121(3):263–8.
63. Rosenbaum S, Wilkerson RG, Winters ME, et al. Clinical practice statement: what is the emergency department management of patients with angioedema secondary to an ACE-Inhibitor? J Emerg Med 2021;61(1):105–12.
64. Simons FER, Gu X, Simons KJ. Epinephrine absorption in adults: intramuscular versus subcutaneous injection. J Allergy Clin Immunol 2001;108(5):871–3.
65. Shaker MS, Wallace DV, Golden DBK, et al. Anaphylaxis—a 2020 practice parameter update, systematic review, and Grading of Recommendations, Assessment, Development and Evaluation (GRADE) analysis. J Allergy Clin Immun 2020;145(4):1082–123.
66. Cardona V, Ansotegui IJ, Ebisawa M, et al. World allergy organization anaphylaxis guidance 2020. World Allergy Organ J 2020;13(10):100472.
67. Pickering RJ, Good RA, Kelly JR, et al. Replacement therapy in hereditary angioedema. Successful treatment of two patients with fresh frozen plasma. Lancet 1969;1(7590):326–30.
68. Winnewisser J, Rossi M, Späth P, et al. Type I hereditary angio-oedema. Variability of clinical presentation and course within two large kindreds. J Intern Med 1997;241(1):39–46.
69. Tang R, Chen S, Zhang HY. Fresh frozen plasma for the treatment of hereditary angioedema acute attacks. Chin Med Sci J 2012 Jun;27(2):92–5.
70. Prematta M, Gibbs JG, Pratt EL, et al. Fresh frozen plasma for the treatment of hereditary angioedema. Ann Allergy Asthma Immunol 2007;98(4):383–8.
71. Wentzel N, Panieri A, Ayazi M, et al. Fresh frozen plasma for on-demand hereditary angioedema treatment in South Africa and Iran. World Allergy Organ J 2019;12(9):100049.
72. Busse PJ, Christiansen SC, Riedl MA, et al. US HAEA Medical Advisory Board 2020 Guidelines for the Management of Hereditary Angioedema. J Allergy Clin Immunol Pract 2021;9(1):132–50, e3.
73. Saeb A, Hagglund KH, Cigolle CT. Using fresh frozen plasma for acute airway angioedema to prevent intubation in the emergency department: a retrospective cohort study. Emerg Med Int 2016;2016(11):6091510–6.

74. Millot I, Plancade D, Hosotte M, et al. Treatment of a life-threatening laryngeal bradykinin angio-oedema precipitated by dipeptidylpeptidase-4 inhibitor and angiotensin-I converting enzyme inhibitor with prothrombin complex concentrates. Br J Anaesth 2012;109(5):827–9.

75. Vázquez-Ramos D, Cordero-Gomez A, Rodríguez-Cintrón W. Recurrent angiotensin-converting enzyme inhibitor-induced angioedema refractory to fresh frozen plasma. Fed Pract 2019;36(12):584–6.

76. Adebayo O, Wilkerson RG. Angiotensin-converting enzyme inhibitor–induced angioedema worsened with fresh frozen plasma. Am J Emerg Med 2016; 35(1):192.e1–2.

77. Chen SX, Hermelin D, Weintraub SJ. Possible donor-dependent differences in efficacy of fresh frozen plasma for treatment of ACE inhibitor-induced angioedema. J Allergy Clin Immunol Pract 2019;7(6):2087–8.

78. Riha HM, Summers BB, Rivera JV, et al. Novel therapies for angiotensin-converting enzyme inhibitor–induced angioedema: a systematic review of current evidence. J Emerg Med 2017;53(5):662–79.

79. Wilkerson RG, Martinelli AN, Oliver WD. Treatment of angioedema induced by angiotensin-converting enzyme inhibitor. J Emerg Med 2018;55(1):132–3.

80. Donaldson VH, Evans RR. A biochemical abnormality in hereditary angioneurotic edema: absence of serum inhibitor of c' 1-esterase. Am J Med 1963;35(1): 37–44.

81. Brackertz D, Kueppers F. Hereditary angioneurotic oedema. Lancet 1973; 2(7830):680.

82. Bork K, Witzke G, Hereditares angioneurotisches Odem. Klinik sowie erweiterte diagnostische und therapeutische Moglichkeiten [Hereditary angioneurotic edema. Clinical aspects and extended diagnostic and therapeutic possibilities] In German. Deutsche medizinische Wochenschrift 1979;104(11):405–9.

83. Gadek JE, Hosea SW, Gelfand JA, et al. Replacement therapy in hereditary angioedema: successful treatment of acute episodes of angioedema with partly purified C1 inhibitor. New Engl J Med 1980;302(10):542–6.

84. Agostoni A, Bergamaschini L, Martignoni G, et al. Treatment of acute attacks of hereditary angioedema with C1-inhibitor concentrate. Ann Allergy 1980;44(5): 299–301.

85. Frank MM. Recombinant and Plasma-Purified Human C1 Inhibitor for the Treatment of Hereditary Angioedema. World Allergy Organ J 2010;3(Suppl 3): S29–33.

86. Craig TJ, Levy RJ, Wasserman RL, et al. Efficacy of human C1 esterase inhibitor concentrate compared with placebo in acute hereditary angioedema attacks. J Allergy Clin Immunol 2009;124(4):801–8.

87. Craig TJ, Bewtra AK, Bahna SL, et al. C1 esterase inhibitor concentrate in 1085 Hereditary Angioedema attacks - final results of the I.M.P.A.C.T.2 study. Allergy 2011;66(12):1604–11.

88. Farrell C, Hayes S, Relan A, et al. Population pharmacokinetics of recombinant human C1 inhibitor in patients with hereditary angioedema. Br J Clin Pharmaco 2013;76(6):897–907.

89. Perza M, Koczirka S, Nomura JT. C1 esterase inhibitor for ace-inhibitor angioedema: a case series and literature review. J Emerg Med 2020;58(3):e121–7.

90. Kovaltchouk U, Zhang B, Jain V, et al. Effectiveness of C1-INH therapy in angiotensin converting enzyme inhibitor induced angioedema. Allergy Asthma Clin Immunol 2021;17(1):18.

91. Available at: https://clinicaltrials.gov/ct2/show/NCT01843530%20. Accessed August 20, 2021.
92. Levy JH, O'Donnell PS. The therapeutic potential of a kallikrein inhibitor for treating hereditary angioedema. Expert Opin Investig Drugs 2006;15(9):1077–90.
93. Levy R, McNeil D, Li H, et al. Results of a 2-Stage, Phase 3 Pivotal Trial, EDEMA3: A Study of Subcutaneous DX-88 (Ecallantide), a Plasma Kallikrein Inhibitor, in Patients with Hereditary Angioedema (HAE). J Allergy Clin Immunol 2008;121(2):S103.
94. Levy RJ, Lumry WR, McNeil DL, et al. EDEMA4: a phase 3, double-blind study of subcutaneous ecallantide treatment for acute attacks of hereditary angioedema. Ann Allergy Asthma Immunol 2010;104(6):523–9.
95. Duffey H, Firszt R. Management of acute attacks of hereditary angioedema: role of ecallantide. J Blood Med 2015;6:115–23.
96. Craig TJ, Riedl M, Li HH, et al. Hypersensitivity reactions to ecallantide: an update of the clinical trial experience and post-market surveillance for treatment of attacks of hereditary angioedema. J Allergy Clin Immunol 2012;129(2):AB220.
97. Bernstein JA, Moellman JJ, Collins SP, et al. Effectiveness of ecallantide in treating angiotensin-converting enzyme inhibitor-induced angioedema in the emergency department. Ann Allergy Asthma Immunol 2015;114(3):245–9.
98. Lewis LM, Graffeo C, Crosley P, et al. Ecallantide for the acute treatment of Angiotensin-converting enzyme inhibitor-induced angioedema: a multicenter, randomized, controlled trial. Ann Emerg Med 2015;65(2):204–13.
99. Bork K, Frank J, Grundt B, et al. Treatment of acute edema attacks in hereditary angioedema with a bradykinin receptor-2 antagonist (Icatibant). J Allergy Clin Immunol 2007;119(6):1497–503.
100. Longhurst HJ. Management of acute attacks of hereditary angioedema: potential role of icatibant 2010;6:795–802.
101. Cicardi M, Banerji A, Bracho F, et al. Icatibant, a new bradykinin-receptor antagonist, in hereditary angioedema. New Engl J Med 2010;363(6):532–41.
102. Lumry WR, Li HH, Levy RJ, et al. Randomized placebo-controlled trial of the bradykinin B$_2$ receptor antagonist icatibant for the treatment of acute attacks of hereditary angioedema: the FAST-3 trial. Ann Allergy Asthma Immunol 2011; 107(6):529–37.
103. Maurer M, Church MK. Inflammatory skin responses induced by icatibant injection are mast cell mediated and attenuated by H1-antihistamines. Exp Dermatol 2012;21(2):154–5.
104. Bas M, Greve J, Stelter K, et al. Therapeutic efficacy of icatibant in angioedema induced by angiotensin-converting enzyme inhibitors: a case series. Ann Emerg Med 2010;56(3):278–82.
105. Schmidt PW, Hirschl MM, Trautinger F. Treatment of angiotensin-converting enzyme inhibitor–related angioedema with the bradykinin B2 receptor antagonist icatibant. J Am Dermatol 2010;63(5):913–4.
106. Bas M, Greve J, Stelter K, et al. A randomized trial of icatibant in ace-inhibitor-induced angioedema. New Engl J Med 2015;372(5):418–25.
107. Straka BT, Stone E, Woodard-Grice A, et al. Effect of bradykinin receptor antagonism on ACE inhibitor-associated angioedema. J Allergy Clin Immunol 2017; 140(1):242–8, e2.
108. Sinert R, Levy P, Bernstein JA, et al. Randomized trial of icatibant for angiotensin-converting enzyme inhibitor–induced upper airway angioedema. J Allergy Clin Immunol Pract 2017;5(5):1402–9, e3.

109. Kieu MCQ, Bangiyev JN, Thottam PJ, et al. Predictors of airway intervention in angiotensin-converting enzyme inhibitor–induced angioedema. Otolaryngol Head Neck Surg 2015;153(4):544–50.
110. McCormick M, Folbe AJ, Lin H-S, et al. Site involvement as a predictor of airway intervention in angioedema. Laryngoscope 2011;121(2):262–6.
111. Chiu AG, Newkirk KA, Davidson BJ, et al. Angiotensin-converting enzyme inhibitor-induced angioedema: a multicenter review and an algorithm for airway management. Ann otology, rhinology, Laryngol 2001;110(9):834–40.
112. Shiga T, Wajima Z, Inoue T, et al. Predicting difficult intubation in apparently normal patients: a meta-analysis of bedside screening test performance. Anesthesiology 2005;103(2):429–37.
113. Long BJ, Koyfman A, Gottlieb M. Evaluation and management of angioedema in the emergency department. West J Emerg Med 2019;20(4):587–600.
114. Ahmad I, El-Boghdadly K, Bhagrath R, et al. Difficult airway society guidelines for awake tracheal intubation (ati) in adults. Anaesthesia 2020;75(4):509–28.
115. Dhooria S, Chaudhary S, Ram B, et al. A randomized trial of nebulized lignocaine, lignocaine spray, or their combination for topical anesthesia during diagnostic flexible bronchoscopy. Chest 2020;157(1):198–204.
116. Driver BE, Mcgill JW. Emergency department airway management of severe angioedema: a video review of 45 intubations. Ann Emerg Med 2017;69(5):635–9.
117. Toh S, Reichman ME, Houstoun M, et al. Comparative risk for angioedema associated with the use of drugs that target the Renin-Angiotensin-aldosterone system. Arch Intern Med 2012;172(20):1582–9.
118. Makani H, Messerli FH, Romero J, et al. Meta-analysis of randomized trials of angioedema as an adverse event of renin-angiotensin system inhibitors. Am J Cardiol 2012;110(3):383–91.
119. Haymore BR, Yoon J, Mikita CP, et al. Risk of angioedema with angiotensin receptor blockers in patients with prior angioedema associated with angiotensin-converting enzyme inhibitors: a meta-analysis. Ann Allergy Asthma Immunol 2008;101(5):495–9.

Hereditary Angioedema

R. Gentry Wilkerson, MD[a],*, Joseph J. Moellman, MD[b]

KEYWORDS

- Hereditary angioedema • C1-inhibitor • Bradykinin • Complement
- Quincke disease • Difficult airway

KEY POINTS

- HAE-C1-INH type I is due to a quantitative deficiency of C1-INH. HAE-C1-INH type II is due to C1-INH that has reduced function. In HAE where there is normal C1-INH, HAE-nl-C1-INH, mutations have been found in the genes that code for factor XII, plasminogen, HMWK, LMWK, and angiopoietin-1.
- In almost all cases of HAE, bradykinin is the final common product that leads to the development of angioedema.
- Clinical findings associated with need for definitive airway management include voice change, hoarseness, stridor, and dyspnea.
- Targeted treatment for acute HAE attacks focuses on decreasing the production of bradykinin through inhibition of kallikrein, and replacement of C1-INH, or by inhibiting the action of bradykinin on the bradykinin B2 receptor.
- In patients who have angioedema involving the tongue, soft palate, or floor of the mouth, the use of fiberoptic nasopharyngoscopy to help identify the presence of swelling of the deeper upper airway structures is recommended.

INTRODUCTION

Hereditary angioedema (HAE) is a rare, potentially life-threatening genetic disorder that presents with episodic swelling of the skin or mucosal tissue of the upper respiratory and gastrointestinal tracts. Heinrich Quincke[1] provided the first description of the disease in 1882, and its heritable nature was documented by William Osler[2] in 1888. Since those first descriptions made more than 100 years ago, there has been remarkable progress made in the classification, diagnosis, and treatment of HAE through a better understanding of the different pathophysiological processes that lead to its multiple types.

This article originally appeared in Emergency Medicine Clinics, Volume 40 Issue 1, February 2022.

[a] Department of Emergency Medicine, University of Maryland School of Medicine, 110 South Paca Street, 6th Floor, Suite 200, Baltimore, MD 21201, USA; [b] Department of Emergency Medicine, University of Cincinnati College of Medicine, 231 Albert Sabin Way, MSB 1654, Cincinnati, OH 45267-0769, USA
* Corresponding author.
E-mail address: gwilkerson@som.umaryland.edu
Twitter: @gentrywmd (R.G.W.); @edmojo (J.J.M.)

Immunol Allergy Clin N Am 43 (2023) 533–552
https://doi.org/10.1016/j.iac.2022.10.012
0889-8561/23/© 2022 Elsevier Inc. All rights reserved.

Because of the risk of airway obstruction and the substantial morbidity that can be associated with attacks of HAE, it is important for the emergency physician to be aware of this disease and the mechanisms that underlie the treatment options that have become available. Since the first disease-specific medication was approved by the United States Food and Drug Administration (FDA) in 2008, there have been major advances in the range of treatment options that are focused on the kallikrein-kinin system, a pathway that leads to the formation of bradykinin. The action of brady-kinin on its specific receptors located on the endothelial layer of blood vessels leads to increased vascular permeability and the extravasation of fluid into the surrounding structures.

It is important to distinguish HAE from other forms of angioedema that may be encountered in the emergency department (ED). Although the skills required for airway management are the same, the potential therapeutic agents used for treatment differ based on the underlying mechanism that leads to the development of angioedema. This article provides a comprehensive review of HAE and the therapeutic options that are now available.

EPIDEMIOLOGY AND TIMING OF DISEASE

The prevalence of HAE has been estimated to be approximately 1:50,000 to 1:100,000 individuals.[3] A recent systematic review of epidemiologic studies found 6 studies that were each focused on an individual country in Europe. The overall prevalence of HAE found in these studies was approximately 1:67,000 individuals.[4] Because of the homo-geneity of the study populations included, it is unknown if this prevalence would hold true for the general worldwide population. If true in the United States, there would be approximately 5000 individuals who have HAE. HAE is classified as an orphan disease because of the fact that it affects fewer than 200,000 people in the United States.[5] HAE type 1 accounts for approximately 85% of cases, whereas type 2 accounts for ~15%. The prevalence of HAE with normal C1-esterase inhibitor (C1-INH) is not known but is likely a small fraction of the prevalence of type 1 and 2. No differences in prevalence have been found based on race and ethnicity.[6]

Patients with HAE are born with the genetic defect that accounts for the disease. In approximately 25% of cases of HAE, the mutation is de novo, and therefore, there will be no family history of the disease.[7] The phenotypic expression varies considerably among those affected. In a recent survey of patients identified through the US Hered-itary Angioedema Association, the mean age of onset of symptoms was 12.5 years, but the mean age of diagnosis was 20.1 years. This suggests that the current delay in diagnosis is 8.6 years.[8] An earlier study found that 7% of patients had symptoms of HAE before age 1 and that those with earlier onset tended to have a more severe course of disease.[9]

CLASSIFICATION AND PATHOPHYSIOLOGY

The genetic defects that cause HAE are inherited in an autosomal dominant fashion. In most forms of HAE, the common mediator for the development of angioedema is bra-dykinin, a nonapeptide that functions as a potent vasodilator leading to increased vascular permeability and subsequent tissue swelling.[10] In the broadest sense, HAE can be classified based on the presence or absence of normal levels of functioning C1-INH. Most cases of HAE are due to reduced levels of normally functioning C1-INH (HAE-C1-INH). There are very rare cases of HAE where there are normal quanti-tative and functional levels of C1-INH (HAE-nl-C1-INH). In the predominant forms of HAE, there is either a quantitative deficiency (HAE-C1-INH type I) or reduced function

(HAE-C1-INH type II) of C1-INH because of a heterogeneous group of mutations of the SERPING1 gene located on chromosome 11 (11q12-q13.1).[11] More than 450 different mutations of the SERPING1 gene that lead to the development of HAE have been reported.[12] C1-INH, which belongs to the superfamily of serine protease inhibitors (serpins), exerts its activity at multiple points in the complement, fibrinolytic, and the contact activating systems (**Fig. 1**). When functional C1-INH decreases to less than a critical threshold of approximately 40%, the risk of an attack of HAE increases.[13] Restoration of C1-INH to levels higher than the 40% threshold has been associated with clinical protection against attacks.[14]

Two independent groups first described HAE with normal C1-INH levels and function in 2000.[15,16] In the past, HAE-nl-C1-INH was referred to as HAE type III; however, it is now known that there are multiple distinct causes of this form of HAE, so the classification HAE type III should not be used. Currently, there are 5 subtypes of HAE-nl-C1-INH based on the underlying genetic mutation that leads to the development of angioedema. These mutations lead to defects in the F12 gene that encodes for coagulation factor XII (FXII), the PLG gene that encodes for plasminogen,[17,18] the KNG1 gene that encodes for high- and low-molecular-weight kininogen,[19] and the ANGPT1 gene that encodes for angiopoietin-1.[20] The fifth subtype of HAE-nl-C1-INH is for patients with a genetic mutation that has not yet been determined. One possible cause of HAE-Unknown is due to a mutation in the MYOF gene that was described recently. This leads to a gain-of-function mutation in the myoferlin protein, an integral membrane protein of endothelial cells that modulates permeability through VEGF signal transduction.[21]

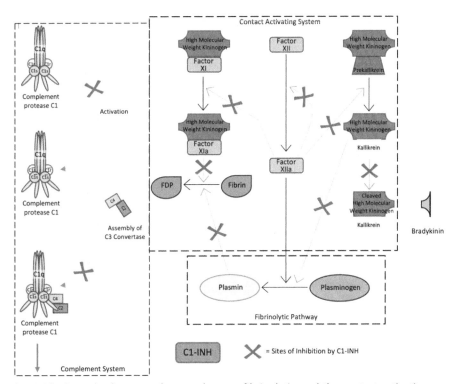

Fig. 1. The interplay between the complement, fibrinolytic, and the contact activating systems with sites of inhibition by C1-INH.

HAE owing to defective production of angiopoietin-1 (HAE-ANGPT1) is unique among the different types of HAE in that the underlying mechanism for the development of angioedema is not associated with overproduction of bradykinin. Instead, defective angiopoietin-1 loses its ability to effectively stabilize vascular endothelium leading to increased vascular permeability. Phenotypic expression is thought to be due to the mechanism of haploinsufficiency in which there is a loss of function in one of the genes coding for a protein that requires both genes to function to have complete function.[22]

In all forms of HAE, except HAE-ANGPT1, bradykinin is the mediator leading to the development of angioedema. Bradykinin binds to and activates the bradykinin B2 receptor on vascular endothelial cells, leading to dissolution of the adherens junctions formed by vascular endothelial-cadherin and loss of integrity of the cell membrane.[23] Under normal conditions, multiple enzymes, collectively known as kininases, quickly metabolize bradykinin. The most important of these enzymes is ACE, which is also known as kininase II. Other kininases include aminopeptidase P, carboxypeptidase M and N, neutral endopeptidase, and dipeptidyl peptidase IV.[24]

CLINICAL PRESENTATION

Clinically, HAE presents with transient asymmetric swelling of subcutaneous and submucosal tissues of the skin as well as the respiratory and gastrointestinal tracts. The subcutaneous swelling is neither pitting nor dependent. HAE is typically not associated with the development of urticaria or pruritus, a feature helpful in distinguishing from angioedema secondary to histamine release. Transient numbness or a tingling sensation in the affected areas has been reported during the prodromal period.[25] Up to one-half of patients with HAE develop a characteristic rash, erythema marginatum, during the prodromal period that is not pruritic but may be confused for an urticarial lesion.[26] Minor trauma and medical procedures, such as dental procedures, may precipitate acute attacks of HAE.[27] Other precipitants include infection and emotional stress. In many instances, an identifiable cause is not found.

The "attacks" of angioedema typically occur earlier in HAE than in acquired C1-INH deficiency (AAE-C1-INH). The symptoms of HAE develop at a median age of 12.5 years,[8] whereas AAE-C1-INH typically develops after the fourth decade of life.[28] In AAE-C1-INH, the lack of appropriate levels of functioning C1-INH develops secondary to the development of some other process, usually an autoimmune or malignant (often B-cell lymphoproliferative disorders or monoclonal gammopathy of undetermined significance) process.

The characteristic presentation of a patient presenting with an attack of HAE is pronounced swelling of the extremities, face, and oropharyngeal structures. Involvement of the upper airway may lead to obstruction and is a significant cause of morbidity and mortality in patients with HAE. Patients may present with complaints of tongue swelling, difficulty speaking and hoarseness, difficulty swallowing, and shortness of breath. Vital sign abnormalities may include tachycardia and hypotension secondary to third spacing. On physical examination, the patient may be noted to have voice change, difficulty tolerating secretions, and difficulty breathing. The extremities and face may be visually swollen. Clinical findings associated with need for definitive airway management include voice change, hoarseness, stridor, and dyspnea.[29,30] Isolated swelling of the genitals may be the only manifestation of an HAE attack.[31,32] Any structure in the oropharynx and deeper upper respiratory tract may show signs of edema, and up to 50% of patients with HAE will experience laryngeal edema at some point.[33] The risk of asphyxiation is higher in patients with undiagnosed HAE than in those that have correctly been diagnosed.[34]

Although HAE is most recognizable for the disfiguring swelling of the face and extremities, abdominal pain is the most commonly encountered symptom.[30,35] Nausea, vomiting, and sometimes diarrhea will often accompany the development of abdominal pain, which may be described as crampy and colicky. Patients may develop abdominal distention and large-volume ascites. Hypotension and tachycardia may develop because of fluid shifts. Small bowel obstruction and intussusception are reported complications of angioedema of the bowel wall.[36,37] Patients with HAE have a higher likelihood than the general population to undergo abdominal surgery. A survey of German patients found that patients with HAE had a rate of appendectomy that was double that of those who did not have HAE (37.7% vs 18.9%).[38] Exploratory laparotomy may be performed when the diagnosis of HAE attack is not considered.[39,40] Recurrent bouts of unexplained abdominal pain may be the presenting feature in some cases of patients who were previously not diagnosed with HAE. The emergency provider should consider HAE in the differential diagnosis of patients presenting with recurrent abdominal pain.

DIAGNOSTIC EVALUATION
Laboratory Testing

In the ED, there is a limited role for laboratory testing. Most laboratory tests that are useful in the setting of HAE have long turnaround times such that the results of these tests are not available during the time that the patient is in the ED. There may be some value in sending certain tests during the ED visit, as the discriminatory value of these tests is best during an acute attack of angioedema. Such tests will be extremely helpful during follow-up appointments with an allergist.

The complement component 4 (C4) level is the most cost-effective screening test for HAE.[41] Decreases in the levels of C4 are not directly responsible for the increases in bradykinin levels that cause angioedema, but it serves as an indicator that there is a problem in the complement pathway. As described in the Classification and Pathophysiology section above, C1-INH is involved in multiple steps of the complement, fibrinolytic, and the contact activating systems. The first step in the classical complement pathway after activation of the C1 complex is the cleavage of C4 and then C2 to generate C4b and C2b, which together form C3 convertase.[42] This step is normally inhibited in the presence of C1-INH. Most cases of HAE are due to mutations in the SERPING1 gene that encodes the C1-INH protein. Therefore, in most cases, the level of C4 will be low during an acute attack; however, during normal periods, the sensitivity of C4 is decreased to between 81% and 96%.[43–45]

Quantitative and functional measurements of C1-INH antigen are used to confirm or exclude the diagnosis of HAE and to differentiate HAE-C1-INH type 1 from type 2. C1-INH antigenic levels are quantified by radial immunodiffusion (RID), turbidimetry, or nephelometry methods.[46] The method of testing is determined by local laboratory test demands and cost considerations. The choice can have substantial impact on the time to result, as the RID method is more time consuming.[47] In HAE-C1-INH type 1, both the quantitative and the functional levels are less than 50% of normal. Results of C1-INH testing in infants and pregnant women should be interpreted with caution, as C1-INH production does not reach normal rates until after the age of 1 year and because of the transient decrease in C1-INH quantity resulting from the increase in plasma volume normally seen during later stages of pregnancy.[48,49] In HAE-C1-INH type II, quantitative levels of C1-INH are normal or elevated;

however, C1-INH function is decreased. In laboratory measurements, C1-INH function is expressed as a percentage of the value found in normal subjects. In the United States, the only test approved by the FDA to measure C1-INH function is an enzyme-linked immunosorbent assay (ELISA) that measures the ability of C1-INH to bind C1s. For the ELISA test, C1-INH function is classified as abnormal if the percentage of mean normal is 40% or less. It is considered equivocal at 41% to 67% and normal at greater than 67% of mean normal.[50] Alternatively, a chromogenic assay directly measures the ability of C1-INH to inhibit the C1 complex. Measurements less than 70% are considered abnormally low.[51] Recent guidelines from the US Hereditary Angioedema Association Medical Board recommend chromogenic testing if initial testing is equivocal.[52] The chromogenic assays are approved for use in Europe, but in the United States, these tests can only be performed for research purposes and in specialist laboratories.[53]

Patients with HAE-nl-C1-INH have normal levels of C4, C1-INH antigen, and C1-INH function. Most cases are due to a genetic defect in the gene encoding for FXII. A commercially available polymerase chain reaction test is available to identify these mutations.[54] Specialized genetic testing is required for cases of HAE-nl-C1-INH due to mutations in the genes for plasminogen, high- and low-molecular-weight kininogen, or angiopoietin-1. Informed consent from the patient is required for all types of genetic testing.

In contrast to HAE, patients who are not born with deficiencies in C1-INH owing to genetics but develop a deficiency later in life are diagnosed with AAE-C1-INH. The underlying cause of this deficiency is due to the development of autoantibodies to C1-INH, increased consumption of C1-INH owing to increased activation of the pathways where C1-INH is involved, or some combination of these 2 mechanisms. At one point, AAE-C1-INH was classified as type I (overconsumption) and type II (destruction by autoantibodies). The subsequent understanding that there was significant contribution by both mechanisms in many cases of AAE-C1-INH has led to this classification falling out of favor.[55] Cases of AAE-C1-INH usually have low levels of C4, C1-INH antigen, and C1-INH function. It can often be distinguished from HAE-C1-INH through testing for concentration of C1q. The level of C1q will be normal in cases of HAE-C1-INH, whereas in AAE-C1-INH the levels are low when there is activation of the classical pathway of the complement system. Detection of autoantibodies to C1-INH is helpful to make the diagnosis of AAE-C1-INH, but they are found in only about 70% of cases.[54]

Radiographic Testing

There is a limited role for radiologic imaging in cases of HAE. Imaging studies may identify the presence of angioedema in locations not visible on physical examination, such as in the case of bowel wall angioedema.[43] This can help establish angioedema as the cause of a patient's presenting complaint. The specific type of angioedema cannot be determined by imaging. In cases of angioedema involving the airway, the use of imaging studies should be done with caution, as the patient may suddenly decompensate while in an area distant from the clinical team and the equipment needed to secure the airway. Use of point-of-care ultrasound imaging has been described for both intestinal[56,57] and upper airway[58] angioedema.

Fiberoptic Nasopharyngoscopy

In patients who have angioedema involving the tongue, soft palate, or floor of the mouth, the use of fiberoptic nasopharyngoscopy to help identify the presence of swelling of the deeper upper airway structures is recommended in consensus guidelines endorsed by the American College of Allergy, Asthma, and Immunology and the Society for Academic Emergency Medicine.[59] Before performing any evaluation of the deeper upper airway structures, preparation for intubation should be performed because of the potential for worsening angioedema from minor trauma. The findings from a nasopharyngoscopic examination help to categorize a patient according to the Ishoo Staging System or Chiu Classification (see section entitled Airway Management).[29,60]

MEDICAL MANAGEMENT

The 3 therapeutic strategies for HAE are focused on long-term prophylaxis, short-term prophylaxis, and on-demand treatment of acute attacks. Before 2009 in the United States, there were no approved treatments for acute attacks of HAE. In the past, long-term prophylaxis was limited to treatment with an attenuated androgen, such as danazol, or an antifibrinolytic, such as ε-aminocaproic acid (EACA). Attenuated androgens and antifibrinolytics are now considered second-line therapies for long-term prophylaxis with the approval of new medications over the last decade.[57] With the approval of a plasma-derived C1-INH concentrate (pd-C1-INH) for HAE prophylaxis in 2008, there have been numerous advances in the treatment of this disease.[61] HAE treatments generally target 3 areas in the pathway of bradykinin formation: replacement of C1-INH, inhibition of bradykinin formation through the inhibition of kallikrein, and antagonism of the bradykinin B2 receptor. Steroids, antihistamines, and epinephrine are considered ineffective in the treatment of bradykinin-mediated angioedema, such as HAE.[62] A major advance in the treatment of HAE is approval of self-administered on-demand treatment. Currently, it is recommended that patients with HAE should have access to 2 doses of on-demand medication that can be self-administered in the event of an acute attacks of HAE.[57]

Replacement of C1-Esterase Inhibitor

The discovery by Donaldson and Evans[63] in 1963 that HAE was the result of a deficiency in C1-INH provided the rationale for replacement therapy to treat this disease. The use of pd-C1-INH was first described in 1973, where it was given to 2 patients with one showing a decrease in the usual time of resolution of an acute attack.[64] Following that, there were multiple other reports demonstrating the efficacy of C1-INH replacement therapy for acute attacks[65–67] as well as for prophylaxis. An intravenous form of pd-C1-INH was first approved for use in Germany in 1979.[68] Currently, there are 3 formulations of pd-C1-INH available in the United States: Berinert (CSL Behring, Marburg, Germany), Cinryze (Takeda, Lexington, MA, USA), and Haegarda (CSL Behring, King of Prussia, PA, USA).

In October 2008, Cinryze became the first of a series of new treatments for HAE when the FDA approved its use in adults and adolescents for prophylaxis against HAE attacks. Initial approval was based on the data from 2 studies that were published in a single article. In the first study, 65 subjects were included for analysis, which showed there was a shorter time to unequivocal relief for Cinryze at a fixed dose of 1000 U versus placebo (2 hours vs 4 hours; $P = .02$). The second study was a cross-over trial that enrolled 22 subjects to receive twice-weekly injections of Cinryze for two 12-week periods whereby the subjects served as their own controls. Patients who were treated with Cinryze had a decrease in the number of attacks per study period (6.26 attacks vs 12.73 attacks; $P<.001$).[69] The FDA expanded the indication for Cinryze to include pediatric patients over the age of 6 in 2018.[70]

The industry-funded IMPACT (International Multi-centre Prospective Angioedema C1-Inhibitor Trials) studies were conducted in the United States to determine the efficacy of Berinert (pd-C1-INH produced by CSL Behring) in the treatment of acute attacks of HAE. The IMPACT-1 trial was a randomized double-blind placebo-controlled study of 125 subjects that compared intravenous Berinert at doses of 10 or 20 U/kg with placebo. The 10-U/kg dose was not found to be effective, but the 20-U/kg dose shortened the time to onset of symptom relief (0.5 hours vs 1.5 hours, $P = .0025$).[71] An open-label, uncontrolled extension study was performed (IMPACT-2) whereby Berinert was used to treat 1085 episodes in 57 patients. The median time to onset of symptom relief was 0.46 hours.[72] Berinert received FDA approval in 2009 for the treatment of acute abdominal, facial, or laryngeal attacks of HAE in adult and adolescent patients. The FDA approved expanded labeling in 2012 to include self-administration of Berinert for the treatment of acute laryngeal attacks.[73]

Conestat alfa, distributed under the brand name Ruconest, is a recombinant human C1-INH (rhC1-INH) made from the milk of transgenic rabbits that undergoes extensive posttranslational glycosylation that decreases the mean plasma half-life from 33 hours to 3 hours as compared with pdC1-INH.[74,75] The decrease in the plasma half-life does not appear to decrease the ability of rhC1-INH to treat acute attacks of HAE, as multiple studies have demonstrated its effectiveness.[76-79] Pooled data from early trials demonstrated that median time to the onset of symptom relief was 67 minutes and that 91.1% of subjects with upper airway symptoms had onset of relief by 4 hours.[80] Ruconest was demonstrated to have a sustained effect despite having a relatively short half-life in a pooled post hoc analysis of 2 trials whereby relapse of symptoms occurred in no patients at 24 hours and 7.1% at 72 hours.[81] The FDA approved Ruconest in 2014 for use in adults and adolescents for acute HAE attacks not involving laryngeal structures. It is contraindicated in patients with an allergy to rabbits or rabbit-derived products.[82] The European requirement that patients are screened with a rabbit-specific immunoglobulin E (IgE) immunoassay before administration of Ruconest was removed in 2016.[83] Additional studies have evaluated the use of rhC1-INH for both short- and long-term prophylaxis of HAE; however, it is not currently approved for this indication in the United States.[84-86]

In 2017, the FDA approved Haegarda for subcutaneous administration as long-term prophylaxis. Evidence supporting this came from the COMPACT (Clinical Study for Optimal Management of Preventing Angioedema with Low-Volume Subcutaneous C1-Inhibitor Replacement Therapy) trial, a randomized, placebo-controlled study with crossover design that enrolled 90 patients to receive pdC1-INH at 40 or 60 IU/kg every 3 to 4 days versus placebo. For the group treated with 60 IU/kg, the normalized attack rate was 0.52 per month, whereas the rate was 4.03 per month in the placebo group.[87] A post hoc analysis of the data from the COMPACT study demonstrated that there were improvements in measures of quality of life for patients receiving either dose of the study drug compared with placebo.[88] An open-label, extension study enrolled patients who completed the COMPACT trial and had high attack frequency before enrollment in the original study. This demonstrated continued efficacy and safety of subcutaneous pdC1-INH.[89] Haegarda is FDA approved for routine prophylaxis to prevent HAE attacks in patients 6 years of age and older.[90]

Kallikrein Inhibition

Ecallantide is a 60-amino-acid recombinant protein produced by the yeast *Pichia pastoris*[91] that functions as a potent and reversible inhibitor of the enzyme kallikrein, preventing it from cleaving bradykinin from HMWK.[92] A series of clinical trials collectively known as the Evaluation of DX-88's Effects in Mitigating Angioedema (EDEMA) studies established the effectiveness of this treatment. The EDEMA0 trial, only published as an abstract, was a phase 2 open-label, dose escalation trial of intravenous ecallantide in 7 patients.[93] The EDEMA1 trial was also a dose escalation trial of intravenous ecallantide but designed as double blind and placebo controlled. Of the different doses of ecallantide studied (5, 10, 20, and 40 mg/m^2), only the 40-mg/m^2 dose was shown to be statistically superior to placebo (P = .0128).[94] The next study, EDEMA2, compared escalating intravenous doses (5, 10, and 20 mg) of ecallantide and a single subcutaneous 30-mg dose. The results of this study were not published but can be obtained in the application to the FDA. The percentage of patients with a response that was considered successful was the highest with the 30-mg subcutaneous dose (82%). The best result for the different intravenous doses was with the 10-mg dose, which had a 68% rate of successful outcomes. Statistical comparisons were not performed.[95] Next, EDEMA3 was a phase 3 randomized, double-blind, placebo-controlled trial whereby patients 10 years of age and older who presented with an acute HAE attack within 8 hours were randomized to receive either ecallantide 30 mg subcutaneously or placebo. Treatment with ecallantide was associated with a significantly higher treatment outcome score at 4 hours compared with placebo.[96] Last, EDEMA4 was also a phase 3 randomized, double-blind, placebo-controlled trial evaluating the use of subcutaneous ecallantide 30 mg versus placebo. The patients who received ecallantide had a greater decrease in the mean symptom complex severity score.[97] A post hoc analysis of multiple ecallantide trials demonstrated that with repeated administration, ecallantide was associated with a 3.5% rate of anaphylaxis.[95] Ecallantide is approved for subcutaneous administration in the United States for the treatment of acute attacks of HAE in patients 12 years of age and older. Because of the risk of anaphylaxis, ecallantide is not approved for self-administration.[98] The application for approval in Europe was withdrawn in 2011.[99]

Lanadelumab, a recombinant human IgG1 monoclonal antibody, is a potent and specific inhibitor of kallikrein that is produced using Chinese hamster ovary cells. Based on the results of a phase 3 trial that showed a reduced frequency of attacks with subcutaneous administration of lanadelumab, it was recently approved in the United States for the prevention of HAE attacks in patients aged ≥12 years. The objective of the Hereditary Angioedema Long-term Prophylaxis (HELP) clinical trial was to determine the efficacy of lanadelumab compared with placebo for preventing attacks of HAE. Three dose regimens were assessed versus placebo: 150 mg every 4 weeks, 300 mg every 4 weeks, and 300 mg every 3 weeks. There was a significant decrease in the number of HAE attacks for each of the 3 lanadelumab doses that were assessed.[100] The benefits were sustained in an open-label extension study. The investigators reported that HAE attack rate was reduced by 87.4% and that 68.9% of subjects treated with 300 mg every 2 weeks had an attack-free period of more than 12 months.[101] The recommended starting dose is 300 mg given subcutaneously every 2 weeks with a reduction in frequency to every 4 weeks if the patient is well controlled without attacks for 6 or more months.[102]

Inhibition of Bradykinin B2 Receptors

Icatibant is a synthetic peptidomimetic drug 10 amino acids in length that is similar in structure to bradykinin, a nonapeptide that functions as a selective inhibitor of the bradykinin B2 receptor, which is responsible for the major effects of bradykinin involved in attacks of HAE. Icatibant has affinity similar to that of bradykinin to the bradykinin B2 receptor but is resistant to enzymatic cleavage because of the substitution of 5 nonproteinogenic amino acids.[103] The efficacy and safety of icatibant were evaluated in 3 randomized, double-blind, controlled clinical trials collectively known as the For Angioedema Subcutaneous Treatment (FAST) studies. The results of the FAST-1 study, which was placebo controlled, and the FAST-2 study, which used the active comparator tranexamic acid (TXA), were published in the same article. The dose of icatibant used for both studies was 30 mg given subcutaneously. In the FAST-2 study, the comparator dose was oral TXA, at a dose of 3 g daily for 2 days. The primary end point for both studies was the median time to clinically significant relief of symptoms. The FAST-1 trial failed to show a statistically significant difference in the primary endpoint for icatibant versus placebo (2.5 hours vs 4.6 hours, P = .014). In the FAST-2 study, the median time to clinically significant relief of symptoms was 2.0 hours for the icatibant group and 12.0 hours for the TXA group (P<.001).[104] The dose chosen for TXA was lower than the dose recommended at that time for use as short-term prophylaxis in HAE.[105] The placebo-controlled FAST-3 study assessed median time to 50% reduction in symptom severity. For the group of patients with cutaneous and abdominal attacks but not involving laryngeal structures, the primary outcome was significantly shorter in the icatibant group compared with placebo (2.0 hours vs 19.8 hours, P<.001). Only 5 patients enrolled in the double-blind study had laryngeal involvement, limiting the comparison to placebo. The 3 patients who received icatibant during this phase of the study had a median time of 2.5 hours to 50% reduction in symptom severity.[106] Icatibant is approved for the treatment of HAE attacks in adult patients 18 years of age and older, including self-administration by the patient.[107] Generic forms of icatibant have now been approved in the United States.[108]

Attenuated Androgens

Attenuated androgens, such as the 17-α-alkylated anabolic steroids danazol and stanozolol, which are dihydrotestosterone derivatives, have been used for decades to reduce the frequency of attacks of HAE. These medications improve the clinical expression of HAE by increasing the amount of C1-INH produced by the liver[109,110] and by increasing expression of C1-INH messenger RNA in circulating monocytes.[111] Because these medications take 1 to 2 days to have any meaningful effect, they are not useful for the treatment of acute attacks.[112] In 1960, Spaulding[113] demonstrated the effectiveness of methyltestosterone therapy. Danazol, which has fewer adverse effects than methyltestosterone, was demonstrated to be effective by Gelfand and colleagues in 1974.[109] Side effects of therapy with attenuated androgens include hirsutism, weight gain, acne, decreased libido, menstrual irregularities, and liver neoplasms.[114] Attenuated androgens should be avoided in prepubescent children because of the risk of premature closure of epiphyseal plates leading to growth retardation.[115] This class should also be avoided in patients with liver disease, patients with androgen-dependent malignancies, and women who are pregnant or lactating.[116] The incidence and severity of side effects are dose dependent, so the lowest clinically effective dose should be used. Protocols have been published to determine the appropriate long-term dosing for danazol.[117,118] A survey of US physicians showed a decrease in the use of attenuated androgens for long-term HAE prophylaxis from 70% in 2010 to 7% in 2019.[119] Attenuated androgens are not recommended for on-demand treatment of an acute attack of HAE.[30]

Antifibrinolytics

The antifibrinolytic medications EACA and its cyclic analogue, TXA, have been used for long-term prophylaxis of HAE, although current data suggest that antifibrinolytics are now rarely used.[8,78] The proposed mechanism of action is inhibition of plasminogen conversion to plasmin leading to decreased activation of FXII.[120] Antifibrinolytics have been used for long-term prophylaxis of HAE since 1972.[121,122] TXA is generally better tolerated than EACA.[73] Because of the possible prothrombotic effect of antifibrinolytics, these should be avoided in patients at increased risk of venous thromboembolism. A report in 2003 of a single center's treatment of HAE patients demonstrated a significant benefit with TXA in only 25% of treated patients.[76] An even more recent study failed to demonstrate any benefit from long-term prophylaxis with TXA.[123] Antifibrinolytics are not recommended for on-demand treatment of an acute attack of HAE.[79]

AIRWAY MANAGEMENT

The major focus of an emergency provider's care of a patient presenting with an HAE attack is ensuring airway patency. In 1999, Ishoo and colleagues[29] proposed a 4-tiered system for use in patients with angioedema owing to any cause to help determine the disposition as well as the need for airway intervention based on the site of swelling (**Table 1**). The stages are based on the anatomic location of the swelling and are not considered sequential. In their study, stridor, change in voice, hoarseness, and dyspnea were found to correlate with a need for airway intervention and admission to an intensive care unit (ICU). Patients with stage I (face, lip) and stage II (soft palate) angioedema were managed as outpatients or hospitalized in non-ICU units. Patients with stage III (tongue) angioedema were managed in the ICU two-thirds of the time. All patients with stage IV (laryngeal) angioedema were treated in an ICU setting. An airway intervention was required in 7% of patients with stage III and 24% of patients with stage IV angioedema. This staging system has not been prospectively validated.[34]

A second classification system was published by Chiu and colleagues[60] in 2001 based on a retrospective analysis of 108 patients with angioedema of any type who presented to 2 tertiary care hospitals (**Table 2**). Most patients included in this analysis had angioedema secondary to ACE inhibitor therapy. There were no patients identified with HAE. Patients were classified as having type 1 if the swelling involved the face and oral cavity but not the floor of the mouth. Type 2 cases had swelling that involved the floor of the mouth and other oropharyngeal structures. In type 3, the oropharyngeal swelling extended to the supraglottic and glottic structures. Rates of intubation were 21.4% and 33.3% for types 2 and 3, respectively.

When a patient with angioedema requires airway management, the treating provider must balance the rapidity with which the airway needs to be secured with the need to prepare for a successful procedure. Before intubation, administration of glycopyrrolate may be useful to decrease secretions, allowing for better visualization of the glottic structures. Rapid sequence intubation, as commonly used by emergency physicians, should not be used initially because paralysis without visualizing the vocal cords could

| Table 1 | | | | | | |
| Ishoo staging of angioedema | | | | | | |
Stage	Site	Episodes (%)	Outpatient (%)	Floor (%)	ICU (%)	Intervention (%)
I	Facial, lip	31	48	52	0	0
II	Soft palate	5	60	40	0	0
III	Tongue	32	26	7	67	7
IV	Laryngeal	31	0	0	100	24

Table 2
Chiu classification of angioedema based on anatomic location[112]

Type	Site	Episodes (%)	Discharged from ED (%)	Floor (%)	ICU (%)	Intubated (%)	Surgical Airway (%)
I	Facial, oral cavity excluding floor of mouth	57.4	69.4	22.6	8.0	0.0	0.0
II	Floor of mouth, oropharyngeal structures (uvula, base of the tongue, and soft palate)	25.9	10.7	28.6	32.1	21.4	7.1
III	Oropharyngeal structures with extension to supraglottic and glottic structures	16.7	5.6	11.1	50.0	33.3	0.0

prove disastrous. Instead, awake intubation allowing the physician to visualize glottic structures may be safer. Noninvasive positive pressure ventilation does not correct a developing anatomic obstruction and should not be considered a temporizing procedure because barotrauma may worsen the angioedema and does not alleviate the underlying problem of airway obstruction. Driver and McGill[124] reviewed the method of intubation for 45 patients with angioedema at a single center. They found that a variety of methods were used, including nasotracheal intubation, video-assisted and direct laryngoscopy, and fiberoptic-assisted nasal and oral methods. A tracheal tube introducer (Bougie) was used in all cases whereby direct and video-assisted laryngoscopy methods were used. The frequency of utilization and success rates of the different methods are likely a reflection of institutional preferences and patient selection bias. The data demonstrate that successful intubation can be performed using a variety of techniques. Physical manipulation of the airway can cause sudden and severe worsening of the swelling. Before any attempt to evaluate or manage the airway, the provider should be prepared to perform a surgical airway, a preparation known as a double setup.[66]

SUMMARY

The ED management of a patient presenting with an acute attack of HAE requires recognition of the disease and careful evaluation for airway involvement. Angioedema itself is a clinical diagnosis of swelling of the subcutaneous and submucosal tissues. Broadly speaking, angioedema is usually caused by either the release of histamine or the presence of bradykinin. Understanding the underlying pathophysiology will help guide medical management with appropriate and effective medications while avoiding treatments that are ineffective and even potentially harmful. There have been major advances in the treatment of HAE since 2008. The cost of these treatments has been very high, so many hospitals may not have HAE-specific medications on formulary. Being aware of what treatment options are available before the critical HAE patient presents to the ED will help with the timely treatment of an acute attack.

CLINICS CARE POINTS

- Patients presenting with recurrent episodes of swelling or unexplained abdominal pain should be considered for evaluation for hereditary angioedema, as there is frequently a multiyear delay in diagnosis from onset of symptoms.

- Patients with hereditary angioedema have a higher likelihood of undergoing abdominal surgeries, which may be avoided if the diagnosis of an acute attack of hereditary angioedema is considered.

- Hereditary angioedema is typically not associated with the development of urticaria or pruritus, a feature helpful in distinguishing from angioedema secondary to histamine release.

- Up to one-half of patients with hereditary angioedema develop a characteristic rash, erythema marginatum, during the prodromal period, which is not pruritic but may be confused for an urticarial lesion.

- Patients with voice change, hoarseness, stridor, and dyspnea are at high risk for needing an airway.

- Patients with acute attacks of hereditary angioedema can be treated with several medications, all of which result in reduced activation of the bradykinin B2 receptor. No study has compared these medications with one another.

- It is recommended to perform fiberoptic nasopharyngoscopy on patients who may be at risk for airway obstruction. The patient should be prepared for intubation, as performing nasopharyngoscopy may result in worsening of the swelling encountered.

DISCLOSURE

The authors have nothing to disclose.

REFERENCES

1. Quincke H. Concerning the acute localized oedema of the skin. Monatsh Prakt Derm 1882;1:129–31.
2. Osler W. Hereditary angio-neurotic oedema. Am J Med Sci 1888;95:362–7.
3. Longhurst H, Cicardi M. Hereditary angio-oedema. Lancet 2012;379(9814): 474–81.
4. Aygören-Pürsün E, Magerl M, Maetzel A, et al. Epidemiology of bradykinin-mediated angioedema: a systematic investigation of epidemiological studies. Orphanet J Rare Dis 2018;13(1):73.
5. Mikami K. Orphans in the market: the history of orphan drug policy. Soc Hist Med 2019;32(3):609–30.
6. Henao MP, Craig TJ, Kraschnewski J, et al. Diagnosis and screening of patients with hereditary angioedema in primary care. Ther Clin Risk Manag 2016;12: 701–11.
7. Tosi M. Molecular genetics of C1 inhibitor. Immunobiology 1998;199(2):358–65.
8. Banerji A, Davis KH, Brown TM, et al. Patient-reported burden of hereditary angioedema: findings from a patient survey in the United States. Ann Allergy Asthma Immunol 2020;124(6):600–7.
9. Bork K, Meng G, Staubach P, et al. Hereditary angioedema: new findings concerning symptoms, affected organs, and course. Am J Med 2006;119(3): 267–74.

10. Nussberger J, Cugno M, Amstutz C, et al. Plasma bradykinin in angio-oedema. Lancet 1998;351(9117):1693–7.
11. Loules G, Zamanakou M, Parsopoulou F, et al. Targeted next-generation sequencing for the molecular diagnosis of hereditary angioedema due to C1-inhibitor deficiency. Gene 2018;667:76–82.
12. Germenis AE, Speletas M. Genetics of hereditary angioedema revisited. Clin Rev Allergy Immunol 2016;51(2):170–82.
13. Späth PJ, Wuthrich B, Bütler R. Quantification of C1-inhibitor functional activities by immunodiffusion assay in plasma of patients with hereditary angioedema–evidence of a functionally critical level of C1-inhibitor concentration. Complement 1984;1(3):147–59.
14. Zuraw BL, Cicardi M, Longhurst HJ, et al. Phase II study results of a replacement therapy for hereditary angioedema with subcutaneous C1-inhibitor concentrate. Allergy 2015;70(10):1319–28.
15. Binkley KE, Davis A. Clinical, biochemical, and genetic characterization of a novel estrogen-dependent inherited form of angioedema. J Allergy Clin Immunol 2000;106(3):546–50.
16. Bork K, Barnstedt SE, Koch P, et al. Hereditary angioedema with normal C1-inhibitor activity in women. Lancet 2000;356(9225):213–7.
17. Bork K, Wulff K, Steinmüller-Magin L, et al. Hereditary angioedema with a mutation in the plasminogen gene. Allergy 2018;73(2):442–50.
18. Dewald G. A missense mutation in the plasminogen gene, within the plasminogen kringle 3 domain, in hereditary angioedema with normal C1 inhibitor. Biochem Biophys Res Commun 2018;498(1):193–8.
19. Bork K, Wulff K, Rossmann H, et al. Hereditary angioedema cosegregating with a novel kininogen 1 gene mutation changing the N-terminal cleavage site of bradykinin. Allergy 2019;343:1286.
20. Bafunno V, Firinu D, D'Apolito M, et al. Mutation of the angiopoietin-1 gene (ANGPT1) associates with a new type of hereditary angioedema. J Allergy Clin Immunol 2018;141(3):1009–17. https://doi.org/10.1016/j.jaci.2017.05.020.
21. Ariano A, D'Apolito M, Bova M, et al. A myoferlin gain-of-function variant associates with a new type of hereditary angioedema. Allergy 2020;75(11):2989–92.
22. D'Apolito M, Santacroce R, Colia AL, et al. Angiopoietin-1 haploinsufficiency affects the endothelial barrier and causes hereditary angioedema. Clin Exp Allergy 2019;49(5):626–35.
23. Bouillet L, PhD TM, Arboleas M, et al. Hereditary angioedema: key role for kallikrein and bradykinin in vascular endothelial-cadherin cleavage and edema formation. J Allergy Clin Immunol 2011;128(1):232–4.
24. Cicardi M, Zuraw BL. Angioedema due to bradykinin dysregulation. J Allergy Clin Immunol Pract 2018;6(4):1132–41.
25. Reshef A, Prematta MJ, Craig TJ. Signs and symptoms preceding acute attacks of hereditary angioedema: results of three recent surveys. Allergy Asthma Proc 2013;34(3):261–6.
26. Maurer M, Magerl M, Ansotegui I, et al. The international WAO/EAACI guideline for the management of hereditary angioedema-the 2017 revision and update. Allergy 2018;73(8):1575–96.
27. Bork K, Hardt J, Staubach-Renz P, et al. Risk of laryngeal edema and facial swellings after tooth extraction in patients with hereditary angioedema with and without prophylaxis with C1 inhibitor concentrate: a retrospective study. Oral Surg Oral Med Oral Pathol Oral Radiol Endod 2011;112(1):58–64.

28. Longhurst HJ, Zanichelli A, Caballero T, et al. Comparing acquired angioedema with hereditary angioedema (types I/II): findings from the Icatibant Outcome Survey. Clin Exp Immunol 2017;188(1):148–53.

29. Ishoo E, Shah UK, Grillone GA, et al. Predicting airway risk in angioedema: staging system based on presentation. Otolaryngol Head Neck Surg 1999;121(3): 263–8.

30. Bentsianov BL, Parhiscar A, Azer M, et al. The role of fiberoptic nasopharyngoscopy in the management of the acute airway in angioneurotic edema. Laryngoscope 2000;110(12):2016–9.

31. Akyuz M, Kaya C, Akdogan MF. A rare cause of recurrent priapism: hereditary angioedema. Andrologia 2015;47(5):600–2.

32. Dhairyawan R, Harrison R, Buckland M, et al. Hereditary angioedema: an unusual cause of genital swelling presenting to a genitourinary medicine clinic. Int J STD AIDS 2011;22(6):356–7.

33. Bork K, Ressel N. Sudden upper airway obstruction in patients with hereditary angioedema. Transfus Apher Sci 2003;29(3):235–8.

34. Bork K, Hardt J, Witzke G. Fatal laryngeal attacks and mortality in hereditary angioedema due to C1-INH deficiency. J Allergy Clin Immunol 2012;130(3):692–7. https://doi.org/10.1016/j.jaci.2012.05.055.

35. Javaud N, Altar A, Fain O, et al. Hereditary angioedema, emergency management of attacks by a call center. Eur J Intern Med 2019;67:42–6.

36. Melendez M, Grosel JM. ACE inhibitor-induced angioedema causing small bowel obstruction. JAAPA 2020;33(8):28–31.

37. Patel N, Suarez LD, Kapur S, et al. Hereditary angioedema and gastrointestinal complications: an extensive review of the literature. Case Reports Immunol 2015;2015(4):1–8.

38. Hahn J, Hoess A, Friedrich DT, et al. Unnecessary abdominal interventions in patients with hereditary angioedema. J Dtsch Dermatol Ges 2018;16(12): 1443–9.

39. De Backer A, De Schepper A, Vandevenne J, et al. CT of angioedema of the small bowel. AJR Am J Roentgenol 2001;176(3):649–52.

40. Fisher AJ, Fleishman MJ, Hancock D. Angioedema of the small bowel: CT appearance. AJR Am J Roentgenol 2000;175(2):554.

41. Manning ME. Hereditary angioedema: differential diagnosis, diagnostic tests, and family screening. Allergy Asthma Proc 2020;41(6):S22–5.

42. Janeway CA Jr, Travers P, Walport M, et al. Immunobiology: the immune system in health and disease. 5th edition. New York: Garland Science; 2001. The complement system and innate immunity. Available at: https://www.ncbi.nlm.nih.gov/books/NBK27100/.

43. Tarzi MD, Hickey A, Förster T, et al. An evaluation of tests used for the diagnosis and monitoring of C1 inhibitor deficiency: normal serum C4 does not exclude hereditary angio-oedema. Clin Exp Immunol 2007;149(3):513–6.

44. Ohsawa I, Honda D, Nagamachi S, et al. Clinical and laboratory characteristics that differentiate hereditary angioedema in 72 patients with angioedema. Allergol Int 2014;63(4):595–602.

45. Zanichelli A, Arcoleo F, Barca MP, et al. A nationwide survey of hereditary angioedema due to C1 inhibitor deficiency in Italy. Orphanet J Rare Dis 2015; 10(1):11–6.

46. Farkas H, Veszeli N, Kajdácsi E, et al. "Nuts and Bolts" of laboratory evaluation of angioedema. Clin Rev Allergy Immunol 2016;51(2):140–51. https://doi.org/10.1007/s12016-016-8539-6.

47. Veronez CL, Grumach AS. Angioedema without urticaria: novel findings which must be measured in clinical setting. Curr Opin Allergy Clin Immunol 2020; 20(3):253–60.
48. Farkas H, Martinez-Saguer I, Bork K, et al. International consensus on the diagnosis and management of pediatric patients with hereditary angioedema with C1 inhibitor deficiency. Allergy 2017;72:300–13.
49. Tanaka H, Tanaka K, Enomoto N, et al. Reference range for C1-esterase inhibitor (C1 INH) in the third trimester of pregnancy. J Perinat Med 2020;49(2):166–9. https://doi.org/10.1515/jpm-2020-0099.
50. Quidel MicroVue C1-Inhibitor Plus EIA Product Insert. Available at: https://www.quidel.com/sites/default/files/product/documents/PIA037003EN00_%2802_20%29_MicroVue_C1_Inhibitor_Plus%20Pkg_Insert.pdf. Accessed December 26, 2020.
51. DiaPharma Technochrom C1-INH Product Insert. Available at: https://diapharma.com/wp-content/uploads/2018/06/5345003-Technochrom-C1-INH-insert-3015600REV020-052018.pdf. Accessed December 26, 2020.
52. Busse PJ, Christiansen SC, Riedl MA, et al. US HAEA Medical Advisory Board 2020 guidelines for the management of hereditary angioedema. J Allergy Clin Immunol Pract 2021;9(1):132–50.e3. https://doi.org/10.1016/j.jaip.2020.08.046.
53. Kaplan AP, Pawaskar D, Chiao J. C1 inhibitor activity and angioedema attacks in patients with hereditary angioedema. J Allergy Clin Immunol Pract 2020;8(3):892–900.
54. Cicardi M, Zanichelli A. Angioedema due to C1 inhibitor deficiency in 2010. Intern Emerg Med 2010;5:481–6.
55. Bouillet-Claveyrolas L, Ponard D, Drouet C, et al. Clinical and biological distinctions between type I and type II acquired angioedema. Am J Med 2003;115(5):420–1.
56. Belkhouribchia J, Backaert T, Neyrinck S. Isolated intestinal angioedema in the emergency department. J Emerg Med 2016;50(4):660–2.
57. Riguzzi C, Losonczy L, Teismann N, et al. Gastrointestinal manifestations of hereditary angioedema diagnosed by ultrasound in the emergency department. West J Emerg Med 2014;15(7):816–8.
58. Schick M, Grether-Jones K. Point-of-care sonographic findings in acute upper airway edema. West J Emerg Med 2016;17(6):822–6.
59. Moellman JJ, Bernstein JA, Lindsell C, et al. A consensus parameter for the evaluation and management of angioedema in the emergency department. Acad Emerg Med 2014;21(4):469–84.
60. Chiu AG, Newkirk KA, Davidson BJ, et al. Angiotensin-converting enzyme inhibitor-induced angioedema: a multicenter review and an algorithm for airway management. Ann Otol Rhinol Laryngol 2001;110(9):834–40.
61. Wilkerson RG. Angioedema in the emergency department: an evidence-based review. Emerg Med Pract 2012;14(11):1–24.
62. Busse PJ, Christiansen SC. Hereditary angioedema. N Engl J Med 2020; 382(12):1136–48.
63. Donaldson VH, Evans RR. A biochemical abnormality in hereditary angioneurotic edema: absence of serum inhibitor of C' 1-esterase. Am J Med 1963; 35(1):37–44.
64. Brackertz D, Kueppers F. Hereditary angioneurotic oedema. Lancet 1973; 2(7830):680.
65. Marasini B, Cicardi M, Martignoni GC, et al. Treatment of hereditary angioedema. Klin Wochenschr 1978;56(16):819–23.

66. Gadek JE, Hosea SW, Gelfand JA, et al. Replacement therapy in hereditary angioedema: successful treatment of acute episodes of angioedema with partly purified C1 inhibitor. N Engl J Med 1980;302(10):542–6.
67. Agostoni A, Bergamaschini L, Martignoni G, et al. Treatment of acute attacks of hereditary angioedema with C1-inhibitor concentrate. Ann Allergy 1980;44(5): 299–301.
68. Aygören-Pürsün E, Bas M, Biedermann T, et al. Guideline: hereditary angioedema due to C1 inhibitor deficiency. Allergo J Int 2019;28(1):1–14.
69. Zuraw BL, Busse PJ, White M, et al. Nanofiltered C1 inhibitor concentrate for treatment of hereditary angioedema. N Engl J Med 2010;363(6):513–22.
70. Package Insert: Cinryze.. Available at: https://www.fda.gov/media/75907/download. Accessed December 28, 2020.
71. Craig TJ, Levy RJ, Wasserman RL, et al. Efficacy of human C1 esterase inhibitor concentrate compared with placebo in acute hereditary angioedema attacks. J Allergy Clin Immunol 2009;124(4):801–8.
72. Craig TJ, Bewtra AK, Bahna SL, et al. C1 esterase inhibitor concentrate in 1085 hereditary angioedema attacks - final results of the I.M.P.A.C.T.2 study. Allergy 2011;66(12):1604–11.
73. Caballero T, Sala-Cunill A, Cancian M, et al. Current status of implementation of self-administration training in various regions of Europe, Canada and the USA in the management of hereditary angioedema. Int Arch Allergy Immunol 2013; 161(Suppl 1):10–6.
74. Martinez-Saguer I, Rusicke E, Aygören-Pürsün E, et al. Pharmacokinetic analysis of human plasma–derived pasteurized C1-inhibitor concentrate in adults and children with hereditary angioedema: a prospective study. Transfusion 2010;50(2):354–60.
75. van Doorn MBA, Burggraaf J, van Dam T, et al. A phase I study of recombinant human C1 inhibitor in asymptomatic patients with hereditary angioedema. J Allergy Clin Immunol 2005;116(4):876–83.
76. Zuraw B, Cicardi M, Levy RJ, et al. Recombinant human C1-inhibitor for the treatment of acute angioedema attacks in patients with hereditary angioedema. J Allergy Clin Immunol 2010;126(4):821–7.
77. Moldovan D, Reshef A, Fabiani J, et al. Efficacy and safety of recombinant human C1-inhibitor for the treatment of attacks of hereditary angioedema: European open-label extension study. Clin Exp Allergy 2012;42(6):929–35.
78. Riedl MA, Bernstein JA, Li H, et al. Recombinant human C1-esterase inhibitor relieves symptoms of hereditary angioedema attacks: phase 3, randomized, placebo-controlled trial. Ann Allergy Asthma Immunol 2014;112(2):163–9.e1.
79. Riedl MA, Levy RJ, Suez D, et al. Efficacy and safety of recombinant C1 inhibitor for the treatment of hereditary angioedema attacks: a North American open-label study. Ann Allergy Asthma Immunol 2013;110(4):295–9.
80. Riedl MA, Li HH, Cicardi M, et al. Recombinant human C1 esterase inhibitor for acute hereditary angioedema attacks with upper airway involvement. Allergy Asthma Proc 2017;38(6):462–6.
81. Bernstein JA, Relan A, Harper JR, et al. Sustained response of recombinant human C1 esterase inhibitor for acute treatment of hereditary angioedema attacks. Ann Allergy Asthma Immunol 2017;118(4):452–5.
82. Package insert: Ruconest. Available at: https://www.fda.gov/media/89212/download. Accessed December 28, 2020.
83. CHMP assessment report on an extension of Marketing Authorisation: Ruconest. Available at: https://www.ema.europa.eu/en/documents/variation-report/

ruconest-h-c-1223-x-0034-epar-assessment-report-variation_en.pdf. Accessed December 28, 2020.

84. Reshef A, Moldovan D, Obtulowicz K, et al. Recombinant human C1 inhibitor for the prophylaxis of hereditary angioedema attacks: a pilot study. Allergy 2012; 68(1):118–24.

85. Valerieva A, Staevska M, Jesenak M, et al. Recombinant human C1 esterase inhibitor as short-term prophylaxis in patients with hereditary angioedema. J Allergy Clin Immunol Pract 2020;8(2):799–802.

86. Riedl MA, Grivcheva-Panovska V, Moldovan D, et al. Recombinant human C1 esterase inhibitor for prophylaxis of hereditary angio-oedema: a phase 2, multi-centre, randomised, double-blind, placebo-controlled crossover trial. Lancet 2017;390(10102):1595–602.

87. Longhurst H, Cicardi M, Craig TJ, et al. Prevention of hereditary angioedema attacks with a subcutaneous C1 inhibitor. N Engl J Med 2017;376(12):1131–40.

88. Lumry WR, Craig TJ, Zuraw B, et al. Health-related quality of life with subcutaneous C1-inhibitor for prevention of attacks of hereditary angioedema. J Allergy Clin Immunol Pract 2018;6(5):1733–41.e.3.

89. Craig TJ, Zuraw B, Longhurst H, et al. Long-term outcomes with subcutaneous C1-inhibitor replacement therapy for prevention of hereditary angioedema attacks. J Allergy Clin Immunol Pract 2019;7(6):1793–802.e2.

90. Package insert: Haegarda. Available at: https://www.fda.gov/media/105611/download. Accessed December 29, 2020.

91. Craig TJ, Li HH, Riedl M, et al. Characterization of anaphylaxis after ecallantide treatment of hereditary angioedema attacks. J Allergy Clin Immunol Pract 2015; 3(2):206–12.e4.

92. Frank MM, Jiang H. New therapies for hereditary angioedema: disease outlook changes dramatically. J Allergy Clin Immunol 2008;121(1):272–80.

93. Cicardi M, Gonzalez-Quevedo T, Caballero T, et al. DX-88 a recombinant inhibitor of human plasma kallikrein. Efficacy and safety in hereditary and acquired angioedema. Mol Immunol 2003;40:197.

94. Schneider L, Lumry W, Vegh A, et al. Critical role of kallikrein in hereditary angioedema pathogenesis: a clinical trial of ecallantide, a novel kallikrein inhibitor. J Allergy Clin Immunol 2007;120(2):416–22.

95. FDA/Center for Drug Evaluation and Research (CDER) application number 125277 summary review.. Available at: https://www.accessdata.fda.gov/drugsatfda_docs/nda/2009/125277s000SumR.pdf. Accessed December 29, 2020.

96. Cicardi M, Levy RJ, McNeil DL, et al. Ecallantide for the treatment of acute attacks in hereditary angioedema. N Engl J Med 2010;363(6):523–31.

97. Levy RJ, Lumry WR, McNeil DL, et al. EDEMA4: a phase 3, double-blind study of subcutaneous ecallantide treatment for acute attacks of hereditary angioedema. Ann Allergy Asthma Immunol 2010;104(6):523–9.

98. Bhardwaj N, Craig TJ. Treatment of hereditary angioedema: a review (CME). Transfusion 2014;54(11):2989–96 [quiz: 2988].

99. Nicola S, Rolla G, Brussino L. Breakthroughs in hereditary angioedema management: a systematic review of approved drugs and those under research. Drugs Context 2019;8:212605–11.

100. Banerji A, Bernstein JA, Martinez-Saguer I, et al. Effect of lanadelumab compared with placebo on prevention of hereditary angioedema attacks: a randomized clinical trial. JAMA 2018;320(20):2108–21.

101. Banerji A, Hao J, Ming Y, et al. Long-term efficacy and safety of lanadelumab: final results from the HELP Open-Label Extension Study. ACAAI 2020.

102. Package insert: Takhzyro. Available at: https://www.accessdata.fda.gov/drugsatfda_docs/label/2018/761090s000lbl.pdf. Accessed December 30, 2020.

103. Charignon D, Späth P, Martin L, et al. Icatibant, the bradykinin B2 receptor antagonist with target to the interconnected kinin systems. Expert Opin Pharmacother 2012;13(15):2233–47.

104. Cicardi M, Banerji A, Bracho F, et al. Icatibant, a new bradykinin-receptor antagonist, in hereditary angioedema. N Engl J Med 2010;363(6):532–41.

105. Bowen T, Cicardi M, Farkas H, et al. International consensus algorithm for the diagnosis, therapy and management of hereditary angioedema. Allergy Asthma Clin Immunol 2010;6(1):24.

106. Lumry WR, Li HH, Levy RJ, et al. Randomized placebo-controlled trial of the bradykinin B2 receptor antagonist icatibant for the treatment of acute attacks of hereditary angioedema: the FAST-3 trial. Ann Allergy Asthma Immunol 2011; 107(6):529–37. https://doi.org/10.1016/j.anai.2011.08.015.

107. Package insert: Firazyr. Available at: https://www.accessdata.fda.gov/drugsatfda_docs/label/2011/022150s000lbl.pdf. Accessed December 30, 2020.

108. FDA 2019 first generic approvals.. Available at: https://www.fda.gov/drugs/first-generic-drug-approvals/2019-first-generic-drug-approvals. Accessed December 30, 2020.

109. Gelfand JAJ, Sherins RJR, Alling DWD, et al. Treatment of hereditary angioedema with danazol. Reversal of clinical and biochemical abnormalities. N Engl J Med 1976;295(26):1444–8.

110. Sheffer AL, Fearon DT, Austen KF. Clinical and biochemical effects of stanozolol therapy for hereditary angioedema. J Allergy Clin Immunol 1981;68(3):181–7.

111. Pappalardo E, Zingale LC, Cicardi M. Increased expression of C1-inhibitor mRNA in patients with hereditary angioedema treated with Danazol. Immunol Lett 2003;86(3):271–6.

112. Zuraw BL. HAE therapies: past present and future. Allergy Asthma Clin Immunol 2010;6(1):23.

113. Spaulding WB. Methyltestosterone therapy for hereditary episodic edema (hereditary angioneurotic edema). Ann Intern Med. 1960;53:739–45.

114. Bowen T, Cicardi M, Farkas H, et al. Canadian 2003 International Consensus Algorithm for the Diagnosis, Therapy, and Management of Hereditary Angioedema. J Allergy Clin Immunol 2004;114(3):629–37.

115. Shahidi NT. A review of the chemistry, biological action, and clinical applications of anabolic-androgenic steroids. Clin Ther 2001;23(9):1355–90.

116. Farkas H. Current pharmacotherapy of bradykinin-mediated angioedema. Expert Opin Pharmacother 2013;14(5):571–86.

117. Cicardi M, Zingale L. How do we treat patients with hereditary angioedema. Transfus Apher Sci 2003;29(3):221–7.

118. Farkas H, Harmat G, Füst G, et al. Clinical management of hereditary angioedema in children. Pediatr Allergy Immunol 2002;13(3):153–61.

119. Riedl MA, Banerji A, Gower R. Current medical management of hereditary angioedema: Follow-up survey of US physicians. Ann Allergy Asthma Immunol. 2021;126(3):264–72.

120. Wahn V, Aberer W, Aygören-Pürsün E, et al. Hereditary angioedema in children and adolescents - a consensus update on therapeutic strategies for German-speaking countries. Pediatr Allergy Immunol 2020;31(8):974–89.
121. Sheffer AL, Austen KF, Rosen FS. Tranexamic acid therapy in hereditary angioneurotic edema. N Engl J Med 1972;287:452–4.
122. Blohmé G. Treatment of hereditary angioneurotic oedema with tranexamic acid. A random double-blind cross-over study. Acta Med Scand 1972;192:293–8.
123. Zanichelli A, Vacchini R, Badini M, et al. Standard care impact on angioedema because of hereditary C1 inhibitor deficiency: a 21-month prospective study in a cohort of 103 patients. Allergy 2010;66(2):192–6.
124. Driver BE, Mcgill JW. Emergency department airway management of severe angioedema: a video review of 45 intubations. Ann Emerg Med 2017;69(5):635–9.

Mimics of Allergy and Angioedema

Scombroid, Mast Cell Activation Disorders, and Hereditary Alpha Tryptasemia

Elizabeth G. Thomas, MD*, Daniel James Thomas, MD

KEYWORDS

- Scombroid • Mastocytosis • Hereditary alpha tryptasemia • Anaphylaxis
- Mast cells • Histamine • Tryptase

KEY POINTS

- Scombroid generally presents 1 to 2 hours after fish ingestion with flushing and a truncal, noncentral clearing rash.
- Anaphylaxis in patients with systemic mastocytosis presents with flushing, hypotension, syncope, and cardiac arrest.
- Patients with systemic mastocytosis with anaphylaxis usually need repeat doses of epinephrine and oftentimes require an epinephrine infusion.
- Several medications commonly used in critical care and emergency medicine should be avoided in patients with systemic mastocytosis because they lead to mast cell degranulation and an anaphylactoid reaction.
- Hereditary alpha tryptasemia is an inherited disorder leading to increased tryptase level and increased allergic events.

INTRODUCTION

True anaphylaxis has several doppelgängers. They so closely resemble true anaphylaxis because they use at least some of the same substrate or product by which symptoms arise. For example, the rash seen with scombroid poisoning is due to the ingestion of exogenous histamine from eating improperly stored fish; the very same effector for the increased vascular permeability and dilation seen with a type I hypersensitivity reaction most often seen in allergic reactions. Hereditary alpha tryptasemia (HaT) is a recently discovered autosomal dominant disorder where there is excess

This article originally appeared in Emergency Medicine Clinics, Volume 40 Issue 1, February 2022.

Department of Emergency Medicine, Ochsner Medical Center, 1514 Jefferson Highway, Jefferson, New Orleans, LA 70121, USA

* Corresponding author.

E-mail address: elizabeth.thomas@ochsner.org

endogenous tryptase, another key player in the innate immune system and hypersensitivity reactions. Systemic mastocytosis (SM) encompasses a wide range of disorders that are due to uncontrolled replication of mast cells and is still being characterized and intensely researched. Because mast cells are the factories that make, store, and release the mediators that lead to allergic reactions' clinical manifestations, it is logical that a disorder based on continuous proliferation of mast cells would lead to a more severe but otherwise similar presentation and requires adjustment in management. It is important for the practicing clinician to be knowledgeable of these mimickers and understand the key distinctions.

SCOMBROID

Scombroid toxicity is a common allergy mimic that results from eating poorly stored fish rich in histamine. The ingestion of high concentration of histamine can lead to severe flushing, rash, headache, and diarrhea. Generally, it presents within an hour of ingestion and is easily treated with antihistamines. Symptoms are rarely fatal. However, it is important to understand and identify this mimic of anaphylaxis and be able to differentiate it from true anaphylaxis.

Epidemiology

Scombroid toxicity is fairly common, with 379 outbreaks noted between 1990 and 2007.[1] In the most recent US report from 2017, scombroid in fish was the most common individual toxin responsible for food-borne outbreaks.[2] That year alone there were 17 outbreaks in the United States with 58 reported cases. There were no deaths. In one of the largest epidemiologic studies done on the subject, of the 61 people surveyed after exposure, only 8 were referred to the emergency department for further care, and none were admitted.[3]

This toxicity is often caused by mackerel, albacore, bonito, and skipjack species of fish.[4] These species are within the Scombroidae family of fish, which is where the disease derives its name. It is also found in other families of fish including salmon, mahimahi, swordfish, and tilapia.[5]

Pathogenesis

Scombroid is caused by improper storage of fish after they are caught. These species of fish are rich in histidine. Several bacteria can produce histamine from histidine via histidine decarboxylase. The most common culprit is *Escherichia coli*, but other agents include Vibrio, Proteus, Serratia, Enterobacter, Klebsiella, Clostridium, Salmonella, and Shigella. When the fish are not properly cooled, there is an overgrowth of these bacteria and thus overproduction of histamine.

The exact role of histamine in scombroid toxicity is not understood. Nevertheless, histamine levels are used as a marker for the level of toxicity, as a more precise measurement has not been discovered.[6] It takes less than 2 hours of storage at temperatures greater than 20 °C to reach levels of histamine that can trigger symptoms.[7] Although cooking the fish kills the bacteria, it does not affect the histamine that is already produced, as histamine is stable to heating and freezing. Many victims report a peppery or spicy taste that is otherwise unexpected.

Presentation and Diagnosis

Normally the patient will present within 1 to 2 hours of eating seafood, which may be discovered from careful history taking. Patients with scombroid poisoning can present with a variety of symptoms, but most commonly present with a rash (**Table 1**). It is an

Table 1 Scombroid signs and symptoms	
Mild	Facial and truncal rash Flushing Headache Nausea and vomiting Diarrhea
Moderate	Palpitations Shortness of breath Headache Blurry vision
Severe (rare)	Bronchoconstriction Hypotension Myocardial ischemia

erythematous, urticarial rash that starts on the head and face and progresses to the trunk.[8] It is without the central clearing which may be seen in classic anaphylaxis (Fig. 1). Patients with scombroid often feel flushing as well as nausea, vomiting, diarrhea, and abdominal cramping. More severe cases can include palpitations, shortness of breath, severe headache, and blurry vision. There have been documented cases of severe hypotension, bronchospasm, and myocardial ischemia related to severe scombroid poisoning.[9–11]

Laboratory tests are generally unrevealing. A serum histamine level will be elevated 2 to 4 times the normal limit; however, this is rarely helpful or available in the acute clinical setting. As such, this is usually a clinical diagnosis. Most symptoms resolve within 24 hours, and there are few long-term side effects. Patients who take antihistamines may have some level of protection. Patients who use monoamine oxidase inhibitors and isoniazid are more vulnerable.[4]

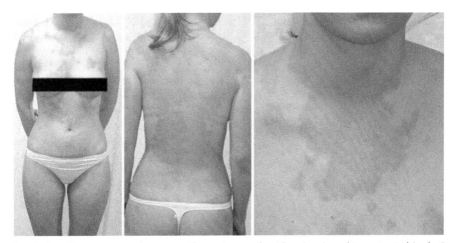

Fig. 1. Exanthem commonly seen with acute scombroid poisoning. (From Jantschitsch C, Kinaciyan T, Manafi M et al. Severe scombroid fish poisoning: An underrecognized dermatologic emergency. Journal of the American Academy of Dermatology, 2011-07-01, Volume 65, Issue 1, Pages 246–247.)

Management

As stated earlier, most cases of scombroid poisoning are nonfatal. Still, it is important to assess ABCs first.

Be prepared for angioedema (in the case of actual anaphylaxis or other mimics) and difficult intubation. If there are symptoms of bronchoconstriction, consider beta agonists. Support any hypotension with fluids and, if necessary, vasopressors.

For most cases of mild scombroid, the patient will improve with supportive care and oral diphenhydramine. Most cases resolve within 30 minutes of treatment. If a patient has severe nausea, cramping, or cannot tolerate oral medications, consider parenteral diphenhydramine.[12] Some patients who continue to have symptoms will benefit from H_2 blockers.[13] If a patient has severe diarrhea, consider intravenous fluids.

If symptoms are controlled, most patients are stable for discharge. Occasionally patients with more severe symptoms or those recalcitrant to treatment may require observation.

Because this toxicity is often due to poorly stored fish, patients are often part of larger outbreaks.[3,7] Clinicians should report any cases to the local health department to help trace the source and prevent further outbreak.

Clinical Care Points

- Scombroid toxicity is related to histamine from improperly stored fish.
- Patients often present 1 to 2 hours after ingestion with flushing, rash, nausea, and vomiting.
- It is usually mild and treatable with antihistamines.
- Occasionally it can be more dangerous, and clinicians should prepare as they do for anaphylaxis.

MAST CELL ACTIVATION DISORDERS
Introduction

Mast cell activation disorders are characterized by excessive mast cells in one or more tissues. SM is the most common form in adulthood, although it is still considered rare. It is thought to be underrecognized because signs and symptoms are often attributed or secondary to another condition. The incidence is ultimately unknown, but it has been estimated to be between 1:1000 and 2:100,000.[14]

Definitions

Until recently, mast cell activation disorders were considered to be a group of myeloproliferative disorders. In 2016, the World Health Organization (WHO) characterized it as its own distinctive group.[15,16] It is now divided into cutaneous mastocytosis (CM), indolent SM (ISM), smoldering SM, SM with an associated hematological neoplasm, aggressive SM, mast cell leukemia, and mast cell sarcoma. Additional subcategories have been further delineated.[16] These divisions and subcategories confer distinct information for an otherwise broad range in morbidity and mortality. Over the last few years, there have been several developments in understanding these differences, their relationship to prognosis, and targeting specific therapies.

Nature of the Problem

These disorders can begin in either childhood or adulthood. The childhood form is generally benign. Involvement typically begins before the age of 2 years, is most often limited to the skin (CM), and most cases will resolve spontaneously by adulthood. If the disease does not resolve by adulthood, the patient will then have the same risk for

Table 2
Features of mastocytosis based on age of onset

	Adult-Onset Mastocytosis	Child-Onset Mastocytosis
Most common form	ISM	CM
Typical course	Chronic	Temporary
Tryptase level (ng/mL)	>20	<20
Typical location of KIT mutation	Exon 17, most frequently D816V	Exon 8, 9, 11, 17, or absent
Most frequent type of skin lesions	Monomorphic maculopapular	Polymorphic maculopapular
Typical size of skin lesions	Small	Large
Typical distribution of skin lesions	Thigh, trunk	Trunk, head, extremities

Adapted from Hartmann K, Escribano L, Grattan C, et al. Cutaneous manifestations in patients with mastocytosis: Consensus report of the European Competence Network on Mastocytosis; the American Academy of Allergy, Asthma & Immunology; and the European Academy of Allergology and Clinical Immunology. *J Allergy Clin Immunol.* 2016;137(1):35 to 45.

developing systemic disease as a person who developed the disease as an adult.[17] Adult onset is more commonly associated with systemic disease and is generally more severe (**Table 2**). In one study of 120 people, cumulative incidence of anaphylaxis in childhood was 9%, and only children with extensive skin involvement experienced this. In the same study, cumulative incidence of anaphylaxis in adulthood was 49% ($P < .01$); of these 48% were characterized as severe anaphylaxis and 38% had associated syncope.[18] Another study of 84 adults showed 43% with at least one episode of anaphylaxis. Most of these cases were characterized as severe and 72% experienced associated syncope.[19]

Life expectancy for adults with SM can be unchanged from the general population in the indolent form to a matter of months with more severe forms. A retrospective study of 342 adults consented from 1976 to 2007 with SM found a survival rate of just 60% at 3 years after diagnosis and 50% after 5 years. After 5 years, the survival curve was similar to that of the general population. Most of these deaths were in the nonindolent SM forms with ISM closely following the normal population curve[20] (**Fig. 2**).

Background

Mast cells differentiate from pluripotent stem cells in the bone marrow and spleen. From here, they go to the epithelium, or just under it, near vessels, smooth muscle cells, and glandular tissue; they do not circulate in peripheral blood.[21] At these sites they are valuable members of the first line of defense in the innate immune system.

Mast cell activation disorders are the result of multiple somatic mutations. Most of the patients with SM share a gain-of-function point mutation of the type III receptor tyrosine kinase, KIT (CD117), which leads to conformational change and continuous activation at the stem cell growth factor binding site and thus unhindered clonal mast cell expansion.[14] Because these are somatic mutations, there is no increased risk of inheritance.

Although the exact relationship between genotype and phenotype is currently being investigated, the location of uncontrolled mast cell growth and their release of diverse mediators can help explain the heterogeneous presentation seen with this group of disorders. Symptoms that are secondary to space-occupying lesions and depend

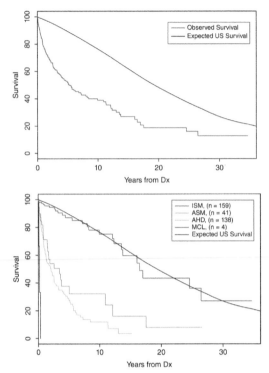

Fig. 2. Kaplan-Meier survival curve for retrospective study of 342 systemic mastocytosis patients compared with the general population. (*From* Lim KH, Tefferi A, Lasho TL, et al. Systemic mastocytosis in 342 consecutive adults: survival studies and prognostic factors. Blood. 2009;113(23):5727 to 5736.)

on location include organomegaly, malabsorption, various cytopenias, and bone pain, among others. On the other hand, mast cell degranulation results in a range of nonspecific symptoms, allergic reactions, spontaneous hemorrhage, or even fatal intractable anaphylactic shock and cardiac arrest (**Table 3**).

Because patients with SM have similar prevalence for immunoglobulin E (IgE)-mediated allergy and atopy to the general population, what distinguishes this group of disorders is the size and therefore severity of response to normal triggers for both IgE- and non-IgE–mediated mast cell degranulation. Mast cell mediator release symptoms can be secondary to either an anaphylactoid nonspecific response or an anaphylactic IgE-mediated pathway. This distinction is irrelevant to the clinician with one exception that is discussed later; otherwise, the term anaphylaxis will be used interchangeably.

Presentation

Most patients will present to the emergency department for symptoms ranging from mild allergic reaction to life-threatening anaphylactic shock. They may note several episodes in the last few years that have otherwise been uncharacteristic for them. Frequently these will be idiopathic, but oftentimes secondary to Hymenoptera stings (wasps, bees, ants, flies), food, or medication.[18]

Prevalence of allergy to Hymenoptera among mastocytosis patients is common, varying between 23% and 47%.[22,23] It should be noted, Hymenoptera stings have

Table 3
Mast cell mediators and their effects by system

Cardiovascular	
1. Prostaglandins	Tachycardia and increased cardiac output lead to flushing
2. Protease (chymase)	Hypertension
3. Histamine	Increased vascular permeability
4. Platelet-activating factor	Arrhythmia
5. Histamine, prostaglandin D2, leukotrienes, and platelet-activating factor	Vasodilation, hypotension
Cutaneous	
1. Histamine	Pruritus
2. Histamine, prostaglandin D2, and platelet-activating factor	Urticaria with or without angioedema
Respiratory	
1. Histamine	Rhinitis
2. Leukotrienes and platelet-activating factor	Pulmonary edema
3. Leukotrienes and prostaglandin D2	Increased mucous production
4. Histamine, prostaglandin D2, leukotrienes, and platelet-activating factor	Bronchoconstriction
Gastrointestinal	
1. Histamine	Increased gastric acid secretion, diarrhea
2. Platelet-activating factor	Abdominal pain
Hematological	
1. Heparin and proteases	Coagulation disturbances
Other	
1. Histamine	Headache
2. Interleukin-6 (IL-6)	Fever
3. Tryptase	Endothelial activation with inflammatory reaction
4. Heparin, IL-6, and tryptase	Osteopenia and osteoporosis
5. Proinflammatory cytokines and chemokines	Fatigue, weight loss, local inflammation, edema

been shown to lead to markedly severe and sometimes fatal anaphylaxis in patients with SM through both allergic IgE-mediated as well as an anaphylactoid non-IgE pathway. These patients can have negative skin tests for Hymenoptera despite associated anaphylaxis and are only later found to have occult mastocytosis.[24] Therefore, a severe systemic reaction to Hymenoptera sting, especially in the setting of reported negative skin tests, should prompt further investigation in someone without a diagnosis of mastocytosis.[25,26]

Flushing and hypotension will be the most common and prominent symptoms in anaphylaxis for patients with SM. Abdominal pain, nausea, vomiting, diarrhea, fatigue, and headache may also be seen with acute mast cell mediator release. Angioedema and urticaria are less common and less prominent symptoms for these patients.

They may report a history of pruritus with or without associated rash. The most common skin finding on examination is a rash composed of several small, tan-yellow to reddish-brown maculopapular lesions. These were traditionally known as urticaria pigmentosa (UP). UP is somewhat of a misnomer though, as they are not true urticaria and are inconsistently hyperpigmented (**Figs. 3** and **4**). The patient may report exacerbation of pruritus with varying medications or behavioral and environmental factors. Darier sign is a finding somewhat specific to mastocytosis but can also be found in scabies. It is elicited by using a tongue depressor to scrape across the top of a skin lesion. Within a few minutes the astute clinician will observe localized erythema (**Fig. 5**). The patient will also report increased pruritus after scraping. Notably, care should be taken to never perform this on a mastocytoma, a yellow-orange maculopapular lesion that is several centimeters in size and more common in the childhood form (**Fig. 6**). Performing Darier sign on a mastocytoma can precipitate severe symptoms.[27]

Diagnosis

Diagnosis of SM can be made by either 1 major and 2 minor or 3 minor WHO criteria . These criteria as well as the WHO classification system have been appropriately modified and externally validated several times over the last 2 decades to account for new research findings.

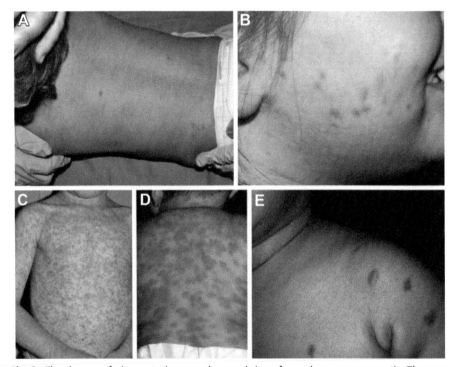

Fig. 3. The degree of pigmentation, number, and size of papules can vary greatly. They can be infrequent and scattered (*A*), several and clustered (*B*), nearly confluent (*C*), or even formed plaques (*D*) or papulonodules (*E*). (*From* Michael D. Tharp and Bryan D. Sofen. Mastocytosis. In: Dermatology, 4th edition. Elsevier Limited: 2018. p. 2102–2112.)

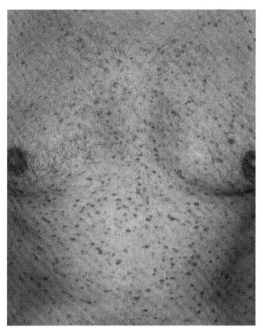

Fig. 4. Pediatric cutaneous mastocytosis with multiple lesions seen with UP. (*From* Michael D. Tharp and Bryan D. Sofen. Mastocytosis. In: Dermatology, 4th edition. Elsevier Limited: 2018. p. 2102–2112.)

Serum tryptase can be obtained in the emergency department or during hospitalization. However, for most providers this test will not be completed at their facility and will thus take a day or more to result.

Furthermore, although obtaining a tryptase level during an episode suggests mastocytosis, it is nondiagnostic. A basal tryptase, taken outside of symptomatic mast cell degranulation, greater than 20 ng/mL qualifies as a minor criterion per WHO guidelines.[16] In addition, it should be noted that an elevated basal serum tryptase is not unique to mastocytosis; it is also seen in acute myeloid leukemia, chronic myeloid

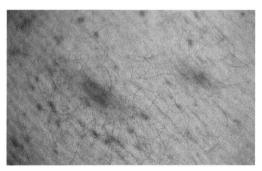

Fig. 5. Darier sign seen after stroking UP in an adult patient with mastocytosis. This should never be done to a solitary mastocytoma because it risks a severe reaction. (*From* Michael D. Tharp and Bryan D. Sofen. Mastocytosis. In: Dermatology, 4th edition. Elsevier Limited: 2018. p. 2102–2112.)

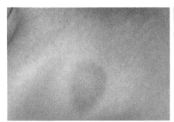 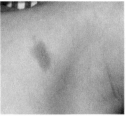 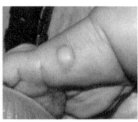

Fig. 6. Solitary mastocytomas in children. These are often a yellow-tan plaque (*A*) and can also have a leathery texture and border on a more pink-tan color (*B*). Occasionally, there can be swelling with an erythematous rim secondary to urtication (*C*). (*From* Michael D. Tharp and Bryan D. Sofen. Mastocytosis. In: Dermatology, 4th edition. Elsevier Limited: 2018. p. 2102–2112.)

leukemia, myelodysplastic syndrome, myeloproliferative neoplasm, chronic eosinophilic leukemia, and HaT.[28–30]

Furthermore, in an external validation study, almost 30% of patients with ISM failed to meet the serum tryptase cut-off, demonstrating another limitation for serum tryptase's helpfulness in diagnosis.[31]

Additional Testing

A standard urinalysis will not be helpful. But if more specific urine studies are available, most patients will have elevated urine histamine, urine *N*-methylhistamine, and urine beta prostaglandin $F2\alpha$.[20]

Standard blood work is usually unremarkable. Although the more aggressive forms may have one or more cytopenias, most will have normal hemoglobin, platelets, and white blood cell count without abnormality on the differential. The most likely abnormality found with liver studies is an elevated alkaline phosphatase.[20]

Outside of the emergency department, bone marrow biopsy with CD25 immunophenotyping is more invasive and specific. It is generally a reliable marker for aggressive systemic disease. But for less aggressive forms such as CM and ISM, nearly 30% did not meet this criterion for diagnosis as detailed by the WHO.[31]

Management

Although angioedema is less common with anaphylaxis in a mastocytosis patient, it is imperative that the airway is first assessed and secured as needed. When there is a known history of, or suspicion for, mastocytosis, care should be taken in selecting medications for rapid sequence intubation that are not associated with mast cell degranulation. Atracurium is especially high risk for mast cell mediator release and should be avoided.

Cis-atracurium, pancuronium, and vecuronium are preferred over succinylcholine and rocuronium, although the risk associated with succinylcholine and rocuronium can be mitigated to an extent with a slower infusion if these are the only paralytics available.[14] Other agents frequently used in emergency and critical care can also be linked to mast cell degranulation (**Table 4**). Radiocontrast media, nonsteroid antiinflammatory medications, and aspirin, among others have also been shown to lead to mast cell mediator release.[14] There are several case reports where mastocytosis first presented with anaphylaxis following regional and general anesthesia.[18,32]

Table 4
Common critical care medications and their expected risk for patients with systemic mastocytosis

	Opioids	Hypnotics	Muscle Relaxants	(Local) Anesthesia	Volatile Anesthetics
Avoid			Mivacurium Atracurium	Nefopam	
Avoid rapid perfusion or use an alternative if possible	Morphine Codeine	Thiopental	Succinylcholine Rocuronium	Lidocaine Bupivacaine	
Low risk	Fentanyl Sufentanil Remifentanil Alfentanil	Midazolam Propofol Etomidate Ketamine	Cis-atracurium Pancuronium Vecuronium	Ropivacaine Paracetamol	Desflurane Sevoflurane Enflurane Isoflurane

Adapted from Hinke Y. van der Weide, David J. van Westerloo, Walter M. van den Bergh. Critical care management of systemic mastocytosis: when every wasp is a killer bee. *Critical Care* 2015;19:238.

Breathing should be assessed next. Although not commonly referenced in the primary literature for SM-related anaphylaxis, if the patient is wheezing or there is concern for bronchospasm, beta agonists or epinephrine can be given.[33]

Attention should then be paid to any hypotension. Treatment is epinephrine, 0.3 mg to 0.5 mg, for adults and 0.01 mg/kg in children intramuscularly; this will not only improve peripheral vasoconstriction and cardiac output, but also through $beta_2$-adrenergic stimulation inhibits additional mast cell degranulation.[34] Often multiple doses repeated every 5 to 15 minutes are required. An intravenous infusion of 1 to 10 μg/min of epinephrine can be given for severe hypotension or cardiac arrest.[33] In addition to epinephrine, one can also place the patient in Trendelenburg position and use fluid resuscitation.

Another potential cause for shock is the possibility of spontaneous hemorrhage. If suspected, but not fully appreciated clinically, this can be confirmed with abnormal coagulation studies. Hemorrhage is a result of the large amount of intrinsic heparin released from massive mast cell degranulation; the treatment is protamine sulfate and plasma coagulation factors.[18]

Standard H_1 and H_2 antihistamine treatments may be used for less severe symptoms. Antihistamines and glucocorticoids are also often given to theoretically prevent a biphasic reaction. In the general population who experience anaphylaxis, there is an increased risk for biphasic reaction with increasing symptom severity; this has not been demonstrated specifically in mastocytosis. A systematic review published in 2020 does not find evidence to support this practice in the general population.[35] Nor is there any data available to support the administration of glucocorticoids to prevent biphasic reactions in mastocytosis anaphylaxis.

Once the patient is stabilized, triggers should be identified and avoided. Most commonly it is Hymenoptera stings (wasps, bees, ants, flies), foods, or medications.[18] Other triggers can include heat, humidity, cold, emotional stress, strenuous exercise, alcohol, spicy food, infections, vaccinations, anesthesia, surgery, and lack of sleep.[36]

Patients should be educated on the potential for life-threatening reactions as well as the need to carry an emergency kit at all times and seek additional emergency medical attention immediately should they have a reaction. Because these patients often require multiple doses of epinephrine, their kits should include 2 doses of self-injecting epinephrine. They should also have a written emergency action plan that identifies their condition and a medical alert bracelet on at all times. In Germany, these kits not only include self-injecting epinephrine but also a fast-acting oral H_1 antihistamine (eg, cetirizine), an oral corticosteroid (eg, betamethasone), as well as a list of medications to avoid.[33]

Clinical Care Points

- SM-related anaphylaxis is secondary to massive mast cell degranulation and mediator release.
- Unsurprisingly, medications used for true anaphylaxis should be used but usually require higher doses.
- Several common medications and agents lead to mast cell degranulation and should be avoided in these patients.
- Patients who present for severe anaphylaxis secondary to Hymenoptera sting should be referred for mastocytosis evaluation.
- It is critical for patients with SM to carry 2 auto-injector epinephrine pens as well as information about their disorder and medications to avoid.

HEREDITARY ALPHA TRYPTASEMIA
Background

HaT is an autosomal dominant disorder causing an increase in total serum tryptase levels and therefore has many similarities with SM. HaT occurs in approximately 4% to 6% of the Western population.[30] The hypothesized mechanism is the formation of heterotetramers composed of alpha and beta tryptase, which increase vascular permeability.[37] There is an increased risk of severe idiopathic anaphylaxis, as well as severe mastocytosis, and hymenoptera-induced anaphylaxis.

Table 5	
Features reported in association with hereditary alpha tryptasemia	
Manifestation	**Reported Prevalence (%)**
Basal serum tryptase >8 ng/mL	100
Chronic gastroesophageal reflux symptoms	56–77
Arthralgia	44–45
Body pain/headache	33–47
Flushing/pruritus	32–55
Irritable bowel syndrome (Rome III)	28–49
Sleep disruption	22–39
Systemic immediate hypersensitivity reaction	21–28
Retained primary dentition	20–33
Systemic venom reaction	14–22
Congenital skeletal abnormality	11–26
Joint hypermobility	0–28
Positive tilt-table test	0–11

Adapted from Lyons JJ. Hereditary Alpha Tryptasemia. Immunol Allergy Clin N America 2018; 38(3):483–95.

Evaluation

Elevated levels of tryptase have been associated with gastrointestinal, cutaneous, atopic, connective tissue, and neuropsychiatric symptoms.[38] Patients with HaT can also have symptoms that manifest as joint hypermobility, vibratory urticaria, dysautonomia such as gastrointestinal hypomobility associated with irritable bowel syndrome, and postural orthostatic tachycardia syndrome[37] (**Table 5**[39]). In addition, there seems to be a gene-dose effect, wherein patients with a duplication had higher levels of tryptase and symptoms compared with those with basal levels, and those with a triplication had higher levels than those with duplication.

Although it has only recently been investigated, serum testing for HaT is a promising biomarker for assessing a patient's risk of developing severe anaphylaxis.[40] Because it is less invasive than the bone marrow biopsy that is sometimes used to diagnose SM, it presents a potentially more appealing option to patients with undifferentiated recurrent allergic reactions. Because it is more prevalent than SM, it may decrease the number of potentially painful diagnostic tests required.[41]

Management

In the acute setting, anaphylactic symptoms should be treated with epinephrine, and evaluation of airway, breathing, and circulation should be paramount. Antihistamines such as diphenhydramine and famotidine, as well as steroids should be given.

Long-term treatment of HaT is similar to treatment of SM. For many symptoms, mast cell stabilizers are beneficial. Because symptoms vary so much between patients, custom approaches are often better than a generalized one. A recent study of omalizumab, which is also used for treatment in SM, demonstrated some benefit in patients experiencing urticaria, nausea, flushing, and fatigue. Patients who exhibited autonomic dysfunction, palpitations, or diarrhea, however, reported no improvement with omalizumab.[42]

Clinical Care Points

- HaT is a hereditary disorder that produces increased basal tryptase levels.
- HaT is often accompanied by manifestations in gastrointestinal, neurologic, or musculoskeletal systems.
- Consider testing patients with recurrent allergic reactions.

SUMMARY

Scombroid toxicity, SM, and HaT present similar to an allergic reaction. Luckily, management is also similar, with a few key differences in choice of medication. Scombroid is usually not life-threatening but SM and HaT can be. Hymenoptera stings resulting in severe anaphylaxis should prompt further investigation into both SM and HaT. Morbidity and mortality can deviate significantly from classic allergic reactions. Therefore, suspicion for and appropriate referral can be life-saving.

DISCLOSURE

The authors declare that they have no relevant or material financial interests that relate to the research described in this article.

REFERENCES

1. Available at handbook of foodborne pathogenic microorganisms and natural toxins. Available at: https://www.fda.gov/media/83271/download. Accessed 11 October 2020.
2. Available at surveillance for foodborne disease outbreaks United States, 2017: Annual Report. Available at: https://www.cdc.gov/fdoss/pdf/2017_FoodBorne Outbreaks_508.pdf. Accessed 11 October 2020.
3. Zapata R, Acevedo K, Verena Mella L, et al. Gastrointestinal and extraintestinal symptoms occurring during a massive outbreak of scombroid fish poisoning in chile: a clinical-epidemiological onsite study. Gastroenterology 2017;152(5): S808-9.
4. Feng C, Teuber S, Gershwin ME. Histamine (Scombroid) fish poisoning: a comprehensive review. Clin Rev Allergy Immunol 2016;50(1):64-9.
5. Nordt SP, Pomeranz D. Scombroid poisoning from tilapia. Am J Emerg Med 2016; 34(2):339.e1-2.
6. Hungerford JM. Scombroid poisoning: a review. Toxicon 2010;56(2):231-43.
7. Centers for Disease Control and Prevention (CDC). Scombroid fish poisoning associated with tuna steaks–Louisiana and Tennessee, 2006. MMWR Morb Mortal Wkly Rep 2007;56(32):817-9.
8. Guergué-Díaz de Cerio O, Barrutia-Borque A, Gardeazabal-García J. Escombroidosis: abordaje práctico. Actas Dermosifiliogr 2016;107:567-71.
9. Ferrazzo G, Andò G, Cerrito M, et al. Non–ST-Elevation Myocardial Infarction-Like Syndrome in Scombroid Tuna Fish Poisoning. Am J Cardiol 2019;124(4):518-21.
10. Iannuzzi M, D'Ignazio N, Bressy L, et al. Severe scombroid fish poisoning syndrome requiring aggressive fluid resuscitation in the emergency department: two case reports. Minerva Anestesiol 2007;73(9):481-3.
11. Wilson BJ, Musto RJ, Ghali WA. A case of histamine fish poisoning in a young atopic woman. J Gen Intern Med 2012;27:878-81.
12. Attaran RR, Probst F. Histamine fish poisoning: a common but frequently misdiagnosed condition. Emerg Med J 2002;19:474-5.
13. Blakesley ML. Scombroid poisoning: prompt resolution of symptoms with cimetidine. Ann Emerg Med 1983;12(2):104-6.
14. Hinke van der Weide Y, David J, van Westerloo, et al. Critical care management of systemic mastocytosis: when every wasp is a killer bee. Crit Care 2015;19:238.
15. Pardanani A. Systemic mastocytosis in adults: 2019 update on diagnosis, risk stratification and management. Am J Hematol 2019;94(3):363-77.
16. Horny HP, Metcalfe DD, Akin C, et al. Mastocytosis. In: Swerdlow SH, et al, editors. WHO classification of tumors of hematopoietic and lymphoid tissues. Lyon, France: International Agency for Research and Cancer (IARC); 2017. p. 62-9.
17. Glick SA, Jakus J, Asrani F, et al. Dermatology. In: Shah BR, Lucchesi M, Amadio J, et al, editors. Atlas of pediatric emergency medicine. 2nd edition.
18. Brockhow K, Jofer C, Behrendt H, et al. Anaphylaxis in patients with mastocytosis: a study on history, clinical features and risk factors in 120 patients. Allergy 2008;63:226-32.
19. Gülen T, Hägglund H, Dahlén B, et al. High prevalence of anaphylaxis in patients with systemic mastocytosis - a single-centre experience. Clin Exp Allergy 2014; 44(1):121-9.
20. Lim KH, Tefferi A, Lasho TL, et al. Systemic mastocytosis in 342 consecutive adults: survival studies and prognostic factors. Blood 2009;113(23):5727-36.

21. Andersen CL, Kristensen TK, Severinsen MT, et al. Systemic mastocytosis–a systematic review. Dan Med J 2012;59(3):A4397.

22. Konrad FM, Unertl KE, Schroeder TH. Provocation of mastocytosis in anaesthesia. Anaesthetist 2009;53:270–1.

23. Van Doormaal JJ, Arends S, Brunekreeft KL, et al. Prevalence of indolent systemic mastocytosis in a Dutch region. J Allergy Clin Immunol 2013;131:1429–30.

24. Kontou-Fili K. Patients with negative skin tests. Curr Opin Allergy Clin Immunol 2002;2(4):353–7.

25. Bonadonna P, Perbellini O, Passalacqua G, et al. Clonal mast cell disorders in patients with systemic reactions to Hymenoptera stings and increased serum tryptase levels. J Allergy Clin Immunol 2009;123(3):680–6.

26. Potier A, Lavigne C, Chappard D, et al. Cutaneous manifestations in Hymenoptera and Diptera anaphylaxis: relationship with basal serum tryptase. Clin Exp Allergy 2009;39:717–25.

27. Hartmann K, Escribano L, Grattan C, et al. Cutaneous manifestations in patients with mastocytosis: Consensus report of the European Competence Network on Mastocytosis; the American Academy of Allergy, Asthma & Immunology; and the European Academy of Allergology and Clinical Immunology. J Allergy Clin Immunol 2016;137(1):35–45.

28. Sperr WR, El-Samahi A, Kundi M, et al. Elevated tryptase levels selectively cluster in myeloid neoplasms: a novel diagnostic approach and screen marker in clinical haematology. Eur J Clin Invest 2009;39:914–23.

29. Valent P, Sperr WR, Sotlar K, et al. The serum tryptase test: an emerging robust biomarker in clinical hematology. Expert Rev Hematol 2014;7(5):683–90.

30. Lyons JJ, Yu X, Hughes JD, et al. Elevated basal serum tryptase identifies a multisystem disorder associated with increased TPSAB1 copy number. Nat Genet 2016 Dec;48(12):1564–9.

31. Sánchez-Muñoz L, Alvarez-Twose I, García-Montero AC, et al. Evaluation of the WHO criteria for the classification of patients with mastocytosis. Mod Pathol 2011;24(9):1157–68.

32. Yunaev M, Hughes ™, Abdul-Razak M. Systemic mastocytosis and surgery a potential disaster. ANZ J Surg 2010;80:860–1.

33. Schuch A, Brockow K. Mastocytosis and anaphylaxis. Immunol Allergy Clin N Am 2017;37(1):153–64.

34. Vaughan ST, Jones GN. Systemic mastocytosis presenting as profound cardiovascular collapse during anaesthesia. Anaesthesia 1998;53:804–9.

35. Shaker MS, Wallace DV, Golden DBK, et al. Anaphylaxis-a 2020 practice parameter update, systematic review, and Grading of Recommendations, Assessment, Development and Evaluation (GRADE) analysis. J Allergy Clin Immunol 2020; 145(4):1082–123.

36. Abid A, Malone MA, Curci K. Mastocytosis *Prim Care* 2016;43(3):505–18.

37. Lyons JJ, Chovanec J, O'Connell MP, et al. Heritable risk for severe anaphylaxis associated with increased α-tryptase-encoding germline copy number at TPSAB1. J Allergy Clin Immunol 2020;6749(20):31029.

38. Lyons JJ, Sun G, Stone KD, et al. Mendelian inheritance of elevated serum tryptase associated with atopy and connective tissue abnormalities. J Allergy Clin Immunol 2014;133(5):1471–4.

39. Lyons JJ. Hereditary Alpha Tryptasemia. Immunol Allergy Clin N America 2018; 38(3):483–95.

40. Greiner G, Sprinzl B, Górska A, et al. Hereditary α tryptasemia is a valid genetic biomarker for severe mediator-related symptoms in mastocytosis. Blood 2021; 137(2):238–47.
41. Carrigan C, Milner JD, Lyons JJ, et al. Usefulness of testing for hereditary alpha tryptasemia in symptomatic patients with elevated tryptase. J Allergy Clin Immunol Pract 2020;8(6):2066–7.
42. Mendoza Alvarez LB, Barker R, Nelson C, et al. Clinical response to omalizumab in patients with hereditary α-tryptasemia. Ann Allergy Asthma Immunol 2020; 124(1):99–100.e1.

Immune-based Therapies— What the Emergency Physician Needs to Know

Sarah B. Dubbs, MD*, Cheyenne Falat, MD, Lauren Rosenblatt, MD

KEYWORDS

- Immunotherapy • Autoimmune • Monoclonal antibody • Checkpoint inhibitor
- Immune-related adverse event

KEY POINTS

- Patients on immune-based therapies are encountered frequently in the emergency department.
- Adverse effects from immunotherapies must be considered in the differential diagnoses for acute illness, although often must be diagnoses of exclusion.
- Key considerations for patients on monoclonal antibody treatment are infusion and hypersensitivity reactions as well as infection.
- Key considerations for patients on cancer immunotherapy include immune-checkpoint inhibitor toxicity, cytokine release syndrome, and chimeric antigen receptor–T-cell therapy neurotoxicity.
- Indications for immune-based therapies continue to expand, including treatment of severe acute respiratory syndrome coronavirus 2 infection.

INTRODUCTION

Immunotherapy refers to a class of biopharmaceutical agents that act by activating or suppressing the immune system. Immunotherapy also is referred to as biologic therapy and has been applied in the treatment of autoimmune disease, malignancies, and infections. Its mechanism can range from being very targeted to very broad, leading to a spectrum of possible side effects and adverse events. Overall, immunotherapies have been effective and well tolerated, leading to exponential growth in their development and use. The cancer immunotherapy market alone generated $75 billion globally in 2019 and is projected to generate more than $143 billion in 2025.[1] Their expanding role in the treatment of many disease processes makes it imperative to have an

This article originally appeared in Emergency Medicine Clinics, Volume 40 Issue 1, February 2022.

Department of Emergency Medicine, University of Maryland School of Medicine, 110 South Paca Street, 6th Floor, Suite 200, Baltimore, MD 21201, USA

* Corresponding author.

E-mail address: sdubbs@som.umaryland.edu

Immunol Allergy Clin N Am 43 (2023) 569–582
https://doi.org/10.1016/j.iac.2022.10.004
0889-8561/23/© 2022 Elsevier Inc. All rights reserved.

immunology.theclinics.com

understanding of the mechanisms, adverse effects, and other considerations for management in the acute care setting.

MECHANISM OF ACTION

In order to understand the mechanisms of action of various immunotherapies, it is important to review the adaptive immune responses, composed of the humoral and cellular immune responses. The humoral immune response consists of antibody production by mature B lymphocytes. Each B lymphocyte expresses an immunoglobulin against exactly 1 antigen on its surface. If the B-lymphocyte immunoglobulin recognizes an antigen, it binds and becomes activated. Once activated, these B lymphocytes differentiate into various cells, including antibody-producing plasma cells and memory cells. Many antigens require costimulation by CD4+ helper T cells for the B lymphocyte to differentiate. Only with T-cell help can the B lymphocytes undergo immunoglobulin gene rearrangements to produce higher-affinity IgG antibodies.[2]

The other component of the immune system, the cellular immune response, consists of cytotoxic (CD8+) and helper (CD4+) T cells. CD8+ T cells are responsible for killing of host cells and are activated via a major histocompatibility complex (MHC) class I process.[3] MHC class I is a molecule expressed on all nucleated cells and is responsible for presenting peptide fragments (including tumor peptides) to the CD8+ T cells to induce a cytotoxic response. CD4+ T cells are responsible for cytokine synthesis and are activated via the MHC class II process. MHC class II is a molecule expressed by antigen-presenting cells (APCs), such as dendritic cells, and is responsible for presenting phagocytosed peptide fragments to the CD4+ T cells to induce cytokine synthesis. T_H1 helper T cells produce cytokines that promote cell-mediated immunity (like interleukin [IL]-2, interferon [IFN]-γ, and tumor necrosis factor α), and T_H2 helper T cells secrete B-cell stimulatory cytokines (like IL-4, IL-5, and IL-10) to help differentiate and proliferate plasma cells. In order for these T cells to become activated (to proliferate and differentiate), they require binding of the antigen-MHC complex by the T-cell receptor (TCR) and binding of a costimulatory molecule (CD28) on the T cell to its B7 ligand (CD80/86) on the APC.[4] Without this costimulation, tolerance to the antigen develops.

The activity of the immune system is regulated by complex pathways. If the immune system is overactive, autoimmune conditions develop. If underactive or evaded, tumors can grow. Some of the mechanisms by which tumors evade the immune system include the loss of MHC class I expression, manipulation of cytokines that inhibit cytotoxic T-cell function and suppress proliferation of CD4+ and CD8+ T cells (secretion of IL-6 and IL-10 and consumption of IL-2), and up-regulated expression of immune checkpoint molecules, such as programmed cell death 1 receptor (PD-1) and programmed cell death ligand 1 (PD-L1).

Immunotherapy is defined as treatments designed to augment, reestablish, or suppress the immune system's ability to prevent and fight disease. These treatments can be accomplished through passive or active immune mechanisms.

Passive immunotherapy includes agents that mediate tumor killing and consists of monoclonal antibody (mAb) administration and adoptive immunotherapy.[5] mAbs, such as rituximab or alemtuzumab, are selective, minimally toxic, and easily mass produced. They can block a target protein's function, trigger downstream signaling of target proteins, or deliver conjugated toxins to cells that express target proteins.[6] Adoptive immunotherapy is the passive administration of cells with antitumor activity to the patient. It can take the form of tumor-infiltrating lymphocytes (TILs), modified TCR therapy, and chimeric antigen receptor (CAR)–T cells. TILs are lymphocytes that are isolated from tumor specimens or blood, expanded ex vivo in the presence of IL-2, and administered back to the patient (often after chemotherapy or radiation).[7] In modified TCR therapy, T cells are transduced with a retrovirus that encodes for TCRs that already recognize the cancer antigens. CAR–T-cell therapy consists of an infusion of T cells with a fusion molecule (intracellular TCR fused to the antigen-binding domain of a B-cell receptor)[8] that recognizes tumor cells with tumor-specific antigens and attack independently of MHC recognition.

Active immunotherapy is the delivery of materials to augment and elicit an immune response. Active immunotherapy can be either specific or nonspecific. Specific active immunotherapy consists of vaccines that initiate and augment an immune response to a specific antigen.[9] They can be tumor-specific peptide or protein antigens, autologous tumor cells (tumor is harvested, altered to be more immunogenic, irradiated, and returned to patient to stimulate a tumor-specific immune response), allogenic vaccines, and APC vaccines. Nonspecific active immunotherapy consists of immunomodulators that augment a preexisting immune response to an antigen. These include checkpoint inhibition and cytokines.

Checkpoint inhibitors interrupt negative feedback loops and re-engage an immune response. Cytotoxic T-lymphocyte–associated antigen 4 (CTLA-4) is expressed by activated T cells, which competes with CD28 for B7 ligands on APCs.[10] By delivering mAbs that bind to CTLA-4 and prevent it from binding to B7, the binding of CD28 to B7 (costimulation) increases, and T-cell responses are enhanced. PD-1 is a receptor expressed on the surface of activated mature T cells, B cells, and other cells. Binding of PD-1 to its ligand, PD-L1, suppresses T-cell function. This helps prevent autoimmune disorders, but some cancers use aberrant expression of PD-L1 to evade immune attack.[11] Delivering anti–PD-1 or anti–PD-L1 antibodies can interrupt this T-cell suppression and restore T-cell function, allowing enhanced antitumor activity.

Cytokine therapy includes IFNs and ILs. IFNs (IFN-α, IFN-β, and IFN-γ) increase MHC/antigen presentation and enhance antibody-dependent cell-mediated cytotoxicity. ILs either can enhance or suppress immune function. IL-2, for instance, is required for the differentiation and proliferation of activated T cells, and high-dose IL-2 promotes cytotoxic T-cell activity.[6] IL-2 therapy, however, carries substantial toxicity because it is not specific against tumor only.

MONOCLONAL ANTIBODIES FOR AUTOIMMUNE DISEASES

The treatment of autoimmune diseases, such as rheumatoid arthritis, multiple sclerosis, lupus, inflammatory bowel disease, and psoriasis, was transformed with the advent of mAb therapy. The first mAb therapy was approved for use in 1986,[12] and, since then, the engineering of antibody therapies has evolved greatly. Many of the current targeted mABs have minimal adverse effects because they have been engineered to be so highly specific. The applications of mABs also have expanded significantly to include onocologic, infectious disease, organ transplant, allergic, and neurologic indications.

Adverse effects from these targeted therapies may precipitate a visit to the emergency department (ED) during or immediately after infusion. Adverse effects include nausea, dizziness, palpitations, and headache as well as serious hypersensitivity, anaphylaxis reactions, and serum sickness.[13-15] Acute reactions occur within 24 hours but occur most often within 10 minutes to 4 hours from the initiation of infusion.[16,17] Treatment of mild to moderate infusion-related reactions is supportive, and patients generally can be discharged home after a period of observation.[14] Delayed reactions manifest as serum sickness-like reactions or type IV hypersensitivity (cell-mediated) mucocutaneous reactions. Serum sickness reactions typically begin 5 days to 7 days after the infusion and may mimic infection and sepsis.[18] From the standpoint of ED management, serum sickness should be a diagnosis of exclusion while infection and other causes on the differential are investigated. The type IV cell-mediated reactions occur between 12 hours and several weeks from the infusion and range from mild maculopapular rash and erythema multiforme to the more serious severe cutaneous adverse reactions, such as Stevens-Johnson syndrome (SJS), toxic epidermal necrolysis (TEN), SJS/TEN overlap syndrome, and drug reaction with eosinophilia and systemic symptoms. Patients experiencing these adverse reactions may experience distress and fear that they cannot continue receiving the inciting therapy; however, they can be reassured that, in most patients, treatment may continue under the guidance of their ordering physician with premedication, adjusted infusion rates, and desensitization.

The other relevant adverse effect of mAB therapy to be considered in the ED is reactivation or increased susceptibility of new infection with rare serious pathogens, including tuberculosis, other mycobacterial infections, herpes simplex virus, varicella zoster virus, hepatitis C, *Pneumocystis jirovecii*, cytomegalovirus, and Epstein-Barr virus.[19] Progressive multifocal leukoencephalopathy due to the John Cunningham (JC) virus also may be triggered by mAB therapy.[19] These infectious complications should be considered in any patient who has undergone recent therapy with mABs.

CANCER IMMUNOTHERAPY

Cancer immunotherapy is evolving rapidly as the most innovative application of immune system-based therapies. As with other immunotherapies, a patient's innate immune system mechanisms are manipulated to act against the target, such as tumor cells or proteins. Multiple mechanisms are employed, including mAB treatment, immune checkpoint inhibition, adoptive cell therapy, and cancer vaccines. They are given as single-therapy treatment or in combination with each other or with traditional cytotoxic chemotherapy, radiation, and/or surgery. In general, this class of cancer treatment has been shown to be well tolerated and provide durable long-term survival for melanoma, lung cancer, and colon cancer. Even so, they are not without adverse effects that prompt ED visits during the acute phase of treatment. A majority of adverse events occur within 6 months of treatment, but long-term effects also should be considered in the ED setting for patients who have undergone immunotherapy treatments up to 2 years prior.[20] A key clinical consideration for those caring for oncology patients in the modern era is recognition of the difference between immunotherapy and traditional chemotherapy. Side effects and complications manifest differently from those in traditional chemotherapy and are referred to as immune-related adverse events (IRAEs).

IFN and IL therapies are used to treat metastatic melanoma and solid tumor malignancies, such as renal cell and non–small cell lung cancer. High-dose IL-2 has been administered in the inpatient setting because it creates a marked systemic inflammatory response, but, because of its high toxicity and low rate of sustained remissions, the application of high-dose IL-2 is decreasing in favor of the recently developed checkpoint inhibitor therapies.

T-cell activation has become a cornerstone of modern cancer immunotherapy. There are 3 main categories or approaches to T-cell immunotherapy: immune checkpoint blockade, adoptive cellular therapy, and cancer vaccines.

Immune checkpoint therapy currently is the most commonly applied type of T-cell immunotherapy. This treatment modality activates the patient's immune response

---

Box 1
US Food and Drug Administration–approved checkpoint inhibitor immunotherapies available as of 2021

CTLA-4 inhibitor
  Ipilimumab (Yervoy)

PD-1 inhibitor
  Nivolumab (Opdivo)
  Pembrolizumab (Keytruda)
  Cemiplimab (Libtayo)

PD-L1 inhibitor
  Avelumab (Bavencio)
  Durvalumab (Imfinzi)
  Atezolizumab (Tecentriq)

---

by inhibiting negative T-cell–regulating molecules—checkpoint molecules that normally serve to limit hyperactivation of the immune system. mAbs are targeted specifically at checkpoint molecules—CTLA-4, PD-1, or PD-L1. **Box 1** lists the US Food and Drug Administration (FDA)-approved checkpoint inhibitor immunotherapies available as of 2021.

T cells interact with tissues throughout the body, leading to the potential for checkpoint inhibitor toxicity to affect any system. The effects tend to be autoimmune/inflammatory in nature, for example, dermatitis, pneumonitis, or colitis. The severity of toxicity also may range from very mild to life-threatening. **Box 2** is a comprehensive listing of IRAEs in patients with cancer treated with immune checkpoint inhibitors. The ED approach to cancer patients on checkpoint inhibitors is challenging because of the variable timing, severity, and vague or nonspecific presentations. Severe IRAEs also can mimic life-threatening disease processes, such as pneumonitis presenting like pneumonia or congestive heart failure.

CAR–T-cell therapy has been approved for use in patients with relapsed or refractory large B-cell lymphoma. It is known to have major side effects systemically with cytokine release syndrome (CRS) as well as CAR–T-cell–associated neurotoxicity, which generally occur early after infusion.[21] Late toxicities of CAR–T-cell therapy include cytopenias and B-cell aplasia.[22] CAR–T-cell therapy traditionally is administered in an inpatient, closely monitored setting, but an increasing number of cancer centers are beginning to administer CAR–T-cell therapy in the outpatient setting.[23] CRS affects up to 90% of patients receiving this therapy and can be severe in 11% to 30%, requiring vasopressors and/or ventilation for supportive care.[24–26] It is marked by a systemic inflammatory response with high cytokine levels (IL-6, IFN-γ, and others). Clinical symptoms range from mild fever and flulike symptoms to hypotension, hypoxia, and organ injury. In addition to supportive care, patients with high-grade CRS may be treated with an antibody that targets the IL-6 receptor, such as tocilizumab. Administration of this treatment must be in conjunction with oncology and intensive care specialists. CAR–T-cell–associated neurotoxicity, also known as immune effector cell-associated neurotoxicity syndrome (ICANS) and previously known as CAR–T-cell–related encephalopathy syndrome, is the second most common acute toxicity of CAR–T-cell therapy, occurring either concurrently with CRS or after CRS has subsided.[22] It presents with symptoms of toxic encephalopathy, beginning with word-finding difficulty, aphasia, and confusion and can progress to depressed level of consciousness, seizures, coma, and cerebral edema. The pathophysiology of the toxicity is actively being researched, and, currently, treatment involves supportive

Box 2
Organ-based classification of immune-related adverse events in patients with cancer treated with immune checkpoint inhibitors

Cardiac
- Myocarditis[a]
  - Autoimmune myocarditis
  - Myocardial fibrosis
- Pericarditis
  - Autoimmune pericarditis
  - Pericardial effusion
  - Pericardial tamponade

Dermatologic
- Alopecia areata/universalis
- Dermatitis herpetiformis
- Erythema multiforme
- Granuloma annulare
- Lichen planopilaris/planus/lichenoid dermatitis
- Panniculitis/erythema nodosum
- Pemphigoid/pemphigus
- Psoriasis
- Pyoderma gangrenosum
- Sweet syndrome
- Vitiligo[a]

Endocrine
- Adrenalitis[a]
  - Adrenal insufficiency
  - Cortisol deficiency
  - Hypercortisolism
  - Hypoadrenalism
  - Isolated adrenocorticotropic hormone deficiency
- Autoimmune diabetes mellitus
- Hyperparathyroidism
- Hypogonadism
- Hypophysitis[a]
  - Autoimmune hypophysitis
  - Hypopituitarism
  - Pan-hypopituitarism
- Thyroiditis[a]
  - Autoimmune thyroiditis
  - Hyperthyroidism
  - Hypothyroidism
  - Graves disease
  - Thyrotoxicosis

Gastrointestinal
- Enterocolitis[a]
  - Ileitis
  - Ileocolitis
  - Ischemic colitis
  - Microscopic colitis
  - Ulcerative colitis
- Hepatitis[a]
  - Autoimmune hepatitis
  - Eosinophilic hepatitis
- Lymphocytic gastritis
- Pancreatitis

Hematological
- Aplastic anemia/pure red cell aplasia

- Autoimmune hemolytic anemia
- Autoimmune neutropenia
- Hemophagocytic lymphohistiocytosis
- Immune thrombocytopenic purpura

Muscular
- Myalgias[a]
- Myositis[a]
  - Antisynthetase syndrome
  - Bulbar myopathy
  - Dermatomyositis
  - Diaphragmatic lymphocytic polymyositis
  - Necrotizing myopathy
  - Orbital myositis

Neurologic
- Aseptic meningitis
- Encephalitis
- Cranial nerve involvement
  - Bilateral hearing loss
  - Facial palsy
  - Oculomotor paresis
- Motor neuropathy
  - Acute generalized motor neuropathy
  - Multifocal motor mock neuropathy
- Myasthenia gravis
- Neuromyelitis optica spectrum disorders
  - Optic neuritis
  - Transverse myelitis
- Polyneuropathies[a]
  - Axonal sensory motor polyneuropathy
  - Multiplex mononeuritis
  - Peripheral sensory neuropathy
- Polyradiculopathies
  - Chronic inflammatory demyelinating polyneuropathy
  - Guillain-Barré syndrome

Ocular
- Conjunctivitis
- Episcleritis/scleritis
- Orbital inflammation
- Uveitis[a]
  - Anterior uveitis
  - Chorioretinopathy
  - Iridocyclitis/iritis
  - Panuveitis
  - Posterior uveitis
- Vogt-Koyanagi-Harada syndrome

Pulmonary
- Interstitial lung disease[a]
  - Alveolitis
  - Organizing pneumonia
  - Pneumonitis
  - Pulmonary fibrosis
  - Pulmonary hemorrhage

Renal
- Acute tubulointerstitial nephritis/renal tubular acidosis
- Glomerulonephritis

Skeletal
- Arthralgia[a]/polyarthralgia

- Arthritis
  - Monoarthritis
  - Oligoarthritis
  - Polyarthritis
- Enthesitis
- Fasciitis/eosinophilic fasciitis
- Jaccoud arthropathy
- Polymyalgia rheumatica
- Psoriatic arthritis
- Rheumatoid arthritis
- Spondyloarthropathy
- Tenosynovitis

Systemic
- Antiphospholipid syndrome
- Lupus
  - Lupus nephropathy
  - Subacute cutaneous lupus erythematosus
  - Systemic lupus erythematosus
- Sarcoidosis
  - Cutaneous sarcoidosis
  - Pulmonary sarcoidosis
  - Renal sarcoidosis
- Sicca syndrome[a]/Sjögren syndrome
- Systemic sclerosis
- Vasculitis[a]
  - Cerebral vasculitis
  - Cryoglobulinemia
  - Cutaneous vasculitis
  - Eosinophilic granulomatosis with polyangiitis
  - Giant cell arteritis
  - Pulmonary vasculitis
  - Henoch-Schönlein purpura

[a] More than 100 cases reported.

With permission, from Ramos-Casals, M., Brahmer, J.R., Callahan, M.K. et al. Immune-related adverse events of checkpoint inhibitors. *Nat Rev Dis Primers* **6**, 38 (2020). https://doi.org/10.1038/s41572-020-0160-6

care with the use of corticosteroids in high-grade cases. Consensus guidelines for grading and treatment of both CRS and ICANS were developed by the American Society for Transplantation and Cellular Therapy in 2018.[27]

NOVEL APPLICATIONS OF IMMUNOTHERAPY IN COVID-19

Since December 2019, the world has been battling a novel viral infection caused by the severe acute respiratory syndrome (SARS)–coronavirus (CoV)-2, which leads to the development of the clinical syndrome, known as COVID-19. As of late summer 2021, there were more than 223 million confirmed cases and 4.6 million documented deaths globally.[28] Cases range from asymptomatic to severe, with many deaths related to progression to severe respiratory failure, acute respiratory distress syndrome (ARDS), and multiorgan failure. The impact of COVID-19 has been profound, prompting a worldwide effort to understand the disease and develop effective treatments and vaccination. Understanding the immunopathogenesis of SARS–CoV-2 has allowed for the opportunity to utilize immunotherapies to target specific immune responses to assist with the management of patients with COVID-19, especially in those with severe disease.

The pathogenesis of viral infection involves first stimulating the innate immune cells to recognize the molecular pattern of the pathogen. The innate immune system consists of cytokine and chemokine of ILs, IFNs, and chemoattractant to activate a response from neutrophils, macrophages, and monocytes to recognize and eliminate the pathogen. Failure to eliminate the virus at this step leads to activation of the adaptive immune system and lymphocyte response. Dysregulation of the immune response can lead to the host's failure to battle a viral infection. SARS–CoV-2 has been noted to be particularly virulent in many people, leading to critical illness and death.[29] The severity of disease presentation is thought to be a result of over-activation of the innate and suppression of the adaptive immune systems.[30]

Based on the available literature, there are several proposed mechanisms leading to the immune system dysregulation. The main causes that have been identified and discussed include host immune system evasion, lymphopenia, T-cell exhaustion, and cytokine storm. These proposed causes often overlap and perpetuate the dysregulation noted in SARS–CoV-2 infections.

Similar to its viral predecessors, SARS-CoV and Middle East respiratory syndrome (MERS)-CoV, SARS–CoV-2 has mechanisms that attempt to evade the host immune detection system.[31] The innate immune response consists of a complicated cascade of receptor presentations, chemokine expression, and pathway activations in an attempt to recognize and eliminate a new pathogen. Type I INF is considered part of that first line of defense by attempting to suppress viral replication and spread. SARS–CoV-2 evades the innate immunity by antagonizing type I INF, suppressing its response and subsequent cascade of events to support the host's immune system. Evasion of the host's innate immune system leads to immunosuppression and unchecked viral replication.

This unchecked viremia progresses to an exaggerated inflammatory response and aggressive production of cytokines, leading to a cytokine storm. As a result of the infection, the body produces high levels of cytokines, leading to influx of immune cells, especially monocytes, macrophages, and neutrophils. These inflammatory cells perpetuate the response by continued and amplified secretion of proinflammatory cytokines, such as IL-2, IL-6, IL-10, and TNF-α. These markers in particular, have been associated with disease severity and specifically cytokine storm. This leads to lung-tissue damage, edema, alveoli fibrosis, and inflammatory exudate, ultimately causing ARDS. The cytokine storm also is associated with development of multiorgan failure.

Along with detection evasion and cytokine storm, SARS–CoV-2 also has affected the adaptive immunity by causing immunosuppression of lymphocytes, affecting $CD8^+$ cells primarily. Lymphopenia has been a hallmark of the clinical presentation of COVID-19 patients, secondary to the dysfunction and exhaustion of T-cells. It is believed that the SARS–CoV-2 virus can infect the T cell directly by invading via angiotensin-converting enzyme 2 receptors, the same receptors that are used to invade the host through respiratory epithelial cells. Additionally, it is believed that the cytokine storm, in particular, elevated levels of IL-2 and IL-6, cause inflammatory dysfunction of T cells. Finally, COVID-19 results in T-cell exhaustion. Studies have found that both $CD4^+$ and $CD8^+$ T cells have increased expression of PD-1 and T-cell immunoglobulin and mucin domain 3 (Tim-3), which are markers for T-cell exhaustion. Expression of PD-1 and Tim-3 were noted to correlate with severity of the disease presentation.

Antivirals along with several immunotherapies are being used in an attempt to treat SARS–CoV-2 infections. These therapies are geared toward targeting the pathways, cell types, cytokines, chemokines, and mechanisms identified as key players in disease progression. As discussed previously, immune system evasion, cytokine storm, lymphopenia, and T-cell exhaustion have been identified as some of the key pathways associated with severe COVID-19. Many of the biologics available specifically attempt to target these mechanisms.

Convalescent plasma was granted emergency use authorization (EUA) by the FDA in August 2020 for patients hospitalized with COVID-19 infection.[32] Plasma from COVID-19 convalescent patients contains antibodies that are postulated to block viral infection and improve clearance of cells infected with the virus.[33–35]

mAbs have developed as a promising treatment modality in COVID-19 infection. LY-CoV555, or bamlanivimab, is a neutralizing antibody against the treat SARS–CoV-2 receptor-binding domain that was developed from the convalescent plasma of infected patients and received EUA from the FDA in November 2020.[36] Another EUA was declared for casirivimab/imdevimab, a combination mAB therapy (REGEN-COV), in late fall 2020.[37] Bamlanivimab's EUA subsequently was revoked in April 2021 and replaced with an EUA for bamlanivimab given in combination with another mAB, etesevimab.[38] The combination therapies are hypothesized to reduce rapid mutation and viral mutant escape.[39] Although these therapies are promising, there remains much to be learned with ongoing investigations.

Inflammatory modulators, such as the IL-6 inhibitor tocilizumab, discussed previously as a treatment of severe CAR–T-cell therapy CRS, are being investigated as a potential therapy for severe COVID-19 infection. Overall evidence appears to show treatment with tocilizumab reduced mortality and led to clinical improvement in patients with severe infection,[40] but further studies are needed to confirm efficacy and safety for this indication.

Several other immune-based therapeutic strategies are being investigated for treatment of COVID-19. These include IFNs, intravenous immunoglobin, and stem cell therapies.[41]

OTHER APPLICATIONS OF IMMUNE-MEDIATED DRUGS

Beyond the use of immunotherapeutics in autoimmune and oncologic conditions, immune-mediated drugs, specifically mAbs, are used for the treatment of numerous conditions. These include, but are not limited to, atopic states, infectious diseases, neurodegenerative diseases, immunosuppression, migraine headaches, hyperlipidemia, osteoporosis, hereditary conditions, and medication neutralization.

Dupilumab is an IL-4 receptor α-antagonist approved for the treatment of moderate to severe atopic dermatitis and uncontrolled asthma (through its reduction of the T_H2 helper T-cell inflammatory response).[42,43] Omalizumab is an IgE antagonist also approved for the treatment of uncontrolled asthma and chronic idiopathic urticaria.[44] Palivizumab is a mAb that binds to respiratory syncytial virus (RSV) and is approved for the prevention of RSV in high-risk infants.[45] Raxibacumab and obiltoxaximab are mAbs approved for the treatment and prophylaxis of inhalational anthrax due to *Bacillus anthracis* spores, and bezlotoxumab is a mAb used to reduce the recurrence of *Clostridium difficile* infections.[46] Ranibizumab and aflibercept are 2 vascular endothelial growth factor inhibitors approved for the treatment of diabetic macular edema, among other ocular conditions.[47] Basiliximab is an IL-2 antagonist approved as immunosuppressive therapy after renal transplantation.[48] Erenumab is a calcitonin gene-related peptide inhibitor approved for once-monthly subcutaneous injection to prevent migraine headaches.[49] Alirocumab and evolocumab are 2 proprotein convertase subtilisin/kexin type 9 inhibitors approved for the reduction of low-density lipoprotein cholesterol.[50] Denosumab is a mAb that binds to RANKL and inhibits the maturation of osteoclasts, approved for the treatment of postmenopausal women with osteoporosis at high risk of fracture.[51] Emapalumab is a mAb that neutralizes IFN-γ and is approved for the treatment of hemophagocytic lymphohistiocytosis through its role in suppression of cytokine release.[52] Lanadelumab is a mAb against plasma kallikrein approved for the prevention of hereditary angioedema.[53] Idarucizumab is a mAb fragment that binds to and neutralizes dabigatran, approved to reverse the anticoagulant effects of dabigatran.[54]

The indications for mAb therapies are vast. Given their widely differing mechanisms, their toxicities differ widely as well. When a patient presents to an ED, it is imperative to review the medication list and the side-effect profile of any immunologic agent prescribed, so that toxicities can be recognized and treated appropriately.

SUMMARY

The intersection of immunology and emergency medicine is not a simple crossroads but a complex weave of overpasses and tunnels. The array of indications for immune-based drugs is immense, and patients on these therapies are encountered daily in the ED. Recognition of the adverse effects allows for improved coordination and care for these complex patients. In addition, understanding the latest developments and indications puts a treatment team in the best position to provide the best care possible.

CLINICS CARE POINTS

- Immune-based therapies are wide ranging, with indications spanning chronic and acute disease, from autoimmune, to oncologic, to infectious, and more.
- mABs currently are the most common type of immune-based therapy and usually are well tolerated.
- Adverse effects of mABs include acute infusion reactions, acute and delayed hypersensitivity responses, and increased risk for severe rare infections.
- Immune checkpoint inhibitors are specific cancer mABs; their IRAEs affect all organ systems. Management is guided by severity of the symptoms.
- Immune-based therapies are actively being investigated for treatment of acute infections, such as SARS–CoV-2. Familiarity with these new treatments is critical.

DISCLOSURE

The authors have nothing to disclose.

REFERENCES

1. Global cancer immunotherapy market analysis & forecast to 2025. Kelly Scientific Publications; 2020. p. 450. Available at: https://kellysci.com/global-cancer-immunotherapy-market-analysis-to-2025/.
2. Coleman RL, Sabbatini PJ. Targeted therapy and immunotherapy. In: Karlan BY, Bristow RE, Li AJ, editors. Gynecologic oncology: clinical practice and surgical atlas. McGraw-Hill Medical; 2015. Available at: http://hemonc.mhmedical.com/content.aspx?aid=1106572124%20. Accessed May 3, 2021.
3. Lake DF, Briggs AD. Immunopharmacology. In: Katzung BG, Vanderah TW, editors. Basic & clinical pharmacology, 15e. McGraw-Hill; 2021. Available at: http://accesspharmacy.mhmedical.com/content.aspx?aid=1176470987%20. Accessed May 3, 2021.

4. Bluestone JA, Anderson M. Tolerance in the age of immunotherapy. N Engl J Med 2020;383(12):1156–66.
5. Galluzzi L, Vacchelli E, Pedro J-MB-S, et al. Classification of current anticancer immunotherapies. Oncotarget 2014;5(24):12472–508.
6. Saibil SD, Wang BX, Butler MO. The immune system and immunotherapy. In: Harrington LA, Tannock IF, Hill RP, et al, editors. The basic science of oncology, 6e. McGraw-Hill Education; 2021. Available at: http://hemonc.mhmedical.com/content.aspx?aid=1179325974%20. Accessed May 3, 2021.
7. Baxevanis CN, Perez SA, Papamichail M. Cancer immunotherapy. Crit Rev Clin Lab Sci 2009;46(4):167–89.
8. Kennedy LB, Salama AKS. A review of cancer immunotherapy toxicity. CA A Cancer J Clin 2020;70(2):86–104.
9. Velcheti V, Schalper K. Basic overview of current immunotherapy approaches in cancer. Am Soc Clin Oncol Educ Book 2016;35:298–308. doi:10.1200/EDBK_156572.
10. Funes SC, Manrique de Lara A, Altamirano-Lagos MJ, et al. Immune checkpoints and the regulation of tolerogenicity in dendritic cells: implications for autoimmunity and immunotherapy. Autoimmun Rev 2019;18(4):359–68.
11. Helmy KY, Patel SA, Nahas GR, et al. Cancer immunotherapy: accomplishments to date and future promise. Ther Deliv 2013;4(10):1307–20.
12. Lu R-M, Hwang Y-C, Liu I-J, et al. Development of therapeutic antibodies for the treatment of diseases. J Biomed Sci 2020;27(1):1.
13. Hansel TT, Kropshofer H, Singer T, et al. The safety and side effects of monoclonal antibodies. Nat Rev Drug Discov 2010;9(4):325–38.
14. Cáceres MC, Guerrero-Martín J, Pérez-Civantos D, et al. The importance of early identification of infusion-related reactions to monoclonal antibodies. Ther Clin Risk Manag 2019;15:965–77.
15. Shivaji UN, Sharratt CL, Thomas T, et al. Review article: managing the adverse events caused by anti-TNF therapy in inflammatory bowel disease. Aliment Pharmacol Ther 2019;49(6):664–80.
16. Calogiuri G, Ventura MT, Mason L, et al. Hypersensitivity reactions to last generation chimeric, humanized [correction of umanized] and human recombinant monoclonal antibodies for therapeutic use. Curr Pharm Des 2008;14(27):2883–91.
17. Khan DA. Hypersensitivity and immunologic reactions to biologics: opportunities for the allergist. Ann Allergy Asthma Immunol 2016;117(2):115–20.
18. Karmacharya P, Poudel DR, Pathak R, et al. Rituximab-induced serum sickness: a systematic review. Semin Arthritis Rheum 2015;45(3):334–40.
19. Salvana EMT, Salata RA. Infectious complications associated with monoclonal antibodies and related small molecules. Clin Microbiol Rev 2009;22(2):274–90. Table of Contents.
20. Haanen JBAG, Carbonnel F, Robert C, et al. Management of toxicities from immunotherapy: ESMO clinical practice guidelines for diagnosis, treatment and follow-up. Ann Oncol 2017;28(suppl_4):iv119–42.
21. Jacobson CA, Farooq U, Ghobadi A. Axicabtagene ciloleucel, an anti-CD19 chimeric antigen receptor T-Cell therapy for relapsed or refractory large B-cell lymphoma: practical implications for the community oncologist. Oncologist 2020;25(1):e138–46.
22. Neelapu SS. Managing the toxicities of CAR T-cell therapy. Hematol Oncol 2019; 37(Suppl 1):48–52.

23. Myers GD, Verneris MR, Goy A, et al. Perspectives on outpatient administration of CAR-T cell therapy in aggressive B-cell lymphoma and acute lymphoblastic leukemia. J Immunother Cancer 2021;9(4):e002056.
24. Shimabukuro-Vornhagen A, Gödel P, Subklewe M, et al. Cytokine release syndrome. J Immunother Cancer 2018;6(1):56.
25. Acharya UH, Dhawale T, Yun S, et al. Management of cytokine release syndrome and neurotoxicity in chimeric antigen receptor (CAR) T cell therapy. Expert Rev Hematol 2019;12(3):195–205.
26. Abramson JS, Lunning M, Palomba ML. Chimeric antigen receptor T-cell therapies for aggressive B-cell lymphomas: current and future state of the art. Am Soc Clin Oncol Educ Book 2019;39:446–53.
27. Lee DW, Santomasso BD, Locke FL, et al. ASTCT consensus grading for cytokine release syndrome and neurologic toxicity associated with immune effector cells. Biol Blood Marrow Transpl 2019;25(4):625–38.
28. WHO COVID-19 Dashboard. Geneva: World Health Organization; 2020. Available at: https://covid19.who.int/. Accessed September 11, 2021.
29. Karthik K, Senthilkumar TMA, Udhayavel S, et al. Role of antibody-dependent enhancement (ADE) in the virulence of SARS-CoV-2 and its mitigation strategies for the development of vaccines and immunotherapies to counter COVID-19. Hum Vaccin Immunother 2020;16(12):3055–60.
30. Chowdhury MA, Hossain N, Kashem MA, et al. Immune response in COVID-19: a review. J Infect Public Health 2020;13(11):1619–29.
31. de Wilde AH, Snijder EJ, Kikkert M, et al. Host factors in coronavirus replication. Curr Top Microbiol Immunol 2018;419:1–42.
32. Available at: https://www.covid19treatmentguidelines.nih.gov/anti-sars-cov-2-antibody-products/convalescent-plasma/. Accessed June 6, 2021.
33. Wang X, Guo X, Xin Q, et al. Neutralizing antibody responses to severe acute respiratory syndrome coronavirus 2 in coronavirus disease 2019 inpatients and convalescent patients. Clin Infect Dis 2020;71(10):2688–94.
34. Garraud O, Heshmati F, Pozzetto B, et al. Plasma therapy against infectious pathogens, as of yesterday, today and tomorrow. Transfus Clin Biol 2016;23(1):39–44.
35. Chen L, Xiong J, Bao L, et al. Convalescent plasma as a potential therapy for COVID-19. Lancet Infect Dis 2020;20(4):398–400.
36. Chen P, Nirula A, Heller B, et al. SARS-CoV-2 neutralizing antibody LY-CoV555 in outpatients with Covid-19. N Engl J Med 2021;384(3):229–37.
37. Available at: https://www.fda.gov/media/145610/download. Accessed June 6, 2021.
38. Available at: https://www.fda.gov/media/145801/download. Accessed June 6, 2021.
39. Baum A, Fulton BO, Wloga E, et al. Antibody cocktail to SARS-CoV-2 spike protein prevents rapid mutational escape seen with individual antibodies. Science 2020;369(6506):1014–8.
40. Samaee H, Mohsenzadegan M, Ala S, et al. Tocilizumab for treatment patients with COVID-19: Recommended medication for novel disease. Int Immunopharmacol 2020;89(Pt A):107018.
41. Salian VS, Wright JA, Vedell PT, et al. COVID-19 transmission, current treatment, and future therapeutic strategies. Mol Pharm 2021;18(3):754–71.
42. Gooderham MJ, Hong HC, Eshtiaghi P, et al. Dupilumab: a review of its use in the treatment of atopic dermatitis. J Am Acad Dermatol 2018;78(3):S28–36.
43. Matsunaga K, Katoh N, Fujieda S, et al. Dupilumab: basic aspects and applications to allergic diseases. Allergol Int 2020;69(2):187–96.

44. Dantzer JA, Wood RA. The use of omalizumab in allergen immunotherapy. Clin Exp Allergy 2018;48(3):232–40.
45. Luna MS, Manzoni P, Paes B, et al. Expert consensus on palivizumab use for respiratory syncytial virus in developed countries. Paediatric Respir Rev 2020;33: 35–44.
46. Raj GM, Priyadarshini R, Murugesan S, et al. Monoclonal antibodies against infectious microbes: so long and too little! Infect Disord Drug Targets 2021; 21(1):4–27.
47. Ozkaya A, Demir G, Kirmaci A. Comparison of aflibercept and ranibizumab in diabetic macular edema associated with subretinal detachment. Eur J Ophthalmol 2020;30(2):363–9.
48. Onrust SV, Wiseman LR. Basiliximab. Drugs 1999;57(2):207–13 [discussion 214].
49. Garland SG, Smith SM, Gums JG. Erenumab: a first-in-class monoclonal antibody for migraine prevention. Ann Pharmacother 2019;53(9):933–9.
50. McDonagh M, Peterson K, Holzhammer B, et al. A systematic review of PCSK9 inhibitors alirocumab and evolocumab. J Manag Care Spec Pharm. 2016;22(6): 641–653q.
51. Deeks ED. Denosumab: a review in postmenopausal osteoporosis. Drugs Aging 2018;35(2):163–73.
52. Vallurupalli M, Berliner N. Emapalumab for the treatment of relapsed/refractory hemophagocytic lymphohistiocytosis. Blood 2019;134(21):1783–6.
53. Syed YY. Lanadelumab: a review in hereditary angioedema. Drugs 2019;79(16): 1777–84.
54. Pollack CV, Reilly PA, Eikelboom J, et al. Idarucizumab for dabigatran reversal. N Engl J Med 2015;373(6):511–20.

Sarcoidosis

Denrick Cooper, MD, MPH[a],*, Salvador Suau, MD[b,c]

KEYWORDS

- Granulomatous • Sarcoidosis • Nongranulomatous

KEY POINTS

- Sarcoidosis has many different manifestations and affects different organ systems.
- Ocular sarcoidosis commonly presents as anterior uveitis, and patients should be seen by an ophthalmologist because of possibility of vision loss.
- Cardiac sarcoidosis carries a poor prognosis and often presents as arrythmias.
- Corticosteroids are the mainstay of treatment of sarcoidosis; however, these medications carry risks with long-term treatment.
- Specialists should be involved early for decompensating patients. If safe for discharge, there must be a plan to see outpatient specialists for diagnoses that hold poorer outcomes (ie, ocular and cardiac sarcoidosis).

INTRODUCTION

Sarcoidosis is a granulomatous disease that affects a multitude of organs. It is often considered a "chameleon" diagnosis because it can masquerade as other diseases. Although classically seen in Black American women with pulmonary complaints, it has a wide array of presentations, some lethal, making it all the more important for emergency physicians to have a deeper understanding of the disease. This review focuses on the acute presentations of sarcoidosis. Pulmonary complaints are most common; however, cardiac, optic, and neurologic manifestations carry high mortality and morbidity. Disease outcomes also have a broad spectrum because of health care disparities. Access to care, socioeconomic status (SES), income, and comorbidities all influence morbidity and mortality.

This article originally appeared in Emergency Medicine Clinics, Volume 40 Issue 1, February 2022.

[a] Department of Emergency Medicine, Ochsner Health System, 1514 Jefferson Hwy, New Orleans, LA 71021, USA; [b] Emergency Medicine Residency, Department of Emergency Medicine, Ochsner Health System, New Orleans, LA, USA; [c] Ochsner Emergency Department, 1514 Jefferson Hwy, New Orleans, LA 71021, USA
* Corresponding author.
E-mail address: Denrick.cooper@ochsner.org

EPIDEMIOLOGY

Sarcoidosis is an inflammatory disease most prevalent in the United States and Scandinavian countries.[1] Sweden and the United States make up the largest proportions of people suffering from sarcoidosis in the world. The exact incidence of the disease in the United States ranges from 7.6 to 8.8 per 100,000.[2] The prevalence of sarcoidosis in the United States is between 150,000 and 200,000.[2] Black Americans have a profoundly increased incidence, and increased mortality and morbidity compared with other ethnicities within the United States. Black American women have the highest incidence of disease of all populations. Patients are typically diagnosed from ages 35 to 50 years old.[3] Some studies show two peaks of incidence at 25 to 29 years old and another at 65 to 69 years.[3]

The disease incidence, mortality, morbidity, and outcomes are skewed based on ethnicity, SES, gender, and income. The incidence in Black Americans is 35.5/100,000 compared with 10.9/100,000 in Whites. Mortality in women compared with men is 3.0 versus 2.3, respectively, whereas Black Americans die at a rate 16 times higher than White Americans.[1] People of African descent in other countries do not have the same burden of disease as Black Americans, hinting at the importance of environmental factors that influence the burden of disease in Black Americans within the United States.

Obesity and occupational status are prominent risk factors of sarcoidosis. A body mass index greater than 30 is associated with a 40% increased incidence of disease.[1] Silica-exposed work environments are associated with increased risk of sarcoidosis.[1] Construction, mining, and agricultural industries have a four-fold increase in the incidence of sarcoidosis.[4] Oddly, multiple studies show a decreased incidence of sarcoidosis in smokers compared with nonsmokers. This is counterintuitive because one would expect the components of cigarettes to increase inflammation rather than serve as a protective factor. Studies have yet to elucidate further confounding factors that may explain the association.

Social determinants of health affect disease severity and resilience. Income, race, and SES are protective or detrimental to disease severity. Patients making less than $35,000 annually have worse long-term outcomes.[4] The disease has an even greater economic impact on individuals because it afflicts patients during their prime wage-earning years, ages 30 to 50. Approximately one-third of individuals reported job loss secondary to the disease.[4] Furthermore, lower SES affects response to treatment regimens. Corticosteroids are the mainstay for treating sarcoidosis; however, those with a lower SES have an increased risk for developing steroid-related complications including sleep apnea and obesity.[4]

CAUSE/PATHOGENESIS

Sarcoidosis is a multisystem disease characterized by granulomatous inflammation throughout the body afflicting different organ systems. It was discovered in 1877 by a dermatologist named Jonathan Hutchinson.[5] The exact cause of sarcoidosis has yet to be discovered, yet many believe that certain genetic predispositions in conjunction with environmental triggers are at the crux of the disease process.

Sarcoidosis has a polygenetic cause made of multiple HLA genes that predispose patients to varying severities and presentations. Familial clusters exist suggesting there are gene mutations associated with the disease. The major histocompatibility complex is a portion of the short arm of chromosome 6 that encodes proteins involved in the human adaptive immune response. One of these proteins, HLA, is responsible for presenting antigens on the surface of antigen-presenting cells to T cells (**Fig. 1**).

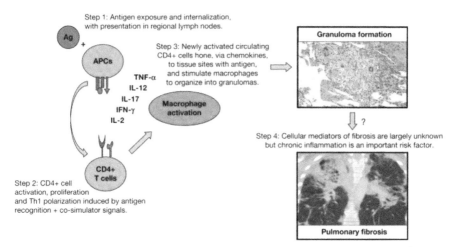

Fig. 1. Antigen presentation to antigen-presenting cells (APC) initiates a cascade of inflammatory markers, leading to the activation and proliferation of CD4$^+$ T cells. Downstream mediators activate macrophages to organize into the granulomas seen in sarcoidosis. Chronic inflammation causes lasting, irreversible fibrotic changes in affected tissues. IFN, interferon; IL, interleukin.

This interaction initiates the host immune response.[6] HLA class II alleles are frequently associated with sarcoidosis, especially more benign forms. Further inflammatory markers, cytokines and chemokines, mediate the granulomatous response seen in the disease state. Tumor necrosis factor (TNF)-α and transforming growth factor-β contribute to the cascade of inflammation. TNF-α is released from macrophages at higher levels, whereas transforming growth factor-β stimulates the deposition of cellular matrices.[7,8]

Sarcoidosis is caused by an inappropriate immune response in conjunction with environmental triggers. Laborers with exposures to silica, insecticides, and agriculture all show increased incidence of sarcoidosis. Additionally, *Mycobacterium* infection and certain cancers (lymphomas) are associated with sarcoidosis.[8]

HISTOLOGY

One mainstay of sarcoidosis is granulomatous inflammation found in biopsy results of affected organ systems. Noncaseating granulomas are hallmark for sarcoidosis.[3] Biopsies are typically taken from lymph nodes, lacrimal glands, or skin lesions because they are more accessible. Antigen-presenting cells presenting antigens to T helper cells initiate the inflammatory cascade (see **Fig. 1**). The interaction serves as the nidus that further inflammatory cells surround. Center portions are noncaseating, meaning without or with little central necrosis. They are clusters of multinucleated giant cells and epithelioid cells surrounded by lymphocytes.[8,9] Histology is a cornerstone for diagnosis and helps to differentiate sarcoidosis from other granulomatous diseases, such as tuberculosis, histoplasmosis, or lymphoma.

DIFFERENTIAL DIAGNOSIS

One of the difficulties of sarcoidosis is its ability to masquerade as other diagnoses. It is diagnosed by a mixture of histopathologic, laboratory, and clinical results, not otherwise explained by other causes (**Table 1**). As such, it is primarily a diagnosis of

Table 1
Differential diagnosis of sarcoidosis

Differential Diagnosis	Histology	Cause	Signs and Symptoms	Epidemiology	Diagnostics
Sarcoidosis	Noncaseating granuloma	Autoinflammatory	Multisystemic	Women, Black American, Scandinavian	Biopsy, CXR, computed tomography scan
Tuberculosis	Caseating granuloma	Mycobacterium	Multisystemic	High-risk groups: homeless, immunosuppressed, endemic countries	AFB sputum staining, QuantiFERON Gold
Lymphoma	Noncaseating granuloma	Proliferation of lymphoid/precursor cells	Lymphadenopathy, B-cell symptoms (night sweats, weight loss, fatigue)	40–70 year old age group	Biopsy, imaging
Cat-scratch disease[12]	Caseating granuloma	Bartonella	Lymphadenopathy (in epitrochlear and axillary nodes), erythematous papule, malaise, myalgia, anorexia	History of cat scratch, animal aggression	IFA, EIA, for IgM and IgG against species, culture
Toxoplasmosis[13–15]	Noncaseating granuloma	Toxoplasmosis gondii	Retinochoroidal inflammation, blindness, seizures, ataxia, AMS, lethargy	Waterborne/foodborne illness, undercooked meats, feline presence, high prevalence in areas of poor water sanitation in South America and Africa, immunocompromised host (AIDS)	T gondii IgM, IgG
Histoplasmosis[16]	Caseating granuloma	Histoplasma capsulatum	Cough, fever, dyspnea, night sweats anorexia, weight loss	Midwestern United States and Central America, immunosuppressed/immunocompromised patients	Cavitary lung lesions, culture, serum antigen, urine antigen
Berylliosis[17]	Noncaseating granulomas	Beryllium exposure	Cough fever, night sweats, fatigue	Beryllium-exposed workers onset 3 mo–30 y of exposure	Serum or BAL + beryllium lymphocyte proliferation test

exclusion. As a non caseating granulomatous disease, other processes with similar histology include *Mycobacterium* disease, and fungal diseases, such as histoplasmosis and coccidiomycosis.[10,11]

PULMONARY SARCOIDOSIS

The lungs are the most commonly affected organ system in sarcoidosis.[3] Patients can present to the emergency department complaining of chest pain, tightness, dyspnea, or cough; however, many patients are asymptomatic. Unfortunately, half of patients do not obtain the correct diagnosis until 3 months after symptoms begin.[18]

Pulmonary sarcoidosis is categorized by stages ranging from I to IV. Stage I is most frequently seen in 40% to 50% of patients. Chest radiograph findings consist of mediastinal and hilar lymphadenopathy without pulmonary infiltrates. The rarest and most severe stage, Stage IV, occurs in 2% to 5% of patients, where there is pulmonary volume loss without adenopathy.[3] Computed tomography is another modality used for diagnosis because some patients do not have salient radiograph findings. Fluorodeoxyglucose (FDG)-PET scans also have a high sensitivity for viewing inflammation in the lung signified by reduced uptake of FDG. Combined with computed tomography scan, FDG-PET is more sensitive than PET scan alone while allowing for the identification of inflammatory loci that can be biopsied for histologic examination.[18]

At times patients further undergo bronchiolar lavage to add more information to the clinical picture. A study found that a ratio of CD4/CD8 greater than 3.5 had a specificity and sensitivity for sarcoidosis of 53% and 94%, respectively.[19]

Most people with pulmonary sarcoidosis do not require treatment.[3] Nevertheless, the first-line treatment of pulmonary sarcoidosis is corticosteroids. All treatment aims to reduce the body's innate inflammatory response. Glucocorticoids are only required for a third of patients with pulmonary sarcoidosis. An initial dose of 20 to 40 mg is effective in acute exacerbations in patients who are naive to the drug.[18] The drug takes 3 to 4 weeks to take effect, therefore if a patient is presenting with an acute exacerbation appropriate disposition into the hospital or outpatient setting is crucial for future follow-up. Steroids are typically tapered to the lowest effective dosage to avoid side effects. Patients often relapse after stopping steroids at a range of 14% to 74% for acute disease and higher, 75%, for chronic disease.

Second-line treatment of pulmonary sarcoidosis is steroid-sparing medications. Methotrexate (MTX) is most commonly used because it is anti-inflammatory and immunosuppressive.[8] MTX is used for patients that are steroid refractory or develop severe steroid side effects. It is started at 5 mg weekly and gradually increased. MTX may require up to 6 months of usage to elicit an effect. Once patients are using the drug, it is prudent to obtain complete blood count and creatine levels on a routine basis.

Severe pulmonary tuberculosis can have detrimental long-term effects on patients. Lung transplantation is needed in end-stage sarcoid patients that fail medical treatment. Patients that undergo transplantation still have poor generalized outcomes. Pulmonary hypertension is seen in 73.8% of patients with pulmonary sarcoidosis.[20]

CARDIAC

Cardiac sarcoidosis is an underreported entity seen in less than 5% of patients; however, autopsies show higher rates.[21] Patients can present with palpitations, syncope, chest pain, or sudden cardiac death, although the latter is rare.[22] The diagnosis of cardiac sarcoidosis requires a mix of invasive and noninvasive testing.

Electrocardiograms are abnormal in 7% of all patients with sarcoidosis,[22] often showing atrioventricular blocks, atrial dysrhythmias, and ventricular dysrhythmias.[23] Echocardiography is useful because it can detect left ventricular systolic dysfunction, dyskinesia, effusion, or valve dysfunction. Cardiac biomarkers are helpful in screening for cardiac sarcoidosis. B-type natriuretic peptide levels greater than 40 pg/mL have a sensitivity for cardiac sarcoidosis of 85.4% and a specificity of 68.1%.[24] Cardiac imaging focuses on FDG-PET scans to look for areas of inflammation, whereas cardiac MRI can assess for scarring, similar to pulmonary sarcoidosis.

First-line medical therapy for cardiac sarcoidosis is corticosteroids with doses starting at 20 to 60 mg/day.[21] MTX in conjunction with steroids is helpful for stabilizing sarcoid-induced congestive heart failure.[25] Refractory sarcoidosis is treated with TNF antagonists, such as infliximab and adalimumab. For patients with severe atrioventricular blocks pacemakers are used alongside implantable cardioverter-defibrillators for patients with poor ejection fractions.

OCULAR SARCOIDOSIS

Ocular sarcoidosis is the second most common extrapulmonary manifestation of sarcoid, after skin. It is most concerning because it can cause blindness if not treated in a timely fashion. Ocular manifestations occur in 10% to 25% of patients.[26] Most present with eye pain, floaters, redness, abnormal discharge, or changes in vision. Different parts of the eye are affected including the anterior and posterior chambers, sclera, conjunctiva, lacrimal gland, and orbit. Anterior uveitis is the most common disease of ocular sarcoidosis.[27] Usually the uveitis is bilateral and overall has a good prognosis.[28] Because ocular sarcoidosis is subclinical or asymptomatic, all patients with sarcoidosis should be screened for ocular involvement.

The gold standard for diagnosing ocular sarcoidosis is biopsy. The lacrimal gland is commonly used because it is easily accessible.

First-line treatment of ocular sarcoidosis is topical steroids. In the setting of anterior uveitis, dosages are started based on the degree of inflammation in the anterior chamber. Prednisolone acetate eight times daily or the more potent difluprednate 4 times daily are both effective.[29] Topical steroids are used for anterior inflammation, whereas posterior inflammation requires local injections. Cycloplegics, such as cyclopentolate, are used to treat pain from ciliary spasms. For severe cases of uveitis, systemic steroids are mainly used.

RENAL

Granulomatous interstitial nephritis is found in 3% of patients with sarcoidosis.[3] Renal sarcoidosis is usually asymptomatic,[22] but associated signs and symptoms include hypercalciuria and nephrocalcinosis. Hypercalcemia is seen in 5% to 10% of patients. 1α-Hydroxylase, responsible for converting 25-hydroxycholecalciferol into 1,25-dihydroxycholecalciferol, is expressed by macrophages in granulomas. Abnormal enzyme expression causes hypercalcemia. Interstitial nephritis is easily treated with corticosteroids or a combination of immunosuppressive drugs.

NEUROLOGIC

Neurosarcoidosis is an uncommon manifestation with cranial nerves (especially II, VII, and VIII), brain parenchyma, and meninges most commonly affected.[3] Granulomatous inflammation of the leptomeninges or of the nerve itself causes facial nerve palsy. The prognosis is favorable, because more than 90% of patients recover function with steroids. The next most common neurologic manifestations are chronic aseptic meningitis, myelitis, and cerebellar parenchymal disease similar to multiple sclerosis.[30] Treatment of neurologic manifestations is similar to other systems in a stepwise fashion from steroids, MTX, and TNF-α inhibitors.

SYNDROMES

Sarcoidosis also manifests as different syndromes. Heerfordt syndrome is a constellation of symptoms characterized by fever, anterior uveitis, CN VII palsy, and parotid gland enlargement.[31] It was first characterized by Dr Christina Heerfordt in 1909.[32] Multiple case reports exist in the literature; however, the exact prevalence of the syndrome is unknown. As with other forms of sarcoidosis, angiotensin-converting enzyme levels are elevated but do not correlate with disease activity.

Löfgren syndrome is another clinical phenotype of sarcoidosis. It was first characterized in 1946 by Dr Sven Löfgren. The syndrome is diagnosed by the presence of erythema nodosum, bilateral hilar lymphadenopathy, and polyarthritis.[33] Younger, female patients of Scandinavian ancestry are commonly afflicted. Löfgren syndrome has a good prognosis with symptoms self-resolving within 1 to 2 years. Nonsteroidal anti-inflammatory drugs are used for arthritic pain. Severe cases are treated with oral steroids until symptom resolution.[33]

CLINICS CARE POINTS

- Cardiac sarcoidosis carries a high mortality and is associated with fatal arrythmias. Electrocardiogram and cardiology consultations should be obtained.

- Untreated or delayed treatment of ocular sarcoidosis confers a high risk of blindness; all patients with sarcoidosis should have at least an outpatient ophthalmology evaluation.

- Corticosteroids are first-line treatment of sarcoidosis.

- Most forms of asymptomatic and less severe pulmonary sarcoidosis do not need treatment and resolve without intervention.

DISCLOSURE

The authors have nothing to disclose.

REFERENCES

1. Arkema EV, Cozier YC. Epidemiology of sarcoidosis: current findings and future directions. Ther Adv Chronic Dis 2018;9(11):227–40.
2. Baughman RP, Field S, Costabel U, et al. Sarcoidosis in America. Analysis based on health care use. Ann Am Thorac Soc 2016;13(8):1244–52.
3. Ungprasert P, Ryu JH, Matteson EL. Clinical manifestations, diagnosis, and treatment of sarcoidosis. Mayo Clin Proc Innov Qual Outcomes 2019;3(3):358–75.
4. Cozier YC, Govender P. Sarcoidosis: an ill-afforded disease. Am J Respir Crit Care Med 2020;201(8):890–1.
5. Llanos O, Hamzeh N. Sarcoidosis. Med Clin North Am 2019;103(3):527–34.
6. Moller DR, Chen ES. Genetic basis of remitting sarcoidosis. Am J Respir Cell Mol Biol 2002;27(4):391–5.

7. Ziegenhagen MW, Benner UK, Zissel G, et al. Sarcoidosis: TNF-alpha release from alveolar macrophages and serum level of sIL-2R are prognostic markers. Am J Respir Crit Care Med 1997;156(5):1586–92.

8. Ramachandraiah V, Aronow W, Chandy D. Pulmonary sarcoidosis: an update. Postgrad Med 2017;129(1):149–58.

9. Myers JL, Tazelaar HD. Challenges in pulmonary fibrosis: 6 problematic granulomatous lung disease. Thorax 2008;63(1):78–84.

10. Prasse A. The Diagnosis, Differential Diagnosis, and Treatment of Sarcoidosis. Deutsches Aerzteblatt Online 2016;113(33-34):565–74.

11. Rosen Y. Pathology of sarcoidosis. Semin Respir Crit Care Med 2007;28(1): 36–52.

12. Mazur-Melewska K, Mania A, Kemnitz P, et al. Cat-scratch disease: a wide spectrum of clinical pictures. Adv Dermatol Allergol Dermatol Alergol 2015;32(3): 216–20.

13. Furtado JM, Smith JR, Belfort R, et al. Toxoplasmosis: a global threat. J Glob Infect Dis 2011;3(3):281–4.

14. Halonen SK, Weiss LM. Toxoplasmosis. Handb Clin Neurol 2013;114:125–45.

15. Toxoplasmosis [Internet]. Available at: https://www.pathologyoutlines.com/topic/lymphnodestoxoplasma.html. Accessed December, 28 2020.

16. Kauffman CA. Histoplasmosis: a clinical and laboratory update. Clin Microbiol Rev 2007;20(1):115–32.

17. Sizar O, Talati R. Berylliosis. In: StatPearls [Internet]. Treasure Island (FL): StatPearls Publishing; 2020. Available at: http://www.ncbi.nlm.nih.gov/books/NBK470364/. Accessed December 28, 2020.

18. Spagnolo P, Rossi G, Trisolini R, et al. Pulmonary sarcoidosis. Lancet Respir Med 2018;6(5):389–402.

19. Nagai S, Izumi T. Bronchoalveolar lavage. Still useful in diagnosing sarcoidosis? Clin Chest Med 1997;18(4):787–97.

20. Duong H, Bonham CA. Sarcoidosis-associated pulmonary hypertension: pathophysiology, diagnosis, and treatment. Clin Pulm Med 2018;25(2):52–60.

21. Ribeiro Neto ML, Jellis CL, Joyce E, et al. Update in cardiac sarcoidosis. Ann Am Thorac Soc 2019;16(11):1341–50.

22. Crouser ED, Maier LA, Wilson KC, et al. Diagnosis and detection of sarcoidosis. An official American Thoracic Society clinical practice guideline. Am J Respir Crit Care Med 2020;201(8):e26–51.

23. Chapelon-Abric C, de Zuttere D, Duhaut P, et al. Cardiac sarcoidosis: a retrospective study of 41 cases. Medicine (Baltimore) 2004;83(6):315–34.

24. Kiko T, Yoshihisa A, Kanno Y, et al. A multiple biomarker approach in patients with cardiac sarcoidosis [Internet]. Int Heart J 2018;59(5):996–1001.

25. Nagai S, Yokomatsu T, Tanizawa K, et al. Treatment with methotrexate and low-dose corticosteroids in sarcoidosis patients with cardiac lesions. Intern Med 2014;53:427–33.

26. Ungprasert P, Tooley AA, Crowson CS, et al. Clinical characteristics of ocular sarcoidosis: a population-based study 1976-2013. Ocul Immunol Inflamm 2019;27:389–95.

27. Heiligenhaus A, Wefelmeyer D, Wefelmeyer E, et al. The eye as a common site for the early clinical manifestation of sarcoidosis. Ophthalmic Res 2011; 46(1):9–12.

28. Rochepeau C, Jamilloux Y, Kerever S, et al. Long-term visual and systemic prognoses of 83 cases of biopsy-proven sarcoid uveitis. Br J Ophthalmol 2017;101(7): 856–61.

29. Sheppard JD, Toyos MM, Kempen JH, et al. Difluprednate 0.05% versus prednisolone acetate 1% for endogenous anterior uveitis: a phase III, multicenter, randomized study. Invest Ophthalmol Vis Sci 2014;55(5):2993–3002.
30. Voortman M, Drent M, Baughman RP. Management of neurosarcoidosis: a clinical challenge. Curr Opin Neurol 2019;32(3):475–83.
31. Tamme T, Leibur E, Kulla A. Sarcoidosis (Heerfordt syndrome): a case report. Stomatologija 2007;9:61–4.
32. Denny MC, Fotino AD. The Heerfordt-Waldenström syndrome as an initial presentation of sarcoidosis. Proc (Bayl Univ Med Cent) 2013;26(4):390–2.
33. Brown F, Modi P, Tanner LS. Lofgren syndrome. In: StatPearls [Internet]. Treasure Island (FL): StatPearls Publishing; 2020. Available at: http://www.ncbi.nlm.nih.gov/books/NBK482315/. Accessed December 1, 2020.

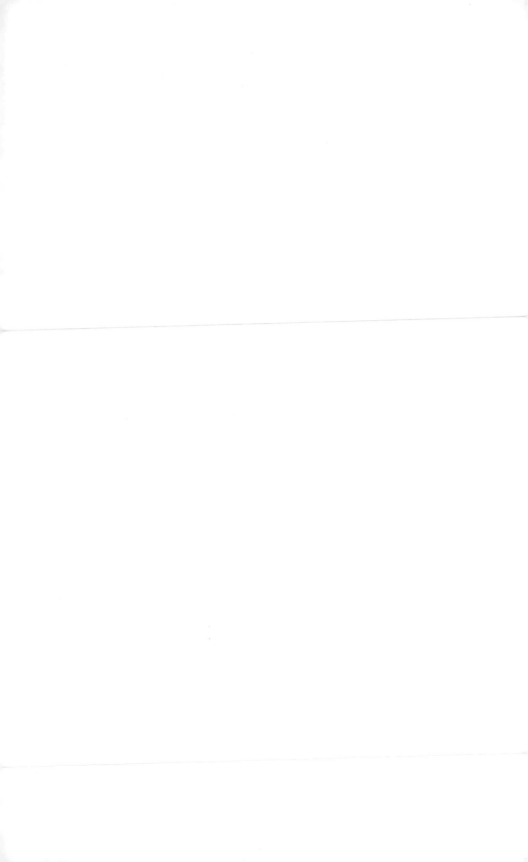

Spondyloarthritides

Hope A. Taitt, MD, Rithvik Balakrishnan, MD*

KEYWORDS

- Spondyloarthritides • Axial spondylitis • Ankylosing spondylitis • Psoriatic arthritis
- Inflammatory bowel disease–associated spondyloarthritis • Reactive arthritis

KEY POINTS

- Evaluation of a patient with a spondyloarthropathy should include consideration of possible complications of the disease as well as its treatments.
- The expanded diagnostic criteria of axial spondylitis allow MRI to diagnose patients with sacroiliitis that may not be apparent on radiograph.
- A trial of nonsteroidal anti-inflammatory drugs can safely be given to patients with suspected spondyloarthritis in the absence of known contraindications and active bowel disease.
- Subsequent treatment should evaluate the axial and peripheral features of spondyloarthritis with attention given to adverse effects.

INTRODUCTION

The term spondyloarthropathy links ankylosing spondylitis (AS), psoriatic arthritis (PsA), reactive arthritis, and inflammatory bowel disease (IBD) -associated arthritis as interrelated disease processes owing to overlapping clinical features and shared genetic predisposition. From early adulthood, these disorders present with musculoskeletal manifestations like inflammatory back pain, enthesitis (inflammation at tendon attachment sites to bone), oligoarthritis (usually of the lower extremities), and dactylitis (sausage digits) as well as extraskeletal manifestations, such as uveitis, psoriasis, and IBD. A patient diagnosed with 1 disease may experience symptoms prominent in another disease process. Genetically, the spondyloarthritides have been associated with the presence of HLA-B27. Despite similar genetics, some disease states are thought to be precipitated by environmental triggers, such as gastrointestinal and genitourinary (GI/GU) infections, whereas others do not appear to have an inciting event.[1,2]

This article originally appeared in Emergency Medicine Clinics, Volume 40 Issue 1, February 2022.

Department of Emergency Medicine, Kings County Hospital, SUNY Downstate Medical Center, Kings County Hospital Center, Room CG65, 451 Clarkson Avenue, Brooklyn, NY 11203, USA
* Corresponding author.
E-mail address: rithvik.balakrishnan@downstate.com

The wide range of signs and symptoms of the spondyloarthritides can make a diagnosis challenging. It has been noted to take 6 to 8 years for most patients to have a definite diagnosis established.[3] This delay can lead to unchecked inflammation, structural damage, and later restriction in physical mobility. Once a diagnosis is made and treatment is started, there are complications the physician should be aware of because of the natural progression of the disease process, and its treatments.

First-line treatment of the spondyloarthritides aims to reduce inflammation with nonsteroidal anti-inflammatory drugs (NSAIDs). Although there is variation in how treatment is escalated, tumor necrosis factor (TNF) inhibitors can generally achieve suppression of symptoms if NSAIDs fail. Conventional disease-modifying antirheumatic drugs (DMARDs) can be used to target specific symptoms, whereas interleukin inhibitors can be used as additional treatment tools.

CLASSIFICATION OF SPONDYLOARTHROPATHIES AND DEFINITIONS

The spondyloarthritides, which are sometimes also referred to as the seronegative spondyloarthropathies owing to the lack of association with a positive rheumatoid factor, are divided into 2 groups: axial spondyloarthritis (SpA) and peripheral SpA. Axial SpA, which refers to patients with predominantly axial spine involvement, is further divided into patients who present with radiographic findings of SpA and patients who lack radiographic Axial SpA findings. Radiographic SpA (also referred to as ankylosing spondylitis) refers to "patients who have already developed structural damage in the sacroiliac joints or spine visible on radiographs while patients without structural damage [are] labelled as non-radiographic SpA."[4] Peripheral SpA consists of PsA, IBD-associated arthritis, and reactive arthritis.

Axial SpA is currently classified by the Assessment in Spondylo-Arthritis International Society (ASAS) criteria developed in 2009 (**Fig. 1**). The ASAS criteria expanded the current (modified New York) definition of sacroiliitis (radiographic finding of grade >2 bilaterally or grade 3–4 unilaterally) to include MRI as a diagnostic modality. An MRI finding of active/acute inflammation highly suggestive of sacroiliitis meets the diagnostic criteria for axial SpA. This addition allows more patients to meet the diagnostic criteria of axial SpA and denotes those without standard radiographic findings of sacroiliitis as nonradiographic SpA.[5–7] Of note, although these 2 processes likely progress along the same spectrum, nonradiographic SpA does not always result in radiographic SpA.[4]

In 2011, the ASAS criteria for peripheral SpA were developed to standardize the diagnoses of patients with peripheral manifestations of SpA (see **Fig. 1**).[8] The presence of arthritis, enthesitis, or dactylitis serves as the basis for making the diagnosis of a peripheral SpA. For the purposes of these disease processes, the ASAS defined the components of these criteria as seen in **Table 1**.

In contrast, reactive arthritis can occur as an oligoarthritis with 5 or fewer joints being inflamed while progressing in either an additive (progressive inflammation without the earlier joint inflammation resolving) or a migratory (joint inflammation in 1 joint resolves as another joint becomes inflamed) pattern, after an inciting GI/GU infection between 1 and 6 weeks prior.[9] Reiter syndrome exists as a subset of reactive arthritis and refers classically to inflammatory arthritis of a large joint, urethritis (men) or cervicitis (women), and either conjunctivitis or uveitis.

There are no classification criteria for reactive arthritis. The diagnostic criteria for the diagnosis of "definite" versus "probable" reactive arthritis are based on major and minor criteria. Definite reactive arthritis is defined as the presence of both major

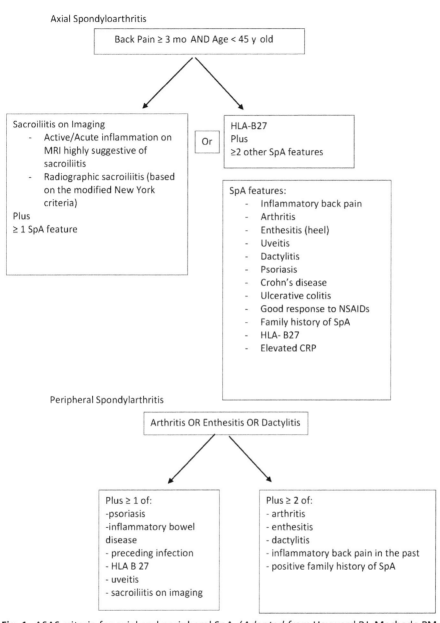

Fig. 1. ASAS criteria for axial and peripheral SpA. (*Adapted from* Hayward RJ, Machado PM. Classification Criteria in Axial Spondyloarthritis: What Have We Learned; Where Are We Going?. Rheum Dis Clin North Am. 2020;46(2):259-274 and the Assessment of Spondyloarthritis International Society)

and relevant minor criteria, whereas a probable diagnosis is made by the presence of both major criteria but no relevant minor criteria (or 1 major and 1 or more minor criteria) (**Box 1**). Of note, there must be identification of an infectious source in order to make any of the above diagnoses. Commonly identified pathogens causing urogenital tract infections include *Chlamydia trachomatis, Neisseria gonorrhoeae,*

Table 1
Definitions of axial spondyloarthritis features for use in Assessment in Spondylo-Arthritis International Society classification of peripheral axial spondyloarthritis

Peripheral Arthritis Symptoms	
Arthritis	Current peripheral arthritis (asymmetric, lower limb predominant)
Enthesitis	Current enthesitis
Dactylitis	Current dactylitis
Additional Spondyloarthritis Symptoms	
Inflammatory back pain	Past history of inflammatory back pain diagnosed by a rheumatologist
Arthritis	Past or present arthritis
Enthesitis	Past or present spontaneous pain or tenderness on examination of an enthesitis
Uveitis	Past or present anterior uveitis, confirmed by an ophthalmologist
Dactylitis	Past or present dactylitis
Psoriasis	Past or present psoriasis
Inflammatory bowel disease	Past or present Crohn disease or ulcerative colitis
Preceding infection	Gastrointestinal (diarrhea) or genitourinary (urethritis, cervicitis) illness 1 mo before onset of the above peripheral arthritis symptoms
Family history of SpA	Presence of axial SpA, psoriasis, acute uveitis, reactive arthritis, or IBD in a first- or second-degree relative
HLA-B27	Positive blood test
Sacroiliitis	Identified on imaging • Modified New York criteria: grade 2–4 bilateral or grade 3–4 unilateral sacroiliitis on radiographs • MRI indicative of acute/active inflammation of the sacroiliac joints

Adapted from the Assessment of Spondyloarthritis International Society.

Mycoplasma genitalium, and Ureaplasma urealyticum. GI illnesses can be caused by Yersinia, Shigella, Salmonella, and Campylobacter jejuni. Less frequently, Clostridium difficile, Chlamydia pneumoniae, and Chlamydia psittaci are found as causative agents.[9,10]

PsA was defined by Moll and Wright[11] in 1973. Previously, PsA had been regarded as 2 distinct entities of psoriasis and arthritis with a possible association with rheumatoid arthritis. Moll and Wright adapted the existing definitions of psoriasis and arthritis to reflect that PsA is psoriasis associated with inflammatory arthritis and usually with a negative serologic test for rheumatoid factor. With this expanded definition, they generated 5 subtypes of PsA. They are as follows:

1. Distal interphalangeal arthritis
2. Arthritis mutilans (a severe, deforming arthritis)
3. Symmetric arthritis (may appear similar to rheumatoid arthritis but has negative serology)
4. Asymmetrical arthritis with only a single or few joints involved (may also include dactylitis as inflammation of the soft tissues between 2 affected joints)
5. Predominant spondylitis with or without peripheral joint involvement[11]

Box 1
Diagnostic criteria for reactive arthritis

Definite Diagnosis requires both major criteria and 1 minor criteria.

Probable Diagnosis requires both major criteria and no minor criteria OR 1 major criterion and 1 or more minor criteria.
   Major criteria:
   1. Arthritis with 2 or 3 of the following:
      a. Asymmetric
      b. Monoarthritis or oligoarthritis
      c. Lower-limb involvement
   2. Preceding symptomatic infection with 1 or 2 of the following:
      a. Enteritis (diarrhea for 1 day minimum; 3 days to 6 weeks before arthritis onset)
      b. Urethritis (dysuria, discharge for 1 day minimum; 3 days to 6 weeks before arthritis onset)
   Minor criteria: Laboratory evidence of infection
   1. Triggering infection
      a. *Chlamydia trachomatis*
         i. Positive urine ligase reaction
         ii. Positive urethral/cervical swab
   2. Persistent synovial infection
      a. Positive immunohistology or polymerase chain reaction for chlamydia

Adapted from Selmi C, Gershwin ME. Diagnosis and classification of reactive arthritis. Autoimmun Rev. 2014;13(4-5):546-549., 2014

In 2006, the Classification Criteria for Psoriatic Arthritis (CASPAR) criteria (**Fig. 2**) were developed based on the evaluation of 1124 patient with PsA, rheumatoid arthritis, AS, undifferentiated arthritis, connective tissue disorders, and other diseases. The goal was to compare the performance of several criteria that had developed since 1973 and to create unified criteria moving forward. For patients with an established inflammatory articular disease (joint, spinal, or entheseal), a score of ≥3 using the CASPAR criteria had a sensitivity of 98.7% and specificity of 91.4% for diagnosis of PsA. (Of note, current psoriasis is assigned a value of 2 points, whereas all other criteria receive 1 point.)[12–15]

IBD-associated SpA, also referred to as enteropathic arthritis, is defined by the presence of peripheral involvement, axial involvement, or both. The diagnosis of IBD-associated peripheral arthritis, which is common in both ulcerative colitis and Crohn disease, is mostly clinical, as peripheral arthritis is nonerosive. There are 2 subtypes of peripheral arthritis associated with IBD. Type 1 is pauciarticular, acute, and usually self-limited. It tends to follow the course of IBD flares. Type 2 peripheral arthritis is polyarticular and chronic in nature. It does not follow the course of IBD. It is known to be strongly associated with uveitis. The axial type of IBD-associated SpA requires the identification of spondylitis or sacroiliitis.[16,17]

EPIDEMIOLOGY

Categorization of the prevalence and incidence of the spondyloarthropathies has been complicated by their considerable overlap, their evolving definitions, and the methodological differences between studies. However, the National Arthritis Data Workgroup estimated in 2008 that the overall SpA prevalence within the United States ranged between 0.34% and 1.3% for adults ≥25 years old.[18] A strong association with the HLA-B27 gene was shown by an analysis of the COMOSPA registry (comprising 3984

Current Psoriasis		2 points

Personal History of Psoriasis	1 point
Family History of Psoriasis	
Psoriatic nail dystrophy	
- Onycholysis	
- Pitting	
- Hyperkeratosis	
Negative Rheumatoid Factor	
Current dactylitis	
History of dactylitis diagnosed by rheumatology	
Radiographic evidence of juxta-articular new bone formation (ill-defined ossification near joint margins)	

Fig. 2. The ClASsification criteria for Psoriatic ARthritis (CASPAR) criteria. (*Adapted from* Rudwaleit M, Taylor WJ. Classification criteria for psoriatic arthritis and ankylosing spondylitis/axial spondyloarthritis. Best Pract Res Clin Rheumatol. 2010;24(5):589-604)

patients from 22 countries in Asia, Africa, Europe, and North America with SpA) demonstrating 78.4% of the patients who met ASAS criteria for axial SpA were also HLA-B27 positive.

Ankylosing Spondylitis

A 2013 review of 29 population-based cross-sectional studies estimated the global prevalence of AS as ranging between 74 (South Africa) and 319 (North America) per 100,000 patients.[19] A review of the NHANES data from 2009 to 2010 using the ESSG criteria estimated the prevalence of AS at 550 per 100,000 patients, and the prevalence of axial spondyloarthritides (which includes AS and nonradiographic SpA) at 1400 per 100,000 patients (ranging from 900 for non-Hispanic blacks to 1500 for Mexican Americans and non-Hispanic whites).[20]

Peripheral Spondyloarthritides

Manifestations of spondyloarthritides are seldom confined to the peripheral skeleton, as demonstrated by an analysis of the COMOSPA registry, which found that, of patients with peripheral manifestations of SpA, 91% also demonstrated concurrent axial or psoriatic symptoms.[21]

Psoriatic

Estimates of the prevalence of PsA range between 20 (China and Mexico) and 420 per 100,000 patients (Italy).[22] Within the United States, an analysis of patients from

Olmsted County, Minnesota who met CASPAR criteria demonstrated a prevalence of 158 per 100,000 patients.[23]

Reactive

Data on incidence of reactive arthritis are generally derived from outbreak studies and questionnaires. Among these, a population study from Oregon and Minnesota of patients with positive cultures for *Escherichia coli* 0157, *Salmonella, Campylobacter, Shigella,* and *Yersinia* estimated an incidence of 0.6 to 3.1 cases of reactive arthritis per 100,000 patients. Risk for rheumatologic sequelae was correlated with GI symptom severity, but not with HLA-B27 prevalence.[24] The overall prevalence of acute reactive arthritis is estimated as ranging between 0.09% and 1%.[22]

Inflammatory Bowel Disease

SpA is a frequently cited extraintestinal manifestation of IBDs, such as Crohn's disease and ulcerative colitis, with a systematic review of available epidemiologic studies finding a prevalence of 13% for peripheral arthritis, 10% for sacroiliitis, and 3% for AS.[25]

CLINICAL MANIFESTATIONS
Musculoskeletal

Low back pain is an extremely common complaint with approximately 25% of US adults reporting 1 day of low back pain in the past 3 months.[26] Its cause is usually intrinsic to the spine ranging from lumbosacral strain and disk herniation to compression fractures, although several factors can suggest a more severe cause to the emergency physician. They include presence of fever, age less than 18 years, age greater than 50 years, GU complications (urinary retention, fecal incontinence), use of steroids or anticoagulants, intravenous drug abuse, recent spinal surgery or epidural injection, and history of malignancy.[27,28] In contrast, the presence of low back pain, before the age of 45, affecting patients for 3 or more months without a mechanical cause should raise suspicion of an SpA prompting imaging and further evaluation.

Inflammatory back pain, as described above, is one of the distinguishing features of SpA. It can be associated also with enthesitis, oligoarthritis (usually of the lower extremities), and dactylitis. Patients may experience nonmusculoskeletal symptoms, such as psoriasis, anterior uveitis, Crohn disease/ulcerative colitis and may report a history of GI/GU illness, a family history of SpA, or presence of the HLA-B27 gene.

IMAGING FINDINGS

The 2 main imaging modalities for the spondyloarthritides are radiographs and MRI of the sacroiliac joint. MRI is more useful for early diagnosis, as it may detect manifestations of the spondyloarthritides before they become visible on plain radiographs.[29]

The common radiographic findings associated with the spondyloarthritides are sacroiliitis and enthesitis. Sacroiliitis involves erosions, sclerosis, and bony bridging. Erosions may be visualized with obscuration of joint outlines that progress to irregular contours in the caudal joint, and finally, to a string-of-pearls appearance with joint space widening.[30] Sclerosis may involve the entire sacroiliac joint, and bony bridging is manifested by blurring of joint outlines on radiograph.

MRI findings associated with sacroiliitis include osteitis (periarticular and subchondral bone marrow edema) and synovitis.

Other radiographic manifestations of AS may include vertebral bone spurs, discitis, and square- or bamboo-shaped vertebrae on plain films. MRI manifestations include capsulitis, enthesitis (inflammation of transitions points between soft tissue and bone), intra-articular enhancement, erosions, and sclerosis.[30]

Radiographic manifestations of PsA are characterized by osteodestructive and osteoproliferative manifestations.[31] Ultrasonography may be used to evaluate for enthesitis at tendon insertion points, which manifests as thickening, loss of uniform linear pattern, blurring of tendon margins, and microcalcifications.[32]

LABORATORY FINDINGS

Although there is no laboratory test or combination of laboratory tests that is diagnostic for the spondyloarthritides, 75% to 95% will carry the HLA-B27 gene, and many will have elevated inflammatory markers, such as C-reactive protein (CRP) (40% of the axial SpA) or erythrocyte sedimentation rate (ESR).[33] However, although the HLA-B27 gene is associated with the spondyloarthritides, it is neither sensitive nor specific for them.

Laboratory findings can be helpful to assess for associated extraskeletal complications, such as IBD. The presence of iron deficiency anemia, leukocytosis, hypokalemia, hypoalbuminemia, or inflammatory markers, such as thrombocytosis, elevated ESR, and elevated CRP, can alert the provider to the presence of concomitant IBD and may prompt a gastroenterology referral.[34]

OUTPATIENT THERAPIES

The treatment options for the spondyloarthritides vary but often overlap because of the similar pathogenesis of these distinct disease states. SpA can be subdivided based on clinical features into axial (back pain and stiffness) and peripheral manifestations (arthritis, dactylitis, and enthesitis). Treatment strategies are summarized in **Fig. 3**.

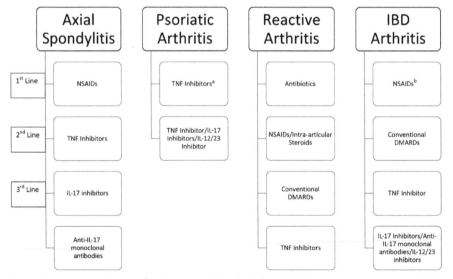

Fig. 3. Treatment pathways for the spondyloarthritides. [a]NSAIDs or conventional DMARDs can be used as first line treatment if PsA is not severe. [b]First line if IBD is stable.

The first-line therapy for all symptoms of axial SpA is NSAIDs, which have demonstrated efficacy when compared with placebo with pain improvement of patients with inflammatory back pain.[35] A 2015 Cochrane review of 39 randomized control trials (RCTs)/quasi-RCTs and cohort studies found that for traditional NSAIDs versus placebo and COX-2 inhibitors versus placebo, NSAIDs and COX-2 inhibitors were more efficacious than placebo in the reduction of pain and improvement in disease activity and functioning. Traditional NSAIDs and COX-2 inhibitors were comparable in efficacy. The most frequently studied NSAID was indomethacin with diclofenac and naproxen as the second and third most evaluated NSAIDs, respectively.[36] The American College of Rheumatology (ACR) does not currently recommend 1 NSAID over another in the treatment of stable or active SpA; they do however recommend continuous NSAID use for active SpA and on-demand NSAID use for stable SpA.[37,38] Dosages for common NSAIDs include naproxen 500 mg twice daily, ibuprofen 800 mg 3 times per day, and celecoxib 200 mg twice per day. Patients often need the maximum dose and benefit from trials of various NSAIDs if the initially selected NSAID is not effective. Each NSAID should be trialed for 2 to 4 weeks before declaring treatment failure. The use of NSAIDs should be paired with nonpharmacologic treatment, such as education, exercise, and physical therapy.

The second-line treatment for axial SpA is biologic DMARDs. Although traditional DMARDs (sulfasalazine, methotrexate) are ineffective for treatment of axial SpA, they have been useful for patients with peripheral manifestations of axial SpA. As TNF and interleukin-17 (IL-17) have been implicated in the pathogenesis of axial SpA, biologic DMARDs (TNF inhibitors and IL-17 antagonists) have been closely examined. There are currently 5 TNF inhibitors approved for use of AS. They are infliximab, etanercept, adalimumab, golimumab, and certolizumab. In patients who have failed NSAID therapy, treatment with these medications has been shown to improve "articular manifestations, CRP levels and MRI-detectable inflammation in the sacroiliac joints or spine in active patients with ankylosing spondylitis."[4] The selection of which TNF inhibitor is used is based on the patient's disease profile, coexisting conditions, and patient/physician preference.

In the event of primary failure to a TNF inhibitor, the ACR recommends trial of an anti-IL-17 monoclonal antibody, such as secukinumab or ixekizumab. If secondary failure occurs, the next drug option should be another TNF inhibitor.[37,38] Of note, the ACR *does not* recommend the routine use of systemic glucocorticoids for the treatment of axial SpA, although they may be considered for peripheral arthritis flares, axial SpA therapy during pregnancy, or an IBD flare.

Tailored treatment for PsA is selected after evaluation of the spectrum of disease manifestation and severity. There are mild discrepancies between the recommendations of the ACR, the European League Against Rheumatism (EULAR), and the Group for Research and Assessment in Psoriasis and Psoriatic Arthritis (GRAPPA) for treatment of PsA, specifically in the order of therapy selection. These discrepancies are also likely due to differences in the approach to treatment targets; the ACR refers to active PsA with the presence of or absence of associated symptoms, whereas GRAPPA and EULAR approach disease processes based on disease domains. The 2018 ACR PsA management guidelines recommend that for treatment-naive patients with active PsA, a TNF inhibitor be tried first over a conventional DMARD, such as methotrexate, leflunomide, sulfasalazine, cyclosporine, or apremilast; if the patient does not have severe PsA or severe psoriasis, NSAIDs or methotrexate (as a conventional DMARD) can be tried first. If TNF inhibitor monotherapy fails to suppress active disease, the ACR recommends trial of either a different TNF inhibitor, IL-17 biologic, or IL-12/23 biologic. It does not delineate order of therapy selection as do the other guidelines.[39–44]

EULAR and GRAPPA both recommend treatment strategies based on clinical manifestations of PsA. For active peripheral arthritis, TNF inhibitors can be used as first-choice agents after conventional DMARDs. GRAPPA recommends IL-12/23 inhibitors and IL-17 inhibitors in addition to TNF inhibitors as first choice after conventional DMARDs.[44] NSAIDs can also be used as treatment. If poor prognostic factors are present, it is preferred that treatment begins with a conventional DMARD. Axial disease involvement can be treated with NSAID therapy first.

Treatment of reactive arthritis should address arthritis symptoms and the precipitant infection. For acute reactive arthritis, NSAIDs are used for symptomatic improvement of peripheral arthritis symptoms. Patients may require a trial of 1 or 2 NSAIDs at maximum dosages to relieve their symptoms. A trial of corticosteroids (intra-articular) can also be considered for the treatment of peripheral arthritis. Systemic steroids can be used at a low/moderate dose if there is incomplete response to NSAIDs or intra-articular steroid injections, although there is little evidence to support their use.

Acute arthritis symptoms that are not completely relieved by NSAIDs can be treated with conventional DMARDs. DMARDs can also be used for chronic (>6 months) reactive arthritis. Sulfasalazine is the DMARD of choice; other DMARDs, such as methotrexate, can be used, but there are limited studies using these medications. Conventional DMARDs can be especially effective if extra-articular manifestations are present. After a 3- to 4-month trial of 1 or 2 conventional DMARDs, treatment-resistant patients can be started on a TNF inhibitor.

The preceding infection of reactive arthritis can be treated with antibiotics provided it is not a self-limited disease. Multiple studies have shown no benefit over placebo in treating self-limited illnesses.[45] Enteric diseases are typically self-limited and do not require antibiotics. Antibiotic treatment can be considered in patients who are of advanced age, patients who are immunocompromised, or if the infection is severe. There are limited data indicating the benefit of treating urogenital disease especially because of the risk of infertility.[45] Patients with GU infections should receive antibiotic treatment. For example, C trachomatis should be treated with azithromycin or doxycycline with empiric treatment for N gonorrhea as indicated. Treatment should be offered to sexual partners. Repeat symptoms should prompt repeat testing. Treatment failure should prompt consideration of alternative causative pathogens of reactive arthritis (ie, Mycoplasma, Ureaplasma) for which antibiotic resistance to first-line agents can occur.[46]

The treatment for IBD-associated arthropathy begins with assessment of the bowel disease. If the IBD is stable and not in flare, NSAIDs can be tried for peripheral and axial disease. NSAIDs, as a first-line therapy, should be given for 2 weeks at inflammatory doses. If there is no improvement and if there are no new GI complaints, a second NSAID can be trialed for 2 weeks. If new or worsening symptoms of bowel disease occur, NSAIDs should be discontinued. If there continues to be peripheral arthritis symptoms in the absence of axial involvement, patients should be given a 3-month trial of a conventional DMARD such as sulfasalazine. If there is no improvement, or if axial disease is present, a TNF inhibitor should be started for at least 3 months. Treatment failure of 1 TNF inhibitor does not reflect the success of this drug class as a whole; a second TNF inhibitor can be trialed before moving on to therapies, such as IL-12/23 inhibitors.

Patients should be treated in collaboration with their gastroenterologist to monitor for active bowel disease that may require treatment. If active bowel disease exists on presentation, NSAID therapy should not be prescribed. Active IBD with axial disease should be started on TNF inhibitors, whereas active IBD with peripheral disease should begin treatment with conventional DMARDs.[34,47]

COMPLICATIONS
Drug-Related

Nonsteroidal anti-inflammatory drugs

Complications owing to NSAID use can be divided into 3 major categories: GI, renal, and cardiovascular. NSAIDs reduce prostaglandin synthesis in the gastric mucosa and can lead to dyspepsia, peptic ulcer disease, and, more seriously, bleeding, perforation, and gastric outlet obstruction (**Table 2**). A review evaluating serious adverse GI events in long-term use of NSAIDs found that there was no significant difference in serious adverse GI events (symptomatic ulcers and ulcer complications) between patients who used COX-2 inhibitors and patients who used nonselective NSAIDs. Several factors increase the risk of NSAID-associated serious GI events: high doses of NSAIDs, age greater than 60 years, history of ulcers and ulcer complications, use of glucocorticoids, anticoagulants, or antiplatelet medications, smoking, and alcohol consumption.[35]

Renal complications of NSAID use include acute renal failure, worsening hypertension, and fluid and electrolyte abnormalities. Acute renal failure, although rare, can occur from lack of prostaglandin-induced vasodilation at the level of the kidneys, resulting in acute renal failure. Hypertension occurs via a similar mechanism; the lack of prostaglandins can ultimately result in sodium and water retention causing hypertension. Hyperkalemia and hyponatremia occur owing to alterations of the RAAS pathway. Of note, acute interstitial nephritis can occur from NSAID use via a different mechanism.

The cardiovascular complications of NSAID use include myocardial infarction and stroke. Several large trials and reviews (PRECISION trial, CNT Collaboration analysis) have indicated that nonselective NSAIDs and COX-2 inhibitors have similar cardiovascular risks over many years.

Table 2 Summary of treatment complications	
Treatment	**Complications**
NSAIDs	Gastrointestinal: • Dyspepsia • Peptic ulcer disease • Bleeding • Perforation • Gastric outlet obstruction Renal: • Acute kidney injury • Acute renal failure • Hypertension • Electrolyte abnormalities (hyperkalemia, hyponatremia) • Acute interstitial nephritis Cardiovascular: • Myocardial infarction • Cerebrovascular accident
DMARDs (select)	Methotrexate: • Gastrointestinal (nausea, vomiting, abdominal pain, decreased oral intake)

(continued on next page)

Table 2
(continued)

Treatment	Complications
	• Hepatotoxicity (elevated liver enzymes) • Nephrotoxicity (elevated creatinine and renal failure) • Interstitial lung disease • Bone marrow toxicity • Infection Sulfasalazine • Dose-dependent reactions (headache, nausea, vomiting, abdominal pain) • Immune-related reactions (hemolytic anemia, agranulocytosis, aplastic anemia, pneumonitis, cutaneous reactions [toxic epidermal necrolysis and Steven-Johnson Syndrome], and hepatotoxicity)
TNF inhibitors	Infection: • Opportunistic infections: Mycobacterium, Pneumocystis pneumonia • Bacterial: S aureus, Listeria, Pseudomonas • Fungal • Viral infections (hepatitis B, hepatitis C, herpes simplex virus) Neutropenia Acute infusion reactions (infliximab) Delayed infusion reactions (infliximab) Injection site reactions Demyelinating disease Congestive heart failure Malignancy Antibody formation (antidrug antibodies and autoimmune)
IL-17 inhibitors (select)	Secukinumab: • Diarrhea • Headache • Nasopharyngitis/upper respiratory tract infections • Inflammatory bowel disease Ixekizumab (include above side effects) • Candida infections
IL-12/23 inhibitors (ustekinumab)	• Headache • Cough • Upper respiratory tract infections • Arthralgias • Injection site erythema • Infection • Malignancy • Cardiovascular events
Steroids	• HPA axis suppression (adrenal insufficiency) • Infection (fungal, bacterial, viral) • Cushingoid features • Catabolic skin changes (high dose) • Weight gain (high dose) • Hyperglycemia (high dose) • Hypertension (high dose) • Cataracts (long-term use) • Osteoporosis

Conventional disease-modifying antirheumatic drugs
Conventional DMARDs include medications such as methotrexate and sulfasalazine. Reported adverse effects are primarily taken from studies in patients with rheumatoid arthritis. Well-known adverse effects of methotrexate include hepatotoxicity, interstitial lung disease, and bone marrow suppression. However, other side effects may occur in patients receiving this treatment. A systematic review by Wang and colleagues[48] found that for methotrexate use in rheumatoid arthritis patients, 20% to 70% of patients experienced adverse GI symptoms, including nausea, vomiting, abdominal pain, and poor appetite. Methotrexate is renally cleared and at low doses can cause a decrease in creatinine clearance; high doses have been shown to cause nephrotoxicity.[49] The risk of infection to patients using methotrexate is not abundantly clear, as it is not an immunosuppressive agent, although concomitant use of steroids or other immunosuppressive agents could lead to higher rates of infection.

Adverse effects owing to sulfasalazine use are generally categorized as either a dose-dependent reaction or an immune-related reaction. Dose-dependent reactions are typically benign and result in headache, nausea, vomiting, and abdominal pain. More serious reactions have been reported as immune-related reactions, such as hemolytic anemia, agranulocytosis, aplastic anemia, pneumonitis, cutaneous reactions (toxic epidermal necrolysis and Steven-Johnson syndrome), and hepatotoxicity.[50,51]

Tumor necrosis factor inhibitors
TNF inhibitors have a wide range of adverse effects that necessitate careful consideration before use. Major adverse effects are infections, mild neutropenia, effects of administration (infusion reactions and local site reactions), and cutaneous reactions.

Infections. A notable risk of TNF inhibitor therapy is immunosuppression and risk for opportunistic infections. TNF inhibitors disrupt the body's natural ability to make granulomas and maintain them. Patients should be screened for latent tuberculosis (TB) infection before initiation of TNF inhibitors, as they are at risk of mycobacterium infections (tuberculous and nontuberculous); latent TB is usually treated if detected before the start of TNF inhibitors.[52]

Patients should also be screened for hepatitis B and C before initiation of a TNF inhibitor and treated for chronic infection before initiation, as hepatitis B can reactivate during TNF inhibitor treatment. Patients with acute hepatitis C should not receive TNF inhibitor therapy.

Opportunistic infections associated with use of TNF inhibitors include fungal (histoplasmosis, coccidioidomycosis, cryptococcosis) infections, common bacterial infections (*Staphylococcus aureus, Listeria, Pseudomonas*), *Pneumocystis jirovecii* pneumonia, and viral infections, such as herpes simplex virus and herpes zoster activation.

Effects of administration. Complications with administration of TNF inhibitors include acute and delayed infusion reactions as well as local site reactions. True anaphylaxis does occur, but many reactions are nonallergic and are not mediated by immunoglobulin E.[53] Delayed infusion reactions occur 1 to 14 days after infusion and mimic serum sickness with the development of fever, rash, myalgias, and arthralgias; they can be treated with supportive care. Local injection site reactions include pain, redness, swelling, and bruising and can be treated with supportive care. Other notable reactions are psoriasis, eczema, and lichen planus.

Other complications. Complications, such as demyelinating disease, heart failure, malignancy, the development of autoantibodies, and other autoimmune illnesses, have been linked temporally to TNF inhibitor use. Briefly, drug-induced demyelinating disease can mimic multiple sclerosis in the wide breadth of presenting symptoms; a potential causal relationship has been identified with use of etanercept and infliximab.[54] The same medications also have been linked to worsening of established heart failure. Many autoimmune conditions can increase one's risk of malignancy, and the use of TNF inhibitors is postulated to further increase that risk, although this requires further investigation. Finally, patients using TNF inhibitors are at an increased risk of developing antidrug antibodies (eg, anti-adalimumab antibody) and autoantibodies (eg, anti-dsDNA), with some going on to develop clinically significant autoimmune illnesses, such as systemic lupus erythematosus.

Monoclonal antibodies

Monoclonal antibodies used against rheumatic diseases include IL-17 inhibitors and IL-12/23 inhibitors. Secukinumab (a fully human monoclonal antibody) and ixekizumab (a humanized monoclonal antibody) target IL-17 and are approved for use for radiographic and nonradiographic SpA as well as PsA and plaque psoriasis. Mild adverse effects of secukinumab include diarrhea, headache, nasopharyngitis, and other upper respiratory tract infections (URIs). A more significant adverse effect is IBD in patients without prior history of GI disease.[55] Ixekizumab has a similar adverse effect profile with additional increased risk for candidal infections.[56]

The IL-12/23 inhibitor ustekinumab has been frequently referenced as a treatment option in the spondyloarthritides. Mild adverse effects include headache, cough, URIs, arthralgias, and injection site erythema. Serious adverse effects, such as infection, malignancy, and cardiovascular events, have been reported at low frequency in long-term trials.[57,58]

Glucocorticoids

The side effects of steroids use are well known, with risk for adverse effects increasing with dosage and duration of use. These side effects include the following:

- Suppression of the hypothalamic-pituitary-adrenal axis leading to loss of cortisol secretion and secondary adrenal insufficiency
- Increased risk of fungal, bacterial, and viral infections owing to immunosuppression
- Development of Cushingoid features and other catabolic skin effects (skin thinning, atrophy, and ecchymosis)
- Weight gain, hyperglycemia, and hypertension at higher doses of glucocorticoids
- Development of cataracts with prolonged usage[59]
- Osteoporosis
- Neuropsychiatric and neurocognitive symptoms

Disease related

Complications owing to each individual spondyloarthropathy are numerous, and a brief overview of extra-articular manifestations and complications is provided in **Box 2**. As the disease processes are interrelated, complications that are listed under 1 disease process can occur in another disease process.

EMERGENCY DEPARTMENT EVALUATION
Suspected New Diagnosis

The emergency department (ED) evaluation of a patient with suspected spondyloarthropathy should begin with assessment of hemodynamic stability. Airway patency, respiratory status, and circulation should be the first 3 items evaluated on presentation in

Box 2
Complications and extra-articular manifestations of the spondyloarthritides

Ankylosing spondylitis
  Cardiovascular disease
    Aortic regurgitation
    Aortic and mitral valve thickening
    Conduction disturbances
    Acute coronary syndrome
    Stroke
    Venous thromboembolism
    Conduction abnormalities
  Pulmonary disease
    Restrictive lung disease due to decreased chest wall and spinal mobility
    Pulmonary fibrosis
  Musculoskeletal
    Osteopenia
    Fractures
    Atlantoaxial subluxation
  Neurologic
    Cord compression
    Spinal nerve compression
  Renal disease
    Immunoglobulin A nephropathy
    Nonspecific glomerulopathy
    Renal amyloidosis

Reactive arthritis
  Ophthalmologic Involvement
    Uveitis
  Cutaneous involvement
    Skin or oral ulcers
    Keratoderma blennorrhagica

Psoriatic arthritis
  Metabolic disease
  Hypertension
  Diabetes
  Atherosclerosis
  Cardiovascular disease (myocardial infarction, stroke, death)

Inflammatory bowel disease–associated arthritis
  Constitutional
    Weight loss
  Gastrointestinal
    Fistulas/abscess
    Colitis complications: GI bleed, toxic megacolon, perforation
  Cutaneous
    Erythema nodosum
    Pyoderma gangrenosum
    Aphthous ulcers
  Ophthalmologic
    Uveitis
    Episcleritis
    Corneal ulcers
  Hepatobiliary
    Fatty liver disease
    Primary sclerosing cholangitis
    Autoimmune liver disease
  Musculoskeletal
    Osteoporosis/osteopenia

that order. Once stability is determined, a careful history and physical examination should be performed. This should include family history and a thorough review of systems to assess for extra-articular manifestations if present. First-line treatment for arthritis symptoms, NSAIDs, can generally be started in the ED unless there is concern for a possible complication of NSAID use. A concern for a new diagnosis should prompt referral to a rheumatologist and additional subspecialist if there is concern for an extra-articular manifestation such as IBD or pulmonary fibrosis.[60]

Suspected Complications

The ED evaluation of a patient with known spondyloarthropathy should include consideration of potential complications of the disorder itself, as well as complications of the medical therapy. The wide range of potentially serious complications associated with individual spondyloarthritides and the used therapeutic modalities necessitates an elevated index of suspicion from the ED physician. Examples would include increased potential for atlantoaxial subluxation in a trauma patient, or opportunistic infection in a febrile patient. Other complications are cataloged in **Table 2** and **Box 2**.

SUMMARY

The spondyloarthritides are a group of chronic rheumatological disorders that include musculoskeletal and extraskeletal manifestations, often share a genetic predisposition, and have overlapping clinical features. Musculoskeletal features can include inflammatory back pain, oligoarthritis, enthesitis, and dactylitis; extraskeletal features can include uveitis, IBD, and skin disorders, such as psoriasis. Patients suffering from the spondyloarthritides can experience complications involving multiple body systems, either as a result of their inherent disease process or as a result of therapeutic modalities. Appropriate ED care for these patients requires maintaining an index of suspicion for the presence of these multisystemic complications.

CLINICS CARE POINTS

- Unless there is a contraindication, nonsteroidal anti-inflammatory drugs should be the first-line treatment for the spondyloarthropathies in the emergency department.
- Clinical suspicion for a spondyloarthropathy should trigger a prompt referral to a rheumatologist.
- The spondyloarthropathies include musculoskeletal and extraskeletal manifestations and have overlapping clinical features.
- Emergency department visits may be prompted by complications of the underlying spondyloarthropathy or of the medical therapies.

DISCLOSURE

None.

REFERENCES

1. Kataria RK, Brent LH. Spondyloarthropathies. Am Fam Physician 2004;69(12): 2853–60.

2. Ehrenfeld M. Spondyloarthropathies. Best Pract Res Clin Rheumatol 2012;26(1): 135–45.
3. van der Linden S, Brown M, Kenna T, et al. Ankylosing spondylitis. In: Firestein GS, Budd RC, Gabriel SE, et al, editors. Kelley and Firestein's textbook of rheumatology. 10th edition. Philadelphia: Elsevier; 2017. p. 1256–79.e5.
4. Sieper J, Poddubnyy D. Axial spondyloarthritis. Lancet 2017;390(10089):73–84.
5. Poddubnyy D. Classification vs diagnostic criteria: the challenge of diagnosing axial spondyloarthritis. Rheumatology (Oxford) 2020;59(Supplement_4):iv6–17.
6. Sieper J, Rudwaleit M, Baraliakos X, et al. The Assessment of SpondyloArthritis international Society (ASAS) handbook: a guide to assess spondyloarthritis. Ann Rheum Dis 2009;68(Suppl 2):ii1–44.
7. Rudwaleit M, van der Heijde D, Landewé R, et al. The development of Assessment of SpondyloArthritis international Society classification criteria for axial spondyloarthritis (part II): validation and final selection [published correction appears in Ann Rheum Dis. 2019 Jun;78(6):e59]. Ann Rheum Dis 2009;68(6): 777–83.
8. Rudwaleit M, van der Heijde D, Landewé R, et al. The Assessment of SpondyloArthritis International Society classification criteria for peripheral spondyloarthritis and for spondyloarthritis in general. Ann Rheum Dis 2011;70(1):25–31.
9. Selmi C, Gershwin ME. Diagnosis and classification of reactive arthritis. Autoimmun Rev 2014;13(4–5):546–9.
10. Bentaleb I, Abdelghani KB, Rostom S, et al. Reactive arthritis: update. Curr Clin Microbiol Rep 2020;7(4):124–32. https://doi.org/10.1007/s40588-020-00152-6.
11. Moll JM, Wright V. Psoriatic arthritis. Semin Arthritis Rheum 1973;3(1):55–78.
12. Taylor W, Gladman D, Helliwell P, et al. Classification criteria for psoriatic arthritis: development of new criteria from a large international study. Arthritis Rheum 2006;54(8):2665–73.
13. Rudwaleit M, Taylor WJ. Classification criteria for psoriatic arthritis and ankylosing spondylitis/axial spondyloarthritis. Best Pract Res Clin Rheumatol 2010;24(5): 589–604.
14. Napolitano M, Caso F, Scarpa R, et al. Psoriatic arthritis and psoriasis: differential diagnosis. Clin Rheumatol 2016;35(8):1893–901.
15. FitzGerald O, Elmamoun M. Psoriatic arthritis. In: Firestein GS, Budd RC, Gabriel SE, et al, editors. Kelley and Firestein's textbook of rheumatology. 10th edition. Philadelphia, PA: Elsevier; 2017. p. 1285–308.e4.
16. Wollheim F. Enteropathic arthritis. In: Firestein GS, Budd RC, Gabriel SE, et al, editors. Kelley and Firestein's textbook of rheumatology. 10th edition. Philadelphia, PA: Elsevier; 2017. p. 1309–28.
17. Holden W, Orchard T, Wordsworth P. Enteropathic arthritis. Rheum Dis Clin North Am 2003;29(3):513–viii.
18. Helmick CG, Felson DT, Lawrence RC, et al, National Arthritis Data Workgroup. Estimates of the prevalence of arthritis and other rheumatic conditions in the United States. Part I. Arthritis Rheum 2008;58(1):15–25.
19. Dean LE, Jones GT, MacDonald AG, et al. Global prevalence of ankylosing spondylitis. Rheumatology (Oxford) 2014;53(4):650–7.
20. Reveille JD, Weisman MH. The epidemiology of back pain, axial spondyloarthritis and HLA-B27 in the United States. Am J Med Sci 2013;345(6):431–6.
21. López-Medina C, Moltó A, Dougados M. Peripheral manifestations in spondyloarthritis and their effect: an ancillary analysis of the ASAS-COMOSPA study. J Rheumatol 2020;47(2):211–7.

22. Stolwijk C, Boonen A, van Tubergen A, et al. Epidemiology of spondyloarthritis. Rheum Dis Clin North Am 2012;38(3):441–76.

23. Wilson FC, Icen M, Crowson CS, et al. Time trends in epidemiology and characteristics of psoriatic arthritis over 3 decades: a population-based study. J Rheumatol 2009;36(2):361–7.

24. Townes JM, Deodhar AA, Laine ES, et al. Reactive arthritis following culture-confirmed infections with bacterial enteric pathogens in Minnesota and Oregon: a population-based study. Ann Rheum Dis 2008;67(12):1689–96.

25. Karreman MC, Luime JJ, Hazes JMW, et al. The prevalence and incidence of axial and peripheral spondyloarthritis in inflammatory bowel disease: a systematic review and meta-analysis. J Crohns Colitis 2017;11(5):631–42.

26. Qaseem A, Wilt TJ, McLean RM, et al. Clinical Guidelines Committee of the American College of Physicians. Noninvasive treatments for acute, subacute, and chronic low back pain: a clinical practice guideline from the American College of Physicians. Ann Intern Med 2017;166(7):514–30.

27. DePalma MG. Red flags of low back pain. JAAPA 2020;33(8):8–11.

28. Will JS, Bury DC, Miller JA. Mechanical low back pain. Am Fam Physician 2018; 98(7):421–8.

29. de Hooge M. The future of imaging in axial spondyloarthritis. Rheum Dis Clin North Am 2020;46(2):297–309.

30. Schorn C. Ankylosing spondylitis. In: Pope T, editor. Musculoskeletal imaging. 2nd edition. Philadelphia: Elsevier Saunders; 2016. p. 691–9.e19.

31. Poggenborg RP, Østergaard M, Terslev L. Imaging in psoriatic arthritis. Rheum Dis Clin North Am 2015;41(4):593–613.

32. Nissman DB, Shankar PV, Pope TL. Reactive Arthritis. In: Pope T, Bloem HL, Beltran J, Morrison WB, Wilson DJ, editors. Musculoskeletal Imaging. 2nd edition. Philadelphia, PA: Elsevier Saunders; 2015. p. 684–90.e2.

33. Hayward RJ, Machado PM. Classification criteria in axial spondyloarthritis: what have we learned; where are we going? Rheum Dis Clin North Am 2020;46(2): 259–74.

34. Ibáñez Vodnizza SE, De La Fuente MPP, Parra Cancino EC. Approach to the patient with axial spondyloarthritis and suspected inflammatory bowel disease. Rheum Dis Clin North Am 2020;46(2):275–86.

35. Song IH, Poddubnyy DA, Rudwaleit M, et al. Benefits and risks of ankylosing spondylitis treatment with nonsteroidal antiinflammatory drugs. Arthritis Rheum 2008;58(4):929–38.

36. Kroon FP, van der Burg LR, Ramiro S, et al. Non-steroidal anti-inflammatory drugs (NSAIDs) for axial spondyloarthritis (ankylosing spondylitis and non-radiographic axial spondyloarthritis). Cochrane Database Syst Rev 2015;(7):CD010952.

37. Ward MM, Deodhar A, Gensler LS, et al. 2019 Update of the American College of Rheumatology/Spondylitis Association of America/Spondyloarthritis Research and Treatment Network Recommendations for the Treatment of Ankylosing Spondylitis and Nonradiographic Axial Spondyloarthritis. Arthritis Care Res (Hoboken) 2019;71(10):1285–99.

38. Ward MM, Deodhar A, Akl EA, et al. American College of Rheumatology/Spondylitis Association of America/Spondyloarthritis Research and Treatment Network 2015 recommendations for the treatment of ankylosing spondylitis and nonradiographic axial spondyloarthritis. Arthritis Rheumatol 2016;68(2):282–98.

39. Singh JA, Guyatt G, Ogdie A, et al. Special article: 2018 American College of Rheumatology/National Psoriasis Foundation guideline for the treatment of psoriatic arthritis. Arthritis Rheumatol 2019;71(1):5–32.
40. Gossec L, Baraliakos X, Kerschbaumer A, et al. EULAR recommendations for the management of psoriatic arthritis with pharmacological therapies: 2019 update. Ann Rheum Dis 2020;79(6):700–12.
41. Coates LC, Kavanaugh A, Mease PJ, et al. Group for Research and Assessment of Psoriasis and Psoriatic Arthritis 2015 treatment recommendations for psoriatic arthritis. Arthritis Rheumatol 2016;68(5):1060–71.
42. Noviani M, Feletar M, Nash P, et al. Choosing the right treatment for patients with psoriatic arthritis. Ther Adv Musculoskelet Dis 2020;12. 1759720X20962623.
43. Mease PJ, Armstrong AW. Managing patients with psoriatic disease: the diagnosis and pharmacologic treatment of psoriatic arthritis in patients with psoriasis. Drugs 2014;74(4):423–41.
44. Ogdie A, Coates LC, Gladman DD. Treatment guidelines in psoriatic arthritis. Rheumatology (Oxford) 2020;59(Supplement_1):i37–46.
45. Rudwaleit M, Braun J, Sieper J. Treatment of reactive arthritis: a practical guide. BioDrugs 2000;13(1):21–8.
46. Manhart LE, Broad JM, Golden MR. Mycoplasma genitalium: should we treat and how? Clin Infect Dis 2011;53(Suppl 3):S129–42.
47. Olivieri I, Cantini F, Castiglione F, et al. Italian Expert Panel on the management of patients with coexisting spondyloarthritis and inflammatory bowel disease. Autoimmun Rev 2014;13(8):822–30.
48. Wang W, Zhou H, Liu L. Side effects of methotrexate therapy for rheumatoid arthritis: a systematic review. Eur J Med Chem 2018;158:502–16.
49. Malaviya AN, Sharma A, Agarwal D, et al. Low-dose and high-dose methotrexate are two different drugs in practical terms. Int J Rheum Dis 2010;13(4):288–93.
50. Watkinson G. Sulphasalazine: a review of 40 years' experience. Drugs 1986; 32(Suppl 1):1–11.
51. Box SA, Pullar T. Sulphasalazine in the treatment of rheumatoid arthritis. Br J Rheumatol 1997;36(3):382–6.
52. Koo S, Marty FM, Baden LR. Infectious complications associated with immunomodulating biologic agents. Infect Dis Clin North Am 2010;24(2):285–306.
53. Cheifetz A, Smedley M, Martin S, et al. The incidence and management of infusion reactions to infliximab: a large center experience. Am J Gastroenterol 2003;98(6):1315–24.
54. Ibrahim WH, Hammoudah M, Akhtar N, et al. Central nervous system demyelination associated with etanercept in a 51 years old woman. Libyan J Med 2007; 2(2):99–102.
55. Fauny M, Moulin D, D'Amico F, et al. Paradoxical gastrointestinal effects of interleukin-17 blockers. Ann Rheum Dis 2020;79(9):1132–8.
56. Huang JX, Lee YH, Wei JC. Ixekizumab for the treatment of ankylosing spondylitis. Expert Rev Clin Immunol 2020;16(8):745–50. https://doi.org/10.1080/1744666X.2020.1803063.
57. Leonardi CL, Kimball AB, Papp KA, et al. Efficacy and safety of ustekinumab, a human interleukin-12/23 monoclonal antibody, in patients with psoriasis: 76-week results from a randomised, double-blind, placebo-controlled trial (PHOENIX 1). Lancet 2008;371(9625):1665–74 [published correction appears in Lancet. 2008 May 31;371(9627):1838].

58. Papp KA, Langley RG, Lebwohl M, et al. Efficacy and safety of ustekinumab, a human interleukin-12/23 monoclonal antibody, in patients with psoriasis: 52-week results from a randomised, double-blind, placebo-controlled trial (PHOENIX 2). Lancet 2008;371(9625):1675–84.

59. Huscher D, Thiele K, Gromnica-Ihle E, et al. Dose-related patterns of glucocorticoid-induced side effects. Ann Rheum Dis 2009;68(7):1119–24.

60. Duba AS, Mathew SD. The seronegative spondyloarthropathies. Prim Care 2018; 45(2):271–87.

Autoimmune Connective Tissue Diseases: Systemic Lupus Erythematosus and Rheumatoid Arthritis

Jonathan Rose, MD, MBA

KEYWORDS

- Rheumatologic emergencies • Systemic lupus erythematosus • Rheumatoid arthritis
- Therapy • Adverse reactions

KEY POINTS

- Signs and/or symptoms considered rheumatic in origin may account for a significant proportion of emergency department visits.
- Absolute or true life- and/or limb-threatening complications associated with autoimmune connective tissue diseases are rare.
- Failing to consider such a diagnosis by virtue of cognitive error, such as availability, may have catastrophic consequences for the patient.
- Underlying stressors and/or concomitant acute or worsening chronic diseases in need of targeted intervention, if left untreated, may contribute to the demise of the patient.
- Patients receiving treatment for autoimmune connective tissue diseases are vulnerable to adverse drug reactions and complications attributable to the deleterious effects of such medications, which can vary widely in their severity, from the mild to lethal.

INTRODUCTION

Systemic lupus erythematosus (SLE) and rheumatoid arthritis (RA) are just 2 of several autoimmune connective tissue diseases that are primarily chronic in nature but can present to the emergency department by virtue of an acute exacerbation of disease. Beyond an acute exacerbation of disease, their predilection for invading multiple organ systems lends itself to the potential for patients presenting to the emergency department with either a single or isolated symptom or a myriad of signs and/or symptoms indicative of a degree of disease complexity and possibly severity that warrants as timely recognition as it does resuscitation.

This article originally appeared in Emergency Medicine Clinics, Volume 40 Issue 1, February 2022.

Department of Emergency Medicine, Memorial Healthcare System, Memorial Hospital West, 703 N Flamingo Road, Pembroke Pines, FL 33028, USA

E-mail address: jonrose@mhs.net

Immunol Allergy Clin N Am 43 (2023) 613–625
https://doi.org/10.1016/j.iac.2022.10.006   immunology.theclinics.com

As many as nearly 9% of all patients presenting to the emergency department do so with symptoms consistent with rheumatic disease.[1] The most common symptoms patients may experience are constitutional, such as fever, fatigue, and weight loss, and musculoskeletal such as neck, back, and/or joint pain and swelling. In general, purely nontraumatic musculoskeletal symptoms account for up to 3% of all patients presenting to the emergency department, approximately 57% of which are back pain related, while approximately 43% are related to a peripheral joint, with 0.6% and 0.3% of these, respectively, being emergent in nature.[2] Beyond the constitutional and musculoskeletal symptoms that may trigger an emergency department visit, the multiorgan system propensity of these conditions yields symptoms that run the gamut of patient experience, the most emergent of which tend to be airway related, cardiovascular, gastrointestinal, hematopoietic, infectious disease, neurologic, pulmonary, and/or renal.

An awareness of autoimmune connective tissues diseases and more specifically the emergent manifestation of their potential presentations is vitally important to the timely recognition of disease states in need of specific, targeted, aggressive intervention that is often multifaceted and multidisciplinary in its approach. Such awareness affords one the opportunity to make the time-sensitive critical decisions that are required to ensure the best possible clinical outcome.

EPIDEMIOLOGY

Both SLE and RA possess a predilection for women. They share a female-to-male ratio of 3:1, but this is only the case in childhood as it relates to SLE, at which time disease tends to be much more severe.[3] During the course of their reproductive years, women are affected by SLE anywhere from 7 to 15 times more often than men, with a median age of onset of 37 to 50 years and 15 to 44 years for white and Black women, respectively and 50 to 59 years and 45 to 64 years for white and Black men, respectively.[4,5] In general, older adults tend to experience a much milder form of disease but men, who are typically older at the time of onset, tend to have a worse outcome with a higher incidence of hematologic, cardiovascular, neurologic, and renal disease and vasculitis among other complicating features.[6–8]

RA tends to affect an older patient population, with a peak incidence in the eighth decade of life, but like SLE, women are oftentimes affected during the latter part of their childbearing years. Unlike SLE, for which, a greater prevalence of disease is found in Asians, African Americans, African Caribbeans and Hispanic Americans, RA has a greater prevalence among Western Europeans and North Americans (Caucasians) and Native Americans.[9–11]

Increased risk associated with SLE and RA has been attributed to lower socioeconomic status[12,13] and education,[14,15] obesity,[16,17] and cigarette smoking.[18,19] The increased morbidity and mortality associated with such socioeconomic, comorbid, and environmental conditions suggests that modifiable risk factor reduction and an improvement in access to medical care may dramatically impact the clinical course of disease for many patients.

PATHOPHYSIOLOGY

SLE and RA are 2 of several autoimmune connective tissue diseases that wreak havoc on one's own self because of a loss of self-tolerance. The identification of self as a threat triggers an immune response, both innate and adaptive, ultimately as dysfunctional as it is destructive, aimed at eliminating the threat by any and all means necessary. The pathogenesis of SLE, like RA, is multifactorial.[20]

Genetic, environmental, immunoregulatory, hormonal, and even epigenetic factors trigger a series of events or events in parallel that promote both B- and T-cell activation. The resultant production of autoantibodies, cytokines and immune complexes, which when deposited in the tissues of target organs, causes local inflammatory destruction via activation of the complement cascade. The damaged tissue of target organs liberates apoptotic cells that when defectively cleared present novel autoantigens. These novel autoantigens when bound to autoantibodies form immune complexes supporting further priming and autoreactivity in a cycle that if left uninterrupted ultimately and irreparably destroys organ systems.[21,22]

EMERGENCY MANIFESTATIONS OF DISEASE

Emergencies in patients with autoimmune connective tissue diseases generally fall into 1 of 5 distinct categories: exacerbations of the diseases themselves, complications known to be associated with the autoimmune connective tissue disease, infections attributable to immunosuppressive therapy, new onset or an exacerbation of a comorbid condition, and adverse drug reactions related to the medications used to treat such conditions.[23] It is important to recognize the potential for not only an acute exacerbation of disease but also a complication of the same in a patient who has not yet had such a diagnosis established in the outpatient setting. Their presentation to the emergency department may be the first disease-related illness of significant enough acuity to warrant emergent medical attention.

AIRWAY-RELATED EMERGENCIES

The potential for life-threatening complications associated with airway-related emergencies in SLE and RA is not limited to acute catastrophic conditions caused by these systemic rheumatic diseases.

Pathologic changes in anatomy create scenarios in which a routine approach to the process of securing an airway in these patients can be fraught with danger and vulnerable to failure. An awareness of these potential procedurally related challenges ensures a level of preparedness including the consideration of alternative, adjunctive techniques and equipment that may prove pivotal in outcome in an emergent situation.

Upper airway obstruction is a potential complication of SLE and RA. Both conditions are associated with cricoarytenoid arthritis but differ in its onset. Acute cricoarytenoid arthritis is a rare but serious cause of upper airway obstruction in patients with SLE. It can be seen in isolation or complicated by secondary bacterial infection such as with epiglottitis or tracheitis. Typical symptoms are to be expected, such as pain in the throat that is exacerbated by speaking and/or swallowing, a sense of fullness or foreign body, change in the sound of speech, shortness of breath, and even stridor. When it occurs, it typically does so in the presence of other associated symptoms and is treated with high-dose corticosteroids, racemic epinephrine, and if indicated, antibiotics. In contrast, chronic cricoarytenoid arthritis is seen in RA and often requires surgical intervention.[24] Although chronic in nature, when associated with laryngeal manipulation or infection, it too can prove acutely fatal.

In a patient with systemic rheumatic disease, a compromised airway, in need of being secured, can prove to be challenging. Temporomandibular joint dysfunction in the setting of RA can significantly reduce opening of the mouth, limiting one's view of the relevant anatomy required for intubation.[23] RA most often affects the cervical spine and in the form of atlantoaxial instability with C1- C2 subluxation or dislocation. Presentation can appear as seemingly mild and benign as being purely radicular in nature but may in fact be caused by myelopathy or as severe as to cause sudden death.[25] Atlantoaxial instability with C1-C2 subluxation or dislocation must be considered in the differential diagnosis for any patient presenting with upper extremity radicular symptoms and/or new occipital pain. A pre-existing diagnosis of RA certainly helps but is not always established, and as consequence, a high index of suspicion is essential. Patients with known RA with or without confirmed atlantoaxial instability with C1-C2 subluxation or dislocation must avoid hyperextension of the cervical spine and maximal passive flexion, which is particularly important to remember when examining a patient after blunt trauma and when positioning a patient for intubation.[26]

At the bedside and beyond, the equipment required for direct laryngoscopy and additional equipment to assist in securing the airway via video laryngoscopy or fiberoptic intubation should be available. In all instances, the possibility of having to resort to a surgical approach must be considered. At the bedside, the equipment necessary to perform a cricothyroidotomy is required, and if appropriate, transfer to the operating room should be considered in patients for whom intubation is anticipated but not immediately necessary.

CARDIOVASCULAR EMERGENCIES

Patients with SLE and RA are vulnerable to the same traditional risk factors for cardiovascular disease (CVD) as those without either of the 2 systemic rheumatic diseases. They are, however, at greater risk overall because of the pathophysiologic mechanisms associated with these conditions and some of the therapeutic agents used to treat them, enabling accelerated atherosclerosis and as a consequence, CVD at a much younger age than the traditional patient. The risk for patients with SLE is at least twice that of the general population, with an acute myocardial infarction (AMI) relative risk of 2.27.[27,28] Patients with RA have an increased risk of acute coronary syndrome (ACS) demonstrated by an overall hazard ratio of 1.41 when compared with the general population.[29] Cardiovascular emergency in the form of ACS secondary to accelerated atherosclerosis in the setting of SLE and RA is by no means the only potential for disaster. Diseases of the electrical conducting system, myocardium, pericardium, valves, and vasculature also have the potential to wreak havoc and in some instances just as or even more lethally.

Arrhythmias are common in SLE and RA and while the most common of these, sinus tachycardia, is typically benign (present in up to 18% of patients with SLE), some can be malignant.[30] High-degree atrioventricular (AV) block, while rare, in the setting of RA is usually complete.[31] Atrial fibrillation is seen in 9% of patients with SLE, and patients with RA have a 40% greater risk of atrial fibrillation than the general population.[30,32] QT prolongation is seen in 17% of patients, increasing the risk for ventricular tachyarrhythmias and as a consequence sudden cardiac death.[30]

Cardiac complications are reported in about 50% of patients with SLE and RA, the most common of which is pericarditis.[31,33] Typically, pericarditis does not occur in isolation but instead with other forms of serositis. More often than not pericarditis is either entirely asymptomatic or benign but can be complicated by pericardial effusion and tamponade and/or be constrictive in its form and as a consequence function impairing cardiac output potentially to the point of collapse.

Myocardial dysfunction to the point of failure is observed in both SLE and RA, the etiology of which is varied. Congestive heart failure may be the direct result of that which has been mentioned previously but may also result from additional cardiac complications associated with SLE and RA such as myocarditis (often with pericarditis), cardiomyopathy, and valvular disease, be it thickening of valve leaflets associated with episodes of valvulitis or endocarditis. Regardless of the cause of valvular disease, it is typically left-sided and regurgitant.[34,35]

Aortic disease, in the form of root abnormality, aortitis, and/or aneurysm, although rare, is more commonly seen in patients with SLE and RA than in the general population.[36] In its most potentially lethal form and via multivariate analyses, patients with SLE and RA have been found to have odds ratios of 2.06 and 1.406 respectively, associating SLE and RA with the coexistence of aortic aneurysms at a significantly higher rate than that seen in the general population.[37,38]

Beyond aortic aneurysm with dissection and/or rupture, thromboembolism is a major cause of morbidity and mortality for patients with rheumatic disease and in particular SLE and RA. All vessels, big and small, arterial and venous, end organ and extremity, are vulnerable. The potential for loss of limb because of peripheral artery ischemia or life because of such potentially catastrophic events as cavernous sinus thrombosis (CST), cerebrovascular accident (CVA), ACS, pulmonary embolism (PE), and the like is much greater than the general population.[39] In some instances, rates of disease, such as venous thromboembolism, are more than 3 times higher than the general population.[40]

In isolation, any organ system compromised by thromboembolism can prove fatal but when multiple organ systems are involved, such as that which occurs in the setting of catastrophic antiphospholipid syndrome (CAPS), half of all patients will die regardless of resuscitative efforts.[41] CAPS is exceedingly rare, representing less than 1% of all patients with APS but is its most severe and rapidly progressing form that in less than 10% of cases is associated with concomitant disease such as SLE and RA, requiring a high index of suspicion. Although absolute confirmation of the diagnosis is beyond the emergency department, requiring an element of histopathological and/or laboratory confirmation, evidence of 3 or more compromised organs, systems, and/or tissues, all having manifested simultaneously or in less than 1 week, in a patient with SLE or RA is highly suspicious.[42] The organ systems involved in decreasing order of frequency include renal (78%), pulmonary (66%), central nervous system (56%), cutaneous (50%), gastrointestinal (38%), hepatic (34%), adrenal (13%), and urogenital (6%).[41]

Once suspected, treatment is to be initiated early and aggressively. Multidisciplinary in its approach, access, ventilatory support, monitoring, fluid resuscitation, electrolyte balance, anticoagulation, and high-dose glucocorticoids are the mainstays of treatment. If these are ineffective, cyclophosphamide and gamma globulin are recommended, and finally, if all else fails, plasmapheresis.[43] Primary as these interventions are in their approach, additional treatment must also be considered in the setting of any underlying or inciting secondary stressor such as antibiotics for infection or operative intervention in the face of organ or extremity necrosis.

GASTROINTESTINAL EMERGENCIES

Both SLE and RA can affect the gastrointestinal (GI) system, with up to 50% of patients with SLE manifesting some form of GI symptomatology during their lifetime; however, actual GI emergencies are rare.[44] Like any other organ system, the GI tract, both hollow and solid, is vulnerable to the same inflammatory and vaso-occlusive dangers associated with SLE and RA and complications associated with their treatment. When caused by the pathophysiologic mechanisms associated with these conditions, most cases can be life threatening if not recognized and treated promptly.[45] Ischemia, infarction, perforation, and end organ failure are on a spectrum of disease carrying a high rate of morbidity and/or mortality. When caused by mesenteric vasculitis, mortality rates are as high as 13%.[46] Prompt administration of glucocorticoids is essential and in refractory cases immunosuppressive agents and biologic agents may be required.[47] Beyond the systemic rheumatic diseases themselves, agents used to treat them, namely glucocorticoids, nonsteroidal anti-inflammatory drugs (NSAIDs), and disease-modifying antirheumatic drugs have been implicated in GI perforations.[48] Regardless of etiology, be it medication or directly disease related, evidence of perforation or end organ compromise including necrosis warrants operative intervention and should not be delayed.[49]

HEMATOPOIETIC EMERGENCIES

Patients with SLE and RA are prone to several hematological disorders, either as a direct consequence of the diseases themselves or the therapeutic agents used to treat them. Of course, one must always consider the possibility of an alternative etiology for the same abnormalities such as infection, malignancy, or some other secondary stressor. In most instances, the hematological findings are nonemergent in nature such as anemia of chronic disease, the most common hematological disorder in SLE and among the most prevalent in RA.[50,51] In rare instances, hematologic emergencies do occur and if unrecognized can prove fatal.

Accelerated loss caused by bleeding, hemolysis, or hypersplenism are potential causes of severe anemia that in the setting of systemic rheumatic disease may not be as simple to address via transfusion alone. Even in the absence of loss, hemolysis, or hypersplenism, severe anemia may occur because of autoimmune bone marrow suppression or may be medication induced. Although bleeding is a risk for patients because of coagulation abnormalities, so too is clotting, as is the case with thrombotic microangiopathies such as CAPS described previously and thrombotic thrombocytopenic purpura. Mortality associated with these conditions is exceedingly high and can be rapid. Approximately 50% of patients with CAPS will die regardless of intervention, and the same percentage of patients with thrombotic thrombocytopenic purpura (TTP) associated with SLE will die if it is not recognized early and treated aggressively via plasma exchange and immunosuppression.[41,52] If untreated, mortality rates approach 90%, and even with aggressive intervention can still be as high as 25%.[53] Delays in initiating plasma exchange increases mortality, furthering the need for early recognition and resuscitation requiring an urgent multidisciplinary approach.[54]

INFECTIOUS DISEASE EMERGENCIES

Any immunocompromising condition, any immunosuppressing treatment, places patients at increased risk of not only serious infection but also its associated increased risk of morbidity and mortality.

Infections are common in patients with systemic rheumatic disease, and the more active the disease, the more serious is the infection, at times yielding a mortality rate that even matches the disease itself.[55] Patients with systemic rheumatic disease are more vulnerable to infections by certain types of pathogens, be they encapsulated, opportunistic or not, but they are still most commonly infected by the same organisms found in the general population, primarily impacting the respiratory and urinary tracts and skin.[56] It is also important to keep in mind that although an acute exacerbation of disease might yield findings consistent with the systemic inflammatory response syndrome not caused by infection, empiric antibiotics are recommended until infection as an etiology of these findings has been ruled out.

Although pulmonary, genitourinary and dermatologic infections are common to both SLE and RA, as they are in the general population, septic arthritis is not as frequently observed in patients with SLE as it is in RA, occurring in less than 1% of hospitalized patients.[57] It is, however, just as dangerous, rapidly leading to joint destruction, quite possibly systemic infection, loss of limb, and possibly life, requiring a high index of suspicion and the prompt initiation of antibiotic treatment following arthrocentesis.[58] Abnormal joint architecture as seen in patients with RA is the most important risk factor, with the therapeutic agents used to treat the disease, in particular glucocorticoids and biologic agents only further increasing this risk.[41,59] It is especially important to recognize that patients actively being treated with such agents are not only more vulnerable because of immunosuppression, but they also might not manifest signs and/or symptoms as intense as those not receiving such treatment.

NEUROLOGIC EMERGENCIES

Although rare, neurologic emergencies, like many other potential threats in SLE and RA, are much more frequently encountered than they are in the general population. As a consequence, there is increased risk because of the pathophysiologic proinflammatory, vaso-occlusive, and coagulopathic nature of these systemic rheumatic diseases and the complications associated with the therapeutic agents used to treat them. An example of this increased risk is observed in patients with SLE who have a two to ten-fold increase in the risk of CVA, with patients less than 50 years of age at greatest risk.[60] Not only are patients at increased risk of CVA, the severity of the event itself tends to be much greater, resulting in not just greater mortality but also morbidity.[61] Vascular catastrophe, be it because of increased risk of thrombosis, embolism, hemorrhage, vasculitis, or dissection, is not the only potential for neurologic disaster; so too is mechanical catastrophe, such as that which occurs in the setting of RA and its associated degenerative disease of the cervical spine, and instability of the atlantoaxial joint and its propensity for subluxation or dislocation as discussed previously. Patients with SLE and RA are at significantly increased risk of sudden death in the setting of either situation.[25,28] These are of course not the only potential threats.

The proinflammatory danger of disease cannot be overstated. Neurologic emergencies such as central nervous system (CNS) vasculitis and transverse myelitis must be considered in the differential diagnosis of any patient presenting with manifestations of neurologic disease, be it brain or cord consistent. The potential for significant morbidity from loss of function and mortality is great, requiring the initiation of early and aggressive treatment including glucocorticoids, immunosuppressive agents, and possibly plasmapheresis.[62]

Timely intervention is, however, not the only concern; so too is possible complication associated with failing to have considered a diagnosis such as cerebral vasculitis as an etiology for a patient's stroke-like presentation or an etiology of Libman-Sacks endocarditis with its associated emboli as a cause of CVA, an absolute contraindication to the administration of tissue plasminogen activator (tPA). Although not an established contraindication, caution must be taken in the setting of CNS vasculitis, as thrombolysis could prove disastrous because of an increased risk of hemorrhage.[63]

PULMONARY EMERGENCIES

As is the case with other organ systems, pulmonary disease in the setting of SLE and RA may be a function of the pathophysiologic nature of the diseases themselves or as a consequence of the therapeutic agents used to treat them. Anatomic changes to the lungs over time yielding interstitial lung disease and pulmonary hypertension, acute events such as thromboembolism or hemorrhage, and infections and comorbidities all contribute to increased morbidity and mortality, with each only further increasing the risk for another. Although pulmonary disease is common in systemic rheumatic disease, acute life-threatening catastrophic pulmonary events are rare; 2 of the most lethal are diffuse alveolar hemorrhage (DAH) and lupus pneumonitis.

Both lupus pneumonitis and DAH are associated with high rates of mortality, approximately 40% and 25%, respectively.[64–66] Patients are typically ill appearing with signs, symptoms, and diagnostic findings seemingly consistent with pneumonia. Disease progression is rapid, often culminating in respiratory failure in need of intubation and mechanical ventilation, an outcome that according to 1 study related to DAH was met with a mortality rate of 62% versus a rate of 0% for patients not requiring such intervention.[67] A firm diagnosis of lupus pneumonitis or DAH is beyond the emergency department, where the primary responsibility is to resuscitate and rule out other potential emergent etiologies for the patient's presentation. Although confirmatory diagnosis is beyond the emergency department, timely diagnosis is essential, as any delay in the administration of glucocorticoids and immunosuppressive therapy such as cyclophosphamide only worsens prognosis.[65]

RENAL EMERGENCIES

Like other organ systems, renal impairment is relatively common in systemic rheumatic disease. Lupus nephritis is present in up to 38% of patients with SLE at the time of initial diagnosis and ultimately impacts up to 50% of patients.[68,69] Although actual emergencies are rare, renal disease is a significant contributor to morbidity and mortality, both chronically and acutely, with 10% to 20% of patients progressing to end-stage renal disease and up to 42.2% of admissions to the intensive care unit (ICU) caused by acute kidney injury.[68,70] Renal impairment in RA is less frequent with the use of methotrexate and newer biologic disease-modifying antirheumatic drugs achieving better control over systemic inflammation and reducing the need for NSAIDs.[71] Acute renal failure is still a potentially dangerous situation for patients with SLE and RA, whether it is caused by flare, vaso-occlusive crisis such as that which occurs in the setting of CAPS, or as an adverse effect of the therapeutic agents used to treat the diseases.

ADVERSE DRUG REACTIONS

Patients with SLE and RA are vulnerable not only to acute exacerbations of the diseases themselves and their associated complications but also adverse drug reactions related to the therapeutic agents used to treat them, which can range from mild to severe and even life-threatening. Although the majority of adverse drug reactions are classified as mild or moderate, 36.6% and 40.7% respectively, 22.7% are classified as severe.[72] Glucocorticoids and disease-modifying antirheumatic drugs are associated with a litany of potentially major adverse drug reactions.[23,73] Major adverse drug reactions associated with glucocorticoids include but are not limited to those that are:

- Ophthalmologic (elevated intraocular pressure)
- Cardiovascular (hypertension, arrhythmias, premature arteriosclerosis)
- GI (peptic ulcer disease, visceral perforation)
- Musculoskeletal (osteoporosis, avascular necrosis)
- Neuropsychiatric (depression, psychosis)
- Metabolic (hyperglycemia, hypothalamic-pituitary-adrenal insufficiency)
- Immune system related (increased risk of infections)

Major adverse drug reactions associated with disease-modifying antirheumatic drugs include but are not limited to anaphylaxis, anemia, leukopenia, thrombocytopenia, and immunosuppression. Patients are susceptible to a host of infections, among them bacterial, fungal, and viral, some newly acquired, others reactivated, and some even opportunistic.

DISCLOSURES

The author has nothing to disclose.

REFERENCES

1. Schlosser G, Doell D, Osterland CK. An analysis of rheumatology cases presenting to the emergency room of a teaching hospital. J Rheumatol 1988;15(2):356–8.
2. Bellan M, Molinari R, Castello L, et al. Profiling the patients visiting the emergency room for musculoskeletal complaints: characteristics and outcomes. Clin Rheumatol 2016;35(11):2835–9.
3. Schaller J. Lupus in childhood. Clin Rheum Dis 1982;8(1):219–28.
4. Lahita RG. The role of sex hormones in systemic lupus erythematosus. Curr Opin Rheumatol 1999;11(5):352–6.
5. Rus V, Maury EE, Hochberg MC. The epidemiology of systemic lupus erythematosus. In: Wallace DJ, Hahn BH, editors. Dubois' lupus erythematosus. Philadelphia: Lippincott Williams and Wilkins; 2002.
6. Boddaert J, Huong DLT, Amoura Z, et al. Late-onset systemic lupus erythematosus: a personal series of 47 patients and pooled analysis of 714 cases in the literature. Medicine (Baltimore) 2004;83(6):348–59.
7. Gilbert EL, Ryan MJ. Estrogen in cardiovascular disease during systemic lupus erythematosus. Clin Ther 2014;36(12):1901–12.
8. Lu LJ, Wallace DJ, Ishimori ML, et al. Review: Male systemic lupus erythematosus: a review of sex disparities in this disease. Lupus 2010;19(2):119–29.
9. Eriksson JK, Neovius M, Ernestam S, et al. Incidence of rheumatoid arthritis in Sweden: a nationwide population-based assessment of incidence, its determinants, and treatment penetration. Arthritis Care Res (Hoboken) 2013;65(6):870–8.
10. Petri M. Epidemiology of systemic lupu erythematosus. Best Pract Res Clin Rheumatol 2002;16(5):847–58.
11. Cross M, Smith E, Hoy D, et al. The global burden of rheumatoid arthritis: estimates from the global burden of disease 2010 study. Ann Rheum Dis 2014; 73(7):1316–22.
12. Fernández M, Alarcón GS, Calvo-Alén J, et al. A multiethnic, multicenter cohort of patients with systemic lupus erythematosus (SLE) as a model for the study of ethnic disparities in SLE. Arthritis Rheum 2007;57(4):576–84.
13. Ghawi H, Crowson CS, Rand-Weaver J, et al. A novel measure of socioeconomic status using individual housing data to assess the association of SES with rheumatoid arthritis and its mortality: a population-based case-control study. BMJ Open 2015;5(4):e006469.
14. Callahan LF, Pincus T. Associations between clinical status questionnaire scores and formal education level in persons with systemic lupus erythematosus. Arthritis Rheum 1990;33(3):407–11.
15. Bengtsson C, Nordmark B, Klareskog L, et al. Socioeconomic status and the risk of developing rheumatoid arthritis: results from the Swedish EIRA study. Ann Rheum Dis 2005;64(11):1588–94.

16. Tedeschi SK, Barbhaiya M, Malspeis S, et al. Obesity and the risk of systemic lupus erythematosus among women in the Nurses' Health Studies. Semin Arthritis Rheum 2017;47(3):376–83.

17. Qin B, Yang M, Fu H, et al. Body mass index and the risk of rheumatoid arthritis: a systematic review and dose-response meta-analysis. Arthritis Res Ther 2015; 17(1):86.

18. Montes RA, Mocarzel LO, Lanzieri PG, et al. Smoking and Its Association With Morbidity in Systemic Lupus Erythematosus Evaluated by the Systemic Lupus International Collaborating Clinics/American College of Rheumatology Damage Index: Preliminary Data and Systematic Review. Arthritis Rheumatol 2016;68(2): 441–8.

19. Sugiyama D, Nishimura K, Tamaki K, et al. Impact of smoking as a risk factor for developing rheumatoid arthritis: a meta-analysis of observational studies. Ann Rheum Dis 2010;69(1):70–81.

20. Tsokos GC. Systemic lupus erythematosus. N Engl J Med 2011;365(22):2110–21.

21. Crampton SP, Morawski PA, Bolland S. Linking susceptibility genes and pathogenesis mechanisms using mouse models of systemic lupus erythematosus. Dis Model Mech 2014;7(9):1033–46.

22. McInnes IB, Schett G. The pathogenesis of rheumatoid arthritis. N Engl J Med 2011;365(23):2205–19.

23. Wolfe RM, Seymore AC, Nelson RD et al. Systemic Rheumatic Diseases. In: Tintinalli JE, Ma O, Yealy DM, et al. editors. Tintinalli's emergency medicine: a comprehensive study guide, 9e.McGraw-Hill.

24. Karim A, Ahmed S, Siddiqui R, et al. Severe upper airway obstruction from cricoarytenoiditis as the sole presenting manifestation of a systemic lupus erythematosus flare. Chest 2002;121(3):990–3.

25. Rawlins BA, Girardi FP, Boachie-Adjei O. Rheumatoid arthritis of the cervical spine. Rheum Dis Clin North Am 1998;24(1):55–65.

26. Slobodin G, Hussein A, Rozenbaum M, et al. The emergency room in systemic rheumatic diseases. Emerg Med J 2006;23(9):667–71.

27. Schoenfeld SR, Kasturi S, Costenbader KH. The epidemiology of atherosclerotic cardiovascular disease among patients with SLE: a systematic review. Semin Arthritis Rheum 2013;43(1):77–95.

28. Vymetal J, Skacelova M, Smrzova A, et al. Emergency situations in rheumatology with a focus on systemic autoimmune diseases. Biomed Pap Med Fac Univ Palacky Olomouc Czech Repub 2016;160(1):20–9.

29. Holmqvist M, Ljung L, Askling J. Acute coronary syndrome in new-onset rheumatoid arthritis: a population-based nationwide cohort study of time trends in risks and excess risks. Ann Rheum Dis 2017;76(10):1642–7.

30. Myung G, Forbess LJ, Ishimori ML, et al. Prevalence of resting-ECG abnormalities in systemic lupus erythematosus:A single-center experience. Clin Rheumatol 2017;36(6):1311–6.

31. Owlia MB, Mostafavi Pour Manshadi SM, Naderi N. Cardiac manifestations of rheumatological conditions: a narrative review. ISRN Rheumatol 2012;2012: 463620.

32. Lindhardsen J, Ahlehoff O, Gislason GH, et al. Risk of atrial fibrillation and stroke in rheumatoid arthritis: Danish nationwide cohort study. BMJ 2012;344:e1257.

33. Kreps A, Paltoo K, McFarlane I. Cardiac manifestations in systemic lupus erythematosus: a case report and review of the literature. Am J Med Case Rep 2018; 6(9):180–3.

34. Roldan CA, Shively BK, Crawford MH. An echocardiographic study of valvular heart disease associated with systemic lupus erythematosus. N Engl J Med 1996;335(19):1424–30.
35. Guedes C, Bianchi-Fior P, Cormier B, et al. Cardiac manifestations of rheumatoid arthritis: a case-control transesophageal echocardiography study in 30 patients. Arthritis Rheum 2001;45(2):129–35.
36. Owlia MB. Clinical spectrum of connective tissue disorders. J Indian Acad Clin Med 2006;7(3):217–24.
37. Guy A, Tiosano S, Comaneshter D, et al. Aortic aneurysm association with SLE - a case-control study. Lupus 2016;25(9):959–63.
38. Shovman O, Tiosano S, Comaneshter D, et al. Aortic aneurysm associated with rheumatoid arthritis: a population-based cross-sectional study. Clin Rheumatol 2016;35(11):2657–61.
39. Tagalakis V, Patenaude V, Kahn SR, et al. Incidence of and mortality from venous thromboembolism in a real-world population: the Q-VTE Study Cohort. Am J Med 2013;126(9):832.e13-8, 32E21.
40. Lee JJ, Pope JE. A meta-analysis of the risk of venous thromboembolism in inflammatory rheumatic diseases. Arthritis Res Ther 2014;16(5):435.
41. Gutiérrez-González LA. Rheumatologic emergencies. Clin Rheumatol 2015; 34(12):2011–9.
42. Asherson RA, Cervera R, de Groot PG, et al. Catastrophic antiphospholipid syndrome: international consensus statement on classification criteria and treatment guidelines. Lupus 2003;12(7):530–4.
43. Ortega-Hernandez OD, Agmon-Levin N, Blank M, et al. The physiopathology of the catastrophic antiphospholipid (Asherson's) syndrome: compelling evidence. J Autoimmun 2009;32(1):1–6.
44. Alves SC, Fasano S, Isenberg DA. Autoimmune gastrointestinal complications in patients with systemic lupus erythematosus: case series and literature review. Lupus 2016;25(14):1509–19.
45. Tian XP, Zhang X. Gastrointestinal involvement in systemic lupus erythematosus: insight into pathogenesis, diagnosis and treatment. World J Gastroenterol 2010; 16(24):2971–7.
46. Yuan S, Ye Y, Chen D, et al. Lupus mesenteric vasculitis: clinical features and associated factors for the recurrence and prognosis of disease. Semin Arthritis Rheum 2014;43(6):759–66.
47. Puéchal X, Gottenberg JE, Berthelot JM, et al. Rituximab therapy for systemic vasculitis associated with rheumatoid arthritis: Results from the AutoImmunity and Rituximab Registry. Arthritis Care Res (Hoboken) 2012;64(3):331–9.
48. Jagpal A, Curtis JR. Gastrointestinal Perforations with Biologics in Patients with Rheumatoid Arthritis: Implications for Clinicians. Drug Saf 2018;41(6):545–53.
49. Gnanapandithan K, Sharma A. Mesenteric Vasculitis. In: StatPearls. Treasure Island (FL): StatPearls Publishing; 2021.
50. Keeling DM, Isenberg DA. Haematological manifestations of systemic lupus erythematosus. Blood Rev 1993;7(4):199–207.
51. Khalaf W, Al-Rubaie HA, Shihab S. Studying anemia of chronic disease and iron deficiency in patients with rheumatoid arthritis by iron status and circulating hepcidin. Hematol Rep 2019;11(1):7708.
52. Kwok SK, Ju JH, Cho CS, et al. Thrombotic thrombocytopenic purpura in systemic lupus erythematosus: risk factors and clinical outcome: a single centre study. Lupus 2009;18(1):16–21.

53. Rock GA, Shumak KH, Buskard NA, et al. Comparison of plasma exchange with plasma infusion in the treatment of thrombotic thrombocytopenic purpura. Canadian Apheresis Study Group. N Engl J Med 1991;325(6):393–7.
54. Perez CA, Abdo N, Shrestha A, et al. Systemic lupus erythematosus presenting as thrombotic thrombocytopenia purpura: how close is close enough? Case Rep Med 2011;2011:267508.
55. Cervera R, Khamashta MA, Font J, et al. Morbidity and mortality in systemic lupus erythematosus during a 10-year period: a comparison of early and late manifestations in a cohort of 1,000 patients. Medicine (Baltimore) 2003;82(5):299–308.
56. Zhou WJ, Yang CD. The causes and clinical significance of fever in systemic lupus erythematosus: a retrospective study of 487 hospitalised patients. Lupus 2009;18(9):807–12.
57. Huang JL, Hung JJ, Wu KC, et al. Septic arthritis in patients with systemic lupus erythematosus: salmonella and nonsalmonella infections compared. Semin Arthritis Rheum 2006;36(1):61–7.
58. Ross JJ. Septic Arthritis of Native Joints. Infect Dis Clin North Am 2017;31(2): 203–18.
59. Salar O, Baker B, Kurien T, et al. Septic arthritis in the era of immunosuppressive treatments. Ann R Coll Surg Engl 2014;96(2):e11–2.
60. Nikolopoulos D, Fanouriakis A, Boumpas DT. Cerebrovascular Events in Systemic Lupus Erythematosus: Diagnosis and Management. Mediterr J Rheumatol 2019; 30(1):7–15.
61. Mikdashi J, Handwerger B, Langenberg P, et al. Baseline disease activity, hyperlipidemia, and hypertension are predictive factors for ischemic stroke and stroke severity in systemic lupus erythematosus. Stroke 2007;38(2):281–5.
62. Kovacs B, Lafferty TL, Brent LH, et al. Transverse myelopathy in systemic lupus erythematosus: an analysis of 14 cases and review of the literature. Ann Rheum Dis 2000;59(2):120–4.
63. Srinivasan G, Boschman C, Roth SI, et al. Unsuspected vasculitis and intracranial hemorrhage following thrombolysis. Clin Cardiol 1997;20(1):84–6.
64. Wan SA, Teh CL, Jobli AT. Lupus pneumonitis as the initial presentation of systemic lupus erythematosus: case series from a single institution. Lupus 2016; 25(13):1485–90.
65. de Prost N, Parrot A, Picard C, et al. Diffuse alveolar haemorrhage: factors associated with in-hospital and long-term mortality. Eur Respir J 2010;35(6):1303–11.
66. Aguilera-Pickens G, Abud-Mendoza C. Pulmonary manifestations in systemic lupus erythematosus: pleural involvement, acute pneumonitis, chronic interstitial lung disease and diffuse alveolar hemorrhage. Reumatol Clin (Engl Ed 2018; 14(5):294–300.
67. Zamora MR, Warner ML, Tuder R, et al. Diffuse alveolar hemorrhage and systemic lupus erythematosus. Clinical presentation, histology, survival, and outcome. Medicine (Baltimore) 1997;76(3):192–202.
68. Menez SP, El Essawy B, Atta MG. Lupus nephritis: current treatment paradigm and unmet needs. Rev Recent Clin Trials 2018;13(2):105–13.
69. Danila MI, Pons-Estel GJ, Zhang J, et al. Renal damage is the most important predictor of mortality within the damage index: data from LUMINA LXIV, a multiethnic US cohort. Rheumatology (Oxford) 2009;48(5):542–5.
70. Dumas G, Géri G, Montlahuc C, et al. Outcomes in critically ill patients with systemic rheumatic disease: a multicenter study. Chest 2015;148(4):927–35.
71. Kapoor T, Bathon J. Renal manifestations of rheumatoid arthritis. Rheum Dis Clin North Am 2018;44(4):571–84.

72. Machado-Alba JE, Ruiz AF, Machado-Duque ME. Adverse drug reactions associated with the use of disease-modifying anti-rheumatic drugs in patients with rheumatoid arthritis. Rev Panam Salud Publica 2014;36(6):396–401.
73. Saag KG, Furst DE. Major side effects of systemic glucocorticoids. In: Post TW, editor. UpToDate. Waltham (MA): UpToDate, Inc; 2020. Available at: https://www.uptodate.com/contents/major-side-effects-of-systemic-glucocorticoids. Accessed November 17, 2020.

Moving?

Make sure your subscription moves with you!

To notify us of your new address, find your **Clinics Account Number** (located on your mailing label above your name), and contact customer service at:

Email: journalscustomerservice-usa@elsevier.com

800-654-2452 (subscribers in the U.S. & Canada)
314-447-8871 (subscribers outside of the U.S. & Canada)

Fax number: 314-447-8029

Elsevier Health Sciences Division
Subscription Customer Service
3251 Riverport Lane
Maryland Heights, MO 63043

*To ensure uninterrupted delivery of your subscription, please notify us at least 4 weeks in advance of move.

Printed and bound by CPI Group (UK) Ltd, Croydon, CR0 4YY

03/10/2024

01040468-0020